Oxford Handbook of
Neuroscience
Nursing

Oxford Handbook of
Neuroscience Nursing

Edited by

Sue Woodward

Lecturer,
Florence Nightingale School of Nursing and Midwifery,
King's College London, UK

Catheryne Waterhouse

Clinical Educator,
Neuroscience Unit,
Royal Hallamshire Hospital,
Sheffield, UK

THE COMET LIBRARY
CLASS No. WY 160.5 WOO
ACC. No. 2168
DATE 9/2010
SUPPLIER TOMS
COST £30

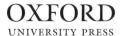

OXFORD
UNIVERSITY PRESS

OXFORD
UNIVERSITY PRESS

Great Clarendon Street, Oxford OX2 6DP

Oxford University Press is a department of the University of Oxford.
It furthers the University's objective of excellence in research, scholarship,
and education by publishing worldwide in

Oxford New York

Auckland Cape Town Dar es Salaam Hong Kong Karachi
Kuala Lumpur Madrid Melbourne Mexico City Nairobi
New Delhi Shanghai Taipei Toronto

With offices in

Argentina Austria Brazil Chile Czech Republic France Greece
Guatemala Hungary Italy Japan Poland Portugal Singapore
South Korea Switzerland Thailand Turkey Ukraine Vietnam

Oxford is a registered trade mark of Oxford University Press
in the UK and in certain other countries

Published in the United States
by Oxford University Press Inc., New York

© Oxford University Press, 2009

The moral rights of the author have been asserted
Database right Oxford University Press (maker)

First published 2009

All rights reserved. No part of this publication may be reproduced,
stored in a retrieval system, or transmitted, in any form or by any means,
without the prior permission in writing of Oxford University Press,
or as expressly permitted by law, or under terms agreed with the appropriate
reprographics rights organization. Enquiries concerning reproduction
outside the scope of the above should be sent to the Rights Department,
Oxford University Press, at the address above

You must not circulate this book in any other binding or cover
and you must impose this same condition on any acquirer

British Library Cataloguing in Publication Data
Data available

Library of Congress Cataloging-in-Publication-Data
Data available

Typeset by Cepha Imaging Private Ltd., Bangalore, India
Printed in China
on acid-free paper through
Asia Pacific Offset

ISBN 978–0–19–954734–0

10 9 8 7 6 5 4 3 2 1

Oxford University Press makes no representation, express or implied, that the drug
dosages in this book are correct. Readers must therefore always check the product
information and clinical procedures with the most up-to-date published product
information and data sheets provided by the manufacturers and the most recent
codes of conduct and safety regulations. The authors and publishers do not accept
responsibility or legal liability for any errors in the text or for the misuse or misap-
plication of material in this work. Except where otherwise stated, drug dosages and
recommendations are for the non-pregnant adult who is not breast-feeding.

Preface

Neuroscience is often perceived to be a difficult topic to get to grips with and does not receive as much coverage as perhaps it should within pre-registration nursing programmes. I can recall as a student nurse my first introduction to neurobiology by our lecturer being less than ideal. Having walked into the room the lecturer stated that she did not understand the nervous system and so was not going to give us a lecture, but instead handed out a guided study sheet so we could go and learn it for ourselves! While I am not going to tell you how many years ago this was, I feel that neuroscience and care of people with neurological problems are not always taught by people who have the relevant knowledge and clinical expertise, and therefore are only dealt with in a superficial manner. This results in students and often qualified nurses who are ill-prepared to deal with the complex needs of people with neurological problems. It is also unlikely that most nursing students will have the opportunity to experience a placement during their training in a specialist neuroscience care setting, although they are highly likely to encounter patients with neurological problems on general medical, elderly care and surgical wards as well as in the community.

It was highlighted in the consultation for the NSF for long-term conditions that when people with neurological problems were being cared for in settings outside of specialist neuroscience centres, their neurological needs were not met. This book aims to dispel the myth that neuroscience nursing is complicated and will provide you with a resource to use when caring for people with neurological problems. Neuroscience nursing often requires rapid or complex decision making, when nurses are required to make sense of considerable amounts of information and act on it. There are few neuroscience nursing textbooks and most of these provide in-depth information about neuroanatomy and physiology, the medical and surgical treatment of patients with neurological conditions, and nursing care plans. While this information and level of detail is important, it is not what is required when you are working on a ward and need to make a decision about care in a particular situation. The *Oxford Handbook of Neuroscience Nursing* will be a resource for you to use when you need relevant and practical clinical guidance in dealing with complex clinical situations or caring for people with neurological problems for the first time. This will enable you to meet the needs of people with neurological problems wherever you encounter them, and will therefore be able to meet the requirements of the NSF.

The book is organised in a way that separates the major neuroscience disciplines, i.e. neurology, neurosurgery, neuroscience critical care, and neurorehabilitation, but there will be a lot of cross-referencing between these sections. This text will provide you with enough information to manage the initial care of the patient, but it is not designed to be an in depth reference for every possible neurological disorder.

Practical guidance is also provided about neurological assessment and investigations, commonly used drugs in neuroscience practice, dealing with neurological emergencies, and legal and ethical issues. A section also covers caring for patients with commonly encountered clinical problems and complementary therapies applied to neuroscience practice are also discussed.

Multidisciplinary team working is essential and commonplace within neuroscience settings; much of the knowledge needed by the different professional groups is shared. This text builds on the very successful *Oxford Handbook of Neurology* but focuses on the issues faced by nurses.

Next time practical guidance is needed on the management of a particular patient, or information is needed about managing a particular situation, then the *Oxford Handbook of Neuroscience Nursing* will provide you with the answers in a succinct and functional way.

Sue Woodward
Catheryne Waterhouse
2009

Contents

Detailed contents

9 Neurosurgery nursing

10 Neuroscience critical care

Contributors

Nadine Abelson-Mitchell
Senior Lecturer,
University of Plymouth,
Plymouth, UK

Sue Beevers
National Service Development
Manager,
Scottish Huntingdon's Association,
Aberdeenshire, UK

Sonja Bellamy
Senior Staff Nurse,
Northern General Hospital,
Sheffield, UK

Mary Braine
Lecturer,
University of Salford,
Salford, UK

Erica Chisanga
Epilepsy Nurse Consultant,
Addenbrooke's Hospital,
Cambridge, UK

Louise L. Clark
Lecturer in Mental Health and
Intellectual Impairment,
Florence Nightingale School of
Nursing and Midwifery,
King's College London,
London, UK

Jan Clarke
Clinical Nurse Specialist for Motor
Neurone Diseases,
National Hospital for Neurology
and Neurosurgery,
London, UK

Gill Cluckie
Stroke Nurse Specialist,
Guy's and St Thomas' NHS
Foundation Trust,
London, UK

Fiona Creed
Senior Lecturer,
University of Brighton,
Brighton, UK

Ben Dorward
Senior Pharmacist,
Royal Hallamshire Hospital,
Sheffield, UK

Alison Forbes
Parkinson's Disease Nurse Specialist,
King's College Hospital,
London, UK

Angus Forbes
Senior Lecturer,
Florence Nightingale School of
Nursing and Midwifery,
King's College London,
London, UK

Lynda Gunn
Nurse Practitioner,
Royal Hallamshire Hospital,
Sheffield, UK

Heather Hale
Clinical Educator,
Royal Hallamshire Hospital,
Sheffield, UK

Paul Harrison
Practice Development Manager,
Spinal Injury Unit,
Northern General Hospital,
Sheffield, UK

Ann Harvey
Senior Chief Clinical,
Physiologist, Neurophysiology,
Ipswich Hospital NHS Trust,
Suffolk, UK

Amanda Hassall
Acting Director of Services,
Headway,
Nottingham, UK

Roni Helliwell
Clinical Educator,
Integra Neurosciences,
Hampshire, UK

Stuart Hibbins
Lecturer in Children's Nursing,
South Bank University,
London, UK

Karen Ibbotson
Macmillan Nurse (Neuroscience),
Royal Hallamshire Hospital,
Sheffield, UK

Susan Jacobs
Parkinson's Disease Nurse
Specialist,
King's College Hospital,
London, UK

Chris Jacobs
Consultant Genetic Counsellor,
Guy's and St Thomas' NHS
Foundation Trust,
London, UK

Katy Judd
Dementia Nurse Consultant,
National Hospital for Neurology
and Neurosurgery,
London, UK

Ehsan Khan
Lecturer,
Florence Nightingale School of
Nursing and Midwifery,
King's College London,
London, UK

Alison Lashwood
Consultant Nurse in Clinical
Genetics and Preimplantation
Genetic Diagnosis,
Guy's and St Thomas' Hospital,
London, UK

Stephen Leyshon
Primary Care Project Lead,
National Patient Safety Agency,
London, UK

Lindy May
Paediatric Nurse Consultant,
Great Ormond Street Hospital for
Children NHS Trust,
London, UK

Jan McFadyen
Nurse Consultant in Non-Cancer
Palliative Care,
South Downs Health NHS Trust,
Brighton and Hove, UK

Amrish Mehta
Consultant Neuroradiologist,
Hammersmith Hospitals,
London, UK

Celia Mostyn
Neurology Liaison Nurse
Specialist,
Great Ormond Street Hospital for
Children NHS Trust,
London, UK

Anne Preece
Professional Development Nurse,
University Hospital Birmingham
Foundation Trust,
Brimingham, UK

Richard Warner
MS Consultant Nurse,
Gloucestershire Hospitals
NHS Trust,
Gloucester, UK

Symbols and abbreviations

📖	cross reference
▶▶	act quickly
⚠	warning
❶	warning
A&E	Accident and Emergency
ABCD	airway, breathing, circulation and disability
ABG	arterial blood gas
ABI	acquired brain injury
Ach	acetylcholine
ACTH	adrenocorticotrophic hormone
AD	autonomic dysreflexia
ADH	anti-diuretic hormone
AED	anti-epileptic drug
AEP	auditory evoked potential
AHP	allied health professionals
AL	activities of living
ALS	amyotrophic lateral sclerosis
ANS	autonomic nervous system
ARDS	acute respiratory distress syndrome
ASDH	acute subdural haematoma
AVM	arteriovenous malformation
BAEP	brainstem auditory evoked potential
BAPEN	British Association of Parenteral and Enteral Nutrition
BBB	blood–brain barrier
BIH	benign intracranial hypertension
BIPAP	biphasic positive airway pressure
BMI	body mass index
BMR	basal metabolic rate
BP	blood pressure
$Ca2+$	calcium
CaO_2	The amount of oxygen carried by aritenal in ml/100ml
CBF	cerebral blood flow
CBT	cognitive behavioural therapy
CBV	cerebral blood volume
CFS	chronic fatigue syndrome
CJO_2	Cerebral oxygen in jugular vien

CMV/IPPV	continuous mandatory or intermittent positive pressure ventilation
CNS	central nervous system
CO2	carbon dioxide
COMT	catechol-o-methyltransferase
COPD	chronic obstructive pulmonary disease
CPAP	continuous positive airway pressure
CPP	cerebral perfusion pressure
CSDH	chronic subdural haematoma
CSF	cerebrospinal fluid
CSW	cerebral salt wasting
CT	computerized tomography
CTA	CT angiography
DBS	deep brain stimulation
DH	Department of Health
DNA	deoxyribonucleic acid
DVT	deep vein thrombosis
ECG	electrocardiogram
ECOG	electrocorticography
EDH	extradural haematoma
EDSS	expanded disability status scale
EEG	electroencephalogram
EMG	electromyography
ESPEN	European Society for Clinical Nutrition and Metabolism
ESR	erythrocyte sedimentation rate
EVD	external ventricular drain
FBC	full blood count
fMRI	functional magnetic resonance imaging
FSH	follicle-stimulating hormone
FVC	forced vital capacity
GA	general anaesthetic
GABA	gamma amino-butyric acid
GBS	Guillain–Barré syndrome
GCS	Glasgow Coma Scale
GP	general practitioner
HAART	highly active antiretroviral therapy
Hb	haemoglobin
HCT	haematocrit
HI	head injury
HIV	human immunodeficiency virus

HRT	hormone replacement therapy
HSV	herpes simplex virus
ICH	intracerebral haematoma
ICP	intracranial pressure
IDEM	intradural–extramedullary
IIH	idiopathic intracranial hypotension
IM	intramuscular
IT	information technology
ITU	Intensive Therapy Unit
IV	intravenous
IVIg	intravenous immunoglobulin
K+	potassium
LH	leuteinizing hormone
LMN	lower motor neurone
LOC	level of consciousness
LP	lumbar puncture
LRECs	Local Research Committees
MAO-B	monoamine oxidase B
MAP	mean arterial pressure
MCI	mild cognitive impairment
ME	myalgic encephalomyelitis
MI	myocardial infarction
MMSE	Mini Mental State Examination
MND	motor neurone disease
MRA	magnetic resonance angiography
MRECs	Multi-centre Research Ethics Committees
MRI	magnetic resonance imaging
MRSA	meticillin-resistant *Staphylococcus Aureus*
MS	multiple sclerosis
Na+	sodium
NAI	non-accidental injury
NBM	nil-by-mouth
NCPC	National Council for Palliative Care
NE	norepinephrine
NG	nasogastric
NICE	National Institute for Health and Clinical Excellence
NMC	Nursing and Midwifery Council
NSAIDs	non-steroidal anti-inflammatory drugs
NSF	National Service Framework
O_2	oxygen

obs	observations
OT	Occupational Therapist
P	pulse
PBP	progressive bulbar palsy
PCT	Primary Care Trust
PD	Parkinson's disease
PE	pulmonary embolus
PEEP	positive end expiratory pressure
PEG	percutaneous endoscopic gastrostomy
PET	positron emission tomography
Physio	physiotherapist/physiotherapy
PICC	peripherally inserted central catheter
PLS	primary lateral sclerosis
PMA	progressive muscular atrophy
PML	progressive multifocal leukoencephalopathy
PNES	psychogenic non-epileptic seizures
PNS	peripheral nervous system
PR	per rectum
PSP	progressive supranuclear palsy
PTA	post-traumatic amnesia
PWP	people with Parkinson's
QoL	quality of life
R	respiratory rate
RCN	Royal College of Nursing
RCP	Royal College of Physicians
REM	rapid eye movement
RICP	raised intracranial pressure
RTA	road traffic addident
SAH	subarachnoid haemorrhage
SCI	spinal cord injury
SDH	subdural haematoma
SE	status epilepticus
SIGN	Scottish Intercollegiate Guidelines Network
SIMV	synchronized intermittent mandatory ventilation
SLE	systemic lupus erythematosis
SLT	Speech and Language Therapist
SMA	spinal muscular atrophy
SPECT	single positron emission computerized tomography
SSEP	somatosensory evoked potential

SUDEP	sudden death in epilepsy
T	temperature
TBI	traumatic brain injury
TSH	thyroid-stimulating hormone
UMN	upper motor neuron
VEP	visual evoked potentials

Chapter 1

Policy influences on neuroscience practice

Introduction

This chapter provides the reader with access to a summary of many recent and relevant UK health policies that underpin and influence neuroscience nursing practice, such as:

- *NSF for Long-term (Neurological) Conditions* (2005)
- NICE Guidelines
- *Saving Lives Delivery Programme* (2007)
- *Our Health, Our Care, Our Say* (2006)
- *Neuroscience Critical Care Report* (2000)
- *Comprehensive Critical Care* (1999)

The chapter also includes an explanation of a number of other key concepts that influence our day-to-day practice. While not government policy or directives, these concepts are equally important to grasp and are regularly encountered by neuroscience nurses, for example:

- Benchmarking
- Role of the voluntary sector
- Expert patients
- Principles of palliative care
- Carers' issues

National Service Frameworks for Long-term (Neurological) Conditions (2005)

National Service Frameworks (NSF) are long-term strategies issued by the Department of Health (DH), aimed at improving standards of care in particular areas of practice. Goals and targets are set for NHS Trusts to meet.

The *NSF for Long-term (Neurological) Conditions* was published by the DH in March 2005 following consultation and is targeted at patients with long-term conditions such as epilepsy, multiple sclerosis (MS), Parkinson's disease (PD) and stroke.

The 11 quality requirements of NSF

The NSF sets out 11 quality requirements to be delivered in the following areas:
- A person-centred service
- Early recognition, prompt diagnosis and treatment
- Emergency and acute management
- Early and specialist rehabilitation
- Community rehabilitation and support
- Vocational rehabilitation
- Providing equipment and accommodation
- Providing personal care and support
- Palliative care
- Supporting family and carers
- Caring for people with neurological conditions in hospital or other healthcare settings

Implementation should be complete by 2015, but no prescriptive elements, monitoring of specific targets or additional funding for implementation have been identified.

Ten Quick Wins

Lack of evidence of implementation led to a relaunch and publication of *10 Quick Wins* by the DH and Care Services Improvement Partnership at the end of 2007. *10 Quick Wins* aim to support, provide tools for and guide implementation of the NSF and include:
- Designate a lead for NSF implementation in the Primary Care Trust (PCT)/Strategic Health Authority (SHA)
- Establish a local implementation group
- Provide appropriate information and advice for service users
- Develop local provision of self-care and self-management for patients with long-term conditions
- Use a single or integrated assessment process
- Appoint practitioners with specialist expertise in neurological conditions
- Implement 18-week referral to treatment pathways

- Establish multi-agency health and social services community rehab
- Improve quality in specialized home care and community services
- Use the care sources improvement partners NSF website

Further information for health professionals and the public

Department of Health (2005) *The national service framework for long-term conditions*. Available from: http://www.dh.gov.uk/en/Publicationsandstatistics/Lettersandcirculars/ Dearcolleagueletters/DH_4106704. Accessed 3 January 2008.

Care Services Improvement Partnership (CSIP) (2007) *10 quick wins to support long-term neurological conditions NSF implementation*. Available from: http://www.longtermconditions.csip.org. uk/articles.asp?action=viewandid=4646. Accessed 3 January 2008.

NICE, Royal College of Physicians and other guidelines

The National Institute for Health and Clinical Excellence (NICE) was set up in 1997 to review evidence and ensure best practice is implemented throughout healthcare settings. Guideline development groups look at clinical evidence of effectiveness and cost-effectiveness before issuing guidelines.

Published guidelines

NICE has published guidelines on a range of neurological conditions:
- Dementia (2006)
- Epilepsy (2004)
- Head injury (revised 2007)
- Multiple sclerosis (MS) (2003)
- Parkinson's disease (PD) (2006)
  Also on other topics relevant to care of neuroscience patients, for e.g.:
- Faecal incontinence (2007)
- Nutrition support in adults (2006)
- Urinary incontinence (2006)

All guidelines are available for download through the NICE website: http:// www.nice.org.uk

Some appeals were made against NICE decisions regarding NHS funding of drugs by patient groups and professionals, i.e. disease-modifying therapies for MS and medication for Alzheimer's disease. Strict criteria are applied for NHS funding of some drugs following NICE recommendations.

The Royal College of Physicians and other guidelines

Some guidelines have been issued by other organizations such as the Royal College of Physicians (RCP).

Guidelines for stroke care are issued by the RCP and are now in their third edition (RCP, 2008).

The Scottish Intercollegiate Guidelines network (SIGN) have also issued guidelines for aspects of stroke care, epilepsy, and head injury that apply to care of patients in Scotland.

Further information for health professionals and the public

Royal College of Physicians (2008) *National clinical guidelines for stroke*, 3rd edn. Prepared by the Intercollegiate Stroke Working Party. London: Royal College of Physicians.
Scottish Intercollegiate Guidelines Network http://www.sign.ac.uk

Saving Lives Delivery Programme (2007)

The *Saving Lives Delivery Programme* was revised in 2007 and stems from the DH initiative to improve cleanliness in hospitals and reduce infection rates, especially aiming to combat methicillin-resistant *Staphyloccccus Aureus* (MRSA) and other healthcare-acquired infections.

This policy is aimed at acute healthcare Trusts and many aspects of the programme are relevant to care of neuroscience patients although they are not mentioned specifically.

Other aspects that have already been implemented from the Cleaner Hospitals Policy since 2000 include:

- Introduction of matrons with responsibility for cleanliness
- National Patient Safety Agency—campaign to promote hand hygiene by healthcare workers
- Hospital deep cleaning programme

Saving Lives: tools available to assist implementation

The DH has made a number of tools available to acute Trusts to assist with implementation. These are for open access by any healthcare professional or NHS Trust and include:

- Self-assessment and action planning tool
- A variety of learning resources
- High-impact interventions and care bundles

Learning resources (see below) and specific guidance of relevance to neuroscience care areas

Guidelines for the following aspects of practice are available for download from the DH website:

- Best practice on isolating patients with healthcare-associated infection
- Infection control in critical care
- MRSA screening
- Antimicrobial prescribing
- Taking blood cultures

High-impact interventions

Care bundles have been produced that relate to specific clinical procedures that carry an increased risk of healthcare-acquired infection if performed incorrectly and not based on best available evidence. This work builds on the systematic reviews produced as part of the evidence based practice in infection control project (Pratt et al., 2007).

- Central venous catheter care
- Peripheral intravenous (IV) cannula care
- Renal catheter care
- Prevention of surgical site infection
- Ventilator and tracheostomy care
- Urinary catheter care
- Reducing risks from *Clostridium difficile*

Further information for health professionals and the public

Department of Health (2008) *Saving lives delivery programme*. Available at http://www.dh.gov.uk/en/ Publichealth/Healthprotection/Healthcareacquiredinfection/Healthcareacquiredgeneralinformation/ ThedeliveryprogrammetoreducehealthcareassociatedinfectionsHCAIincludingMRSA/index.htm. Accessed 31 March 2008.

Pratt RJ, Pellowe CM, Wilson JA, Loveday HP *et al.* (2007) EPIC2: National evidence-based guidelines for preventing healthcare-associated infections in NHS Hospitals in England. *Journal of Hospital Infection*, 65: S1–S64. Available from http://www.epic.tvu.ac.uk/PDF%20Files/epic2/ epic2-final.pdf.

Our Health, Our Care, Our Say (2006)

This white paper was published in January 2006 by the DH. It aims to reform community-based health and social care services to make them more personalized and give patients more choice.

Key elements of the reforms

- Introduction of health checks for over 40s (a health MOT) to identify people at risk of stroke, heart disease and diabetes, for example, and encourage them to make healthier choices based on risk assessment
- Give patients more information and choice regarding general pracitioner (GP) registration (e.g. a patient with epilepsy or migraine may choose to register with a GP with a special interest in their condition)
- Guaranteed registration at a GP practice and longer opening hours
- Reduce inequalities in access to services in deprived areas and for those patients who are most vulnerable (e.g. people with ongoing care needs and long-term neurological conditions with disabilities)
- Help people with long-term conditions to manage their own condition by giving information and allowing them to make informed choices about treatment options
- Increasing investment in Expert Patient Programmes
- For social care, individual budgets will be piloted, bringing together funding from a variety of sources to make it easier for people with disability to access support
- Develop personal health and social care plans for people with complex needs, such as many neuroscience patients, to ensure more joined up care—links to the quality requirements of the NSF
- More support for carers
- Introduce practice-based commissioning of services and pilot individual patient budgets—increase focus on personalized purchasing and give patients more control over services
- Shift care provision from acute hospital to community and home-based care
- Increase joint commissioning of health and social care services between PCTs and local authorities
- In areas of poor provision increase access to GP and other services by allowing PCTs to award contracts to the private sector

Three years on we are beginning to see the impact of some of these changes, with the first contracts awarded to commercial companies to provide GP services in inner cities and the national roll-out of the health screening programme in early 2008.

Further information for health professionals and the public

Department of Health (2006) *Our health, our care, our say: a new direction for community services.* available from: http://www.dh.gov.uk/en/Publicationsandstatistics/Publications/PublicationsPolicyAndGuidance/Browsable/DH_4127552. Accessed 31 March 2008.

Neuroscience Critical Care Report (2000)

The report *Comprehensive Critical Care* (2000) outlined a far-reaching modernization programme for the development of critical care services. Patients requiring specialized neurocritical care were identified for a further detailed review which was undertaken by an expert multiprofessional group.

Main areas identified for consideration

- Improving access to care:
  - Lack of equity in the geographical distribution of services
  - Poor communication/lack of clear guidelines
- Capacity:
  - Inadequate number of funded and staffed level 2 and 3 neuroscience critical care beds
- Outreach services:
  - Required to cover the whole of the patient pathway
- Referral to a tertiary neuroscience centre:
  - Access
  - Inconsistent advice
  - Delayed transfers
- Repatriation:
  - Lack of appropriate neuroscience rehabilitation services
  - Lack of discharge planning leading to bed blocking
  - Cancellation of elective procedures
- Transfers:
  - Time-consuming and costly with lack of agreed standards
- Neuro-radiology services:
  - Lack of 24hr facilities
- The workforce:
  - Lack of appropriately skilled staff
  - Significant increase in workload over the last ten years
  - Special needs of neuroscience patients
- The role of allied health professionals (AHP) and healthcare scientists (HCS)

Recommendations

- Patients developing acute symptoms should have access to a specialist neuroscience opinion in an appropriate time frame—normally within 24hrs.
- Patients with potentially life-threatening insults should expect immediate admission to a specialist neuroscience centre
- Neuroscience networks should be developed to ensure all patients can access a quality neuroscience critical care facility in an appropriate timescale
- Tertiary neuroscience centres should be fully equipped and optimally staffed with multiprofessional teams trained and competent in the management of these conditions

- A neuroscience critical care service should be provided by a consultant with expertise in neuroscience critical care at all times
- Medical staff responsible for these patients in Accident and Emergecny (A&E) and primary care should be competent in the management of patients with acute neurological conditions
- Develop communication and information technology (IT) strategies to reduce the number of inappropriate transfers and facilitate discharges from neuroscience centres
- Tertiary centres should provide agreed multiprofessional guidelines/ policies for referral/transfer
- To develop appropriately resourced outreach services
- Define the current true capacity, determine levels of met and unmet need to facilitate sensible commissioning
- Tertiary centres should have 24 hr access to computerized tomography (CT), magnetic resonance imaging (MRI), cerebral angiography and plain films
- Neuroradiology should be co-located within the neuroscience department
- AHPs and HCSs need to be included in the development of a neuroscience service as a more coordinated and resourced multidisciplinary team can ensure equality in care delivery

Further information for health professionals and the public

Department of Health (2000) *Comprehensive critical care: a review of adult critical care services.* London: Department of Health.

Department of Health (2004) *Neuroscience critical care report: progress in developing services.* London: Department of Health. http://www.doh.gov.uk/nhsexec/compcritcare.htm

Comprehensive Critical Care (1999)— a review of adult critical care services

In 1999 a government review of adult critical care services recommended a far-reaching modernization programme which would be a patient-focused comprehensive service encompassing the whole patient pathway and inclusive of all professions and specialties.

Critical care services had previously developed in a haphazard and unplanned way with little consistency in the organization and capacity and a wide variation between NHS Trusts.

Characteristics of the modernized service are to encompass:
- Integration
- Networks
- Workforce development
- Data-collecting culture—promoting an evidence base

Classification of critical care patients

The existing division of critical care patients into high dependency and intensive care was replaced by a classification focusing on the level of care required by the patient rather than their location.

Level 0	Patients whose needs can be met through normal ward care in an acute hospital
Level 1	Patients at risk of their condition deteriorating, or those recently relocated from higher levels of care, whose needs can be met on an acute ward with additional advice and support from the critical care team
Level 2	Patients requiring more detailed observation or intervention including support for a single failing organ system or post-operative care and those 'stepping down' from higher levels of care
Level 3	Patients requiring advanced respiratory support alone or basic respiratory support together with support of at least two organ systems. This level includes all complex patients requiring support for multi-organ failure

- Hospitals admitting emergency patients are expected to have all levels of care available.
- Hospitals carrying out elective surgery are expected to have at least up to level 2 facilities.
- If level 3 facilities are not available, suitable protocols must be in place for the safe transfer to a level 3 facility if required.

Recommendations

- Organization within Trusts:
  - Establishment of Trust-wide critical care delivery groups
  - Participation in national data-collection projects to provide direct comparison of outcomes between units
  - Outreach services to be established to avert admissions, enable discharges and share critical care services
  - Flexibility of bed usage
  - Discharge/transfers
  - Long-term support and follow-up
- Organization between Trusts
- The establishment of critical care networks is recommended to:
  - Plan services to meet the needs of the critically ill
  - Encourage general and specialist critical care services to develop
  - Agree common standards and protocols to work to
  - Commissioners to ensure resources available
- Human resources. Recommendations on recruitment, retention, education and training, workforce planning and leadership are identified:
  - Nurse staffing to be based on patient dependency, not bed numbers
  - Competency-based modular training to be developed to include therapy services
  - A review of the balance of staff to ensure work is undertaken by the appropriate staff
  - Every critical care unit is to be led by a doctor trained in specialist intensive care medicine and every weekday session to be covered by a consultant
- Standards and guidelines. The development of multiprofessional, interagency guidelines, standards and protocols to include:
  - Admissions and discharges
  - Transfer and transport of critically ill patients
  - Timely information for patients, relatives etc.
  - Organization of organ donation

Further information for health professionals and the public

Department of Health (2000) *Comprehensive critical care: a review of adult critical care services.* London: Department of Health. http://www.doh.gov.uk/nhsexec/compcritcare.htm

Benchmarking neuroscience practice

The concept of benchmarking originates from industry and provides one method of scrutinizing care delivery and re-examining performances. It is an integral part of quality assurance and is a structured process that links theory to practice.

Benchmarking identifies and shares current 'best practice' and involves continuously reviewing and evaluating care in light of new, emerging best evidence, thus providing an impetus for change.

Definitions are varied but essentially it is: a continuous process that searches for best practices, sets standards for comparison and through action planning leads to a superior performance.

The five main types of benchmarking

- Internal: within your organization/centre —most common
- External: outside your organization/centre —prevents 'reinventing the wheel'
- International: guiding national health policy priorities
- Strategic: comparing organization's strategies
- Process: address processes and functions within organization's delivery of services

Neuroscience benchmarking group

The group commenced in the UK and Ireland in the early 1990s and membership includes nurses from clinical practice and education. It is divided into regional groups, providing an active network to share knowledge and expertise, promoting a learning culture.

- Groups aim to standardize, advance and improve practice
- Each benchmark contains:
  - an overall statement
  - four factors to achieve the outcomes—staff education, patient education, policy, and documentation
  - key resources
  - the actual benchmark itself, and a scoring continuum for each factor
- Benchmarks are:
  - clinically varied: medical, surgical, rehabilitation e.g., neurological observations
  - reviewed every 2 years
  - issues/problems that arise from practice

Four main stages of the benchmarking process

- Plan—decide what to benchmark
- Measure—collect data
- Analyse—make comparisons, share information, integrate results into action plan
- Implement—action plans, monitoring, and reviewing

Benchmarking can help to:

- Monitor services
- Scrutinize care delivery and identify gaps in practice and opportunities for research
- Learn from others
- Facilitate cross-hospital discussions and networking
- Identify the need for additional resources
- Reduce complacency
- Reduce misconceptions by those outside your department/unit
- Demonstrate the nursing contribution to patient outcomes
- Build teams—work towards common goal
- Bring about an innovative bottom-up approach to change
- Provide service users with a direct indicator of performance

Key issues to consider

- Benchmark—relevance, importance, scope availability of resources
- Long-term effects requires involvement of all concerned
- Requires—commitment, motivation, time, and resources
- Communication—effective, timely, and transparent
- Leadership
- Education—methods, process

Further information for health professionals and the public

The National Neuroscience Benchmarking Group is now under the umbrella of the British Association of Neuroscience Nurses. Published benchmarks can be accessed via the website: http://www.nnbg.org.uk

Paediatric Neuroscience Benchmarking Group

Paediatric neuroscience comprises approximately 10% of all neuroscience workload, with a mixture of dedicated paediatric neuroscience wards, and paediatric wards with a number of neuroscience beds. The group has been running for 11 years and has proved an essential method of comparing and sharing practice across these centres, assisting uniformity of practice, and providing support and advice.

Best practice is achieved by:
- Collaborative agreement
- Professional consensus
- Research and evidence-based practice
- Monitoring practice
- Encourages networking

Many areas have been benchmarked but examples that differ vastly from adult practice include:
- Paediatric Glasgow Coma Scale (GCS)
- EVD management
- Intracranial pressure (ICP) management
- Procedural sedation
- Pain management
- Management of the child with spinal dysraphism

The group meets every three months and the venue is rotated, the chair and secretarial duties are rotated every 18 months, responsibility for literature searches is shared, and multicentred audit is encouraged.

In addition to the benchmarking process, the host centre invites a guest speaker to talk on an innovative subject, and various projects are undertaken including producing parent information leaflets on many procedures, and the production of a spinal neurological observation chart.

The group has held several conferences, published articles, and individuals have spoken at international and national conferences on paediatric neuroscience benchmarking.

Further information for health professionals and the public

British Association of Neuroscience Nurses http://www.bann.org.uk

Neuroscience nurse specialists

Neuroscience nurse specialists work with patients with a range of different neurological conditions, such as MS, PD, stroke and epilepsy. The specialist nursing roles evolved to address the complex self-care needs of patients and the wide range of different physical and emotional problems which they encounter.

Specialist roles were first established in North America in the 1970s and they are now well-established in the UK. While specialist nurses were traditionally employed in hospital neurology settings, their roles have now diversified and they can be found in primary care trusts, rehabilitation and palliative care settings.

The focus of their roles has also shifted with cross-boundary working, particularly supporting primary and continuing care settings, being increasingly central. More recently there has been a strong focus in using the roles to help prevent or minimize hospital admissions.

Key functions of the neuroscience nurse specialist roles

- Information provision for patients and carers
- Psychological, social, and physical assessment and intervention
- Specialist disease-specific assessment and intervention
- Coordination and care management
- Managing the diagnosis
- Patient education (individual and group)
- Medicines management and support
- Self-care behaviour support
- Symptom prevention or resolution
- Education of other health professionals
- Developing care systems (guidelines and care pathways)
- Care planning and case management
- Research and audit

These components relate closely to the needs of patients with enduring neurological health problems who require support:

- During the diagnosis
- In lifelong adjustment and coping
- In dealing with depression
- In maintaining personal autonomy
- In meeting daily living needs
- In managing symptoms
- In dealing with stigma
- In resolving relationship problems
- To maintain their social support system
- With financial employment problems (Forbes *et al*, 2003).

Resource allocation and specialist nurse provision

Unfortunately there are many areas in the UK that are still poorly provided for with neuroscience nurse specialists. This lack of equity has led many disease charities to set up posts in partnership with the NHS. Other posts are supported by pharmaceutical companies to help support patients using therapies that demand complex administration or self-care behaviours, such as interferon. The evidence base for the impact of these roles is very underdeveloped reflecting the broad and multifaceted nature of the roles.

Specialist nursing associations

Many disorders now have their own specialist nurse associations: these are a useful point of contact for information about the disorders and the specialist roles. These associations also identify levels of competencies within the roles linked to clinical expertise and continuing professional development.

The Parkinson's disease and MS associations have, for example, identified a career development pathway from registered practitioner to nurse consultant. The MS specialist nurse association has also developed a competency document detailing all the core facets of the role delineating novice, competent and expert level practice (MS Trust 2003).

References

Forbes A., While A., Dyson L., Grocott T. and Griffiths P. (2003) Impact of clinical nurse specialists in multiple sclerosis—synthesis of the evidence. *Journal of Advanced Nursing*, 42(5): 442–62.

MS Trust, UKMSSNA, Royal College of Nursing (RCN) (2009) *Competencies for MS specialist services*. London: MS Trust.

Further information for health professionals and the public

Epilepsy nurses association http://www.esna-online.org.uk.
Parkinson's disease nurse specialist association http://www.pdnsa.net/events.html.
MS specialist nurse association http://www.ukmssna.org.uk.

The role of the voluntary sector

The voluntary sector, or third sector as it has more recently become known, plays an increasingly important role in the neurological care pathway.

A number of different services are offered and provided at little or no cost to the statutory authorities. The sector is primarily made up of a number of small, medium and large charities, community-based groups, and 'not-for-profit' organizations, which have been set up because statutory services do not currently exist to support and fund such services. They have been set up to meet needs identified on a local and national level.

Primarily statutory monies go toward 'front line' services. However, the voluntary sector would argue that many of the services they provide ought to be treated as front line.

Those who have experience of working in other sectors recognize the increasing pressures put on those in the statutory sector and empathize with them; however as well as providing the hands-on support that our colleagues do, those of us working in the voluntary sector have pressures of a different sort and spend a lot of time working as fundraisers, employers, marketing executives, publishers, volunteers, holiday organizers, budget holders, employment law experts, public speakers and administrators in our spare time.

Services include:
- Information/advice
- Advocacy
- Bereavement
- Counselling
- Hospice care
- Long-term care
- Rehabilitation (vocational/ physical/cognitive)
- Respite care
- Day Services including providing physiotherapy, occupational therapy (OT), speech and language therapy (SLT), and neuropsychology support
- Carer support/advice
- Outreach
- Housing/transitional/independent living
- Benefit advice

Specialized services also exist and can be as diverse as providing 'Support Dogs' that instinctively know when their owner is going to have a seizure. Those in the voluntary sector are also often involved in campaigning for equality and improvement in services.

When patients have been through the front line services, the voluntary sector steps in to continue that care and support. Few people know that the majority of these services are provided by charities and not-for-profit organizations.

Like the statutory sector, the voluntary sector employs staff but would not be able to provide the services that it does without the support of volunteers who spend hours of their own time working for nothing. Without them, the voluntary sector would not exist or survive.

Expert patients programme

More people are now living longer with chronic illness. This programme was launched by the DH in 1999 with the first programmes being piloted in 2002.

Their aim is to support people to increase confidence, improve quality of life and better manage their condition (Department of Health, 2006).

Programme structure

Delivered as courses locally by 'volunteer tutors' with chronic conditions, where patients are taught skills to help them self-manage their condition including:

- Problem-solving
- Decision-making
- Resource utilization
- Developing effective partnerships with healthcare providers and taking action (Department of Health, 2006)

Patients can find a course in their area by searching online through the DH website.

Specific programmes are also available for marginalized communities and young people, for carers to help them learn to look after themselves and online programmes are available for those who are not able to get to a local course.

Outcomes from the programme

- Patients are able to improve their communication skills and confidence—enables them to better interact with the healthcare system and professionals
- Helps patients plan for the future
- Helps patients manage day-to-day activities
- Patients learn how to manage symptoms better, e.g. fatigue, depression, pain, spasticity

Reference

Department of Health (2006) *The expert patients programme*. Available from: http://www.dh.gov.uk/en/Aboutus/MinistersandDepartmentLeaders/ChiefMedicalOfficer/ProgressOnPolicy/ProgressBrowsableDocument/DH_4102757. London: Department of Health. Accessed 07 January 2008.

Intellectual impairment and neuroscience

Intellectual impairment is an umbrella term which covers a variety of conditions including what was traditionally known as learning disability, dementia, long term and enduring mental health problems where cognition is affected, pervasive developmental disorders (including autism, Asperger's syndrome, other childhood disintegrative disorders and Retts syndrome), and acquired brain injury. Another group of individuals who fall in to this category are those who function on the borderline of learning disability and may have additional mental health problems that affect their every day functioning. Many of these people remain officially undiagnosed.

Prevalence

Prevalence figures for these groups are estimations only.

- *Learning disability*, mild to moderate; 1.2 million in England (25 per 1000 population)
- *Learning disability*, severe or profound; 210,000 in England
- *Acquired brain injury*; 170,000 in the UK suffering from long-term effects with 12,000 needing long-term care
- *Dementia*; 165,000 new cases diagnosed in England and Wales each year with Alzheimer's disease being responsible for 70% of all cases.

For people with long-term mental health problems where cognition is affected, and for those on the borderline of having a learning disability and additional mental health problems, there are no figures available.

Diagnosis

Diagnosis is dependent on the cause of the impairment.

Some forms of learning disability may be identified prior to birth, for example when there is a genetic condition. More mild forms of learning disability are often picked up later in childhood.

Dementia risk increases with age but there are 18,000 people under the age of 65 with dementia in the UK.

Acquired brain injury and the lasting impact on the individual often occurs some time after the original trauma.

The effects of long-term mental health problems on cognition increases with age and those with borderline learning disabilities appear to be more prone to developing mental health problems in young adulthood.

Effects of intellectual impairment

These vary enormously depending on the individual and the cause and severity of the impairment, but in general more common problems include:

- Communication problems
- Difficulty with aspects of daily living including self-care
- Mobility issues
- Epilepsy
- Increased risk of mental health problems
- Social isolation
- Increased risk of dementia
- Increased risk of either obesity or malnutrition

- Dehydration and urinary tract infections
- Constipation
- Syndrome-specific problems
- Behaviour that may challenge
- Increased risk of cancer, especially gastrointestinal

Aims of care

Mainstream NHS care for all these patient groups is the aim, with specialist services kept to a minimum.

Predominantly social care is provided.

Caring for someone with intellectual impairment in a health environment

- Employ a biopsychosocial approach to care
- Use simple language avoiding metaphors and similes
- Use open body language and a friendly approach
- Include carers in the investigative process but don't ignore the patient
- Ensure they understand what you are saying to them
- Give prompts if needed to remind them to eat, drink, go to the toilet etc
- Develop risk assessments if the patient exhibits behaviours which are challenging
- Interpret challenging behaviours as they are usually a mode of communication

Further information for health professionals and the public

National Autistic Society http://www.nas.org.uk

Palliative care

Palliative care is the active, holistic care of patients with advanced progressive illness. Management of pain and other symptoms, and provision of psychological, spiritual, and social support is paramount. The goal of palliative care is the achievement of the best quality of life for patients and their families. Many aspects of palliative care are also applicable earlier in the course of the illness, in conjunction with active treatment.

Contribution of palliative care to people with neurological conditions

- Control or amelioration of symptoms such as pain, muscle spasm, drooling, and breathlessness
- Social support by facilitating participation in interactions with others in hospice settings of care
- Familiarity in communicating with people who are trying to make sense of their life as it draws to a close
- Advance care planning to support decision-making around end of life issues
- Supporting death in the individual's place of choice
- Care through the dying process
- Bereavement support for families and friends left behind

Collaborative working

Palliative practitioners work within multiprofessional teams, usually consisting of specialist nurses (the largest group), doctors, and social workers. They often include chaplains and other spiritual advisers, occupational therapists and physiotherapists.

This should enable good cross-boundary working with neurological nurses and doctors and rehabilitation professionals.

Phases of intervention

There are four significant points during a journey with any progressive neurological illness that might suggest the usefulness of a palliative approach, sometimes with the collaboration of a palliative practitioner.

- The time of diagnosis, when the person and family are likely to have fears and questions about the nature of dying and what the future might hold. Although the neurological team is the main source of care and support, there may be much to be learnt from the palliative care team around communicating about decline and death, and the support available.
- Living with advancing illness, as the symptom control burden increases and function declines. The difficulty of living with increasing uncertainty can be a heavy burden; palliative teams have considerable expertise in supporting people along this journey. This may also be the time when spiritual concerns come to the fore, as people seek to find meaning in their lives.
- The process of dying, when expertise in end of life care and knowledge of local resources and end of life programmes is invaluable.
- Support in bereavement, which can be challenging after what may have been years of immersion in the caring experience.

Palliative care and the individual journey

Each experience of living with a long-term neurological condition is unique. Nevertheless, there are some factors that are common to everyone. The National Council for Palliative Care (NCPC) and neurological partners have summarized this journey in a pathway, demonstrating points when collaborative working with a palliative team is appropriate. These are:

- Intractable symptoms causing suffering, especially pain, but also nausea and breathlessness
- Difficulties with care coordination/management of complex needs
- Lifespan is likely to be limited
- Issues of communication and competence arise
- There is a need for care planning/advance decisions (Brown and Sutton, 2007).

Family support

Families and friends of people with progressive neurological conditions face particular challenges as they learn to live with personality and cognitive changes in their loved ones, along with increased physical dependency. As the person nears the end of life, a mixture of emotions is frequently prevalent in informal carers. Palliative care teams have considerable experience and expertise in exploring and validating these emotions.

And finally...

It is important not to make false claims that all will be well, but, rather, to offer hope of amelioration and to dispel fear of abandonment.

Reference

Brown J and Sutton L (2007) *A neurological pathway*. London: National Council for Palliative Care. Available at http://www.ncpc.org.uk/download/policy/NeuroPathway/pdf.

Further information for health professionals and the public

Help the Hospices http://www.hospiceinformation.info
National Council for Palliative Care http://www.ncpc.org.uk

National Council for Palliative Care: Neurological Conditions Policy Group

The National Council for Palliative Care (NCPC) Neurological Conditions Policy Group was established in March 2005.

It aims to develop a palliative care pathway for people with neurological conditions, but initially has focused on a few specific neurological conditions.

The work of the group is underpinned by the NSF for long-term neurological conditions.

Aims of the pathway

- Provide a template for ideal care, promoting the key worker concept
- For use by professionals
- Keeping the patient/family at the centre of care decisions
- Recognizing the need for local variation
- Supporting the proactive interface between pivotal services, e.g. neurology, palliative care, geriatric care, rehabilitation, voluntary agencies, social care (NCPC, 2007a)

Comments on the pathway are invited through the NCPC website.

Dementia project

The NCPC have also launched a project aimed specifically at palliative care for people with dementia in early 2007. This work is being led by the Older People Policy Group.

Project objectives

- Map current provision of palliative care services for people with dementia
- Highlight gaps in provision within different care settings
- Understand user and carers' needs of palliative care services
- Identify and share notable practice
- Develop practical guidance to promote palliative care for people with dementia (NCPC, 2007b)

References

NCPC (2007a) Neurological Conditions Policy Group. Available from: http://www.ncpc.org.uk/
   policy_unit/neuro_pg.html. Accessed 31 March 2008.
NCPC (2007b) Dementia project. Available from: http://www.ncpc.org.uk/policy_unit/
   dementiawg.html. Accessed 31 March 2008.

Further information for health professionals and the public

National Council for Palliative Care: http://www.ncpc.org.uk

Carers

There are two main types of carer:
- Paid
- Unpaid

Paid carers

Carers who are paid are normally employed by statutory services, or voluntary organizations. They can be employed as care workers, support workers, or buddies, who provide friendship or companionship.

In extreme cases, however, someone who has sustained a brain injury (or medical negligence) might be in receipt of a compensation/insurance payout and may be able to 'employ' their own carer workers. However, becoming an employer has its own pressures. For example, issues such as contracts, holiday entitlement, sick pay, work rotas and training have to be considered—as indeed does the importance of maintaining a professional relationship. To counter this, many victims of road traffic incidents who receive compensation monies employ a case manager to look after this work.

Unpaid carers

Family members often become carers by default, sometimes having been pushed into the situation due to a feeling of obligation and an inability to say no brought on by guilt.

It is often expected that family members take on the mantle of carer when their relative leaves hospital. Sometimes this is totally inappropriate as the unpaid carer finds themselves having to give up their own work and identity in order to care for their relative. More importantly, they may not have the requisite skills or physical health to adequately take on the role.

At Headway, which helps both those with brain injuries and also their carers, we know that relationships regularly break down because of the physical, psychological, and social pressures caring for a family member puts on people; e.g., it is sometimes not appropriate for a partner to be the main physical carer—the romance side of a relationship suffers whereas a 'paid' carer remains detached from the situation.

If a family carer is in paid employment, employers will understandably only allow limited time off work and eventually the carer has to make the decision whether to give up work and the income that comes with it in order to become a full time carer.

Carers assessment

It is important that the unpaid carer has a carers' assessment to assess their own needs before any discharge. Just as the patient must never be discharged into the community without adequate support, similarly the 'unpaid carer' must never be put into the position where they feel vulnerable and at risk. They must also have a strong network of support.

Underpinning neuroanatomy and physiology

Divisions of the nervous system

The nervous system is divided into a central and a peripheral nervous system. The central nervous system consists of the brain and spinal cord. The peripheral nervous system is made up of the 12 cranial nerves and the spinal nerves.

The central nervous system

The brain is further subdivided.

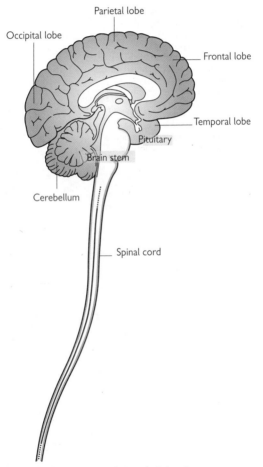

Fig. 2.1 The central nervous system: brain and spinal cord.

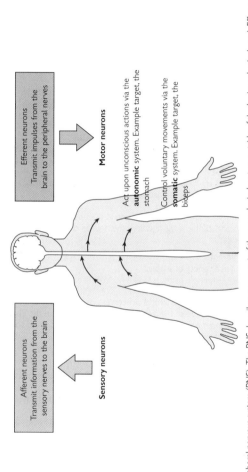

Fig. 2.2 The peripheral nervous system (PNS). The PNS describes every part of the neurological system outside of the brain and spinal cord. Efferent neurons are sometimes further divided into the sympathetic (generally stimulates function, e.g. increases heart rate) and parasympathetic (generally inhibits functioning of target, e.g. decreases heart rate) systems.

Cells of the nervous system

There are two distinct cell populations: neurons and neuroglia.

Neurons

The neuron is the functional cell of the brain and nervous system and consists of:

- A soma (cell body).
  - The typical soma contains a prominent nucleus. There are no centrioles and therefore the cell is incapable of mitosis that would enable them to repair themselves when damaged.
  - The soma also contains mitochondria, ribosomes and rough endoplasmic reticulum, known as *Nissl* bodies, that give the cytoplasm a coarse, grey appearance.
- Several branching dendrites that receive incoming signals.
- An elongated axon that transmits outgoing signals.
  - The base of the axon is attached to the soma at the axon hillock. Action potentials begin at the boundary between the axon hillock and the axon. Branches of the axon are called collaterals.
  - The axons travel in tracts or clusters throughout the brain, providing extensive interconnections between areas.
- One or more synaptic knobs.
  - Expanded synaptic knobs are found at the tips of each branch and forms part of the synapse where the neuron communicates with other cells.

Neuronal shapes

Neurons have a variety of shapes:

- Multipolar—multiple processes extend from the cell body, e.g. motor neurons controlling skeletal muscle.
- Unipolar—dendritic and axonal processes are continuous and the cell body lies to one side of the axon, e.g. sensory neurons in the PNS.
- Bipolar—consist of one dendrite and one axon with a central soma, e.g. cranial nerves innervating the eye and ear.

Types of neurons

There are three types of neurons:

- Sensory (afferent)—convey information from external and internal environments.
- Motor (efferent)—convey information from CNS to other tissues, organs or systems.
- Interneurons—connect with multiple neurons within the brain and spinal cord.

Neuroglia

Glial cells regulate the environment around the neurons, providing a supporting framework for neural tissue.

CNS glial cells

- Astrocytes. These cells are the largest and most numerous glial cells within the CNS that secrete essential chemicals for the maintenance of the blood–brain barrier, protecting the CNS from toxins in the general circulation. They provide a structural framework for neurons and other cells and repair other damaged neural tissue.

- Oligodendrocytes. Oligodendrocytes secrete the white, lipid-rich, myelin sheath surrounding axons within the CNS, improving the speed and conduction of impulses along the axon. The gaps between adjacent cell processes are called Nodes of Ranvier.
- Ependymal cells. These cells line the central canal of the spinal cord and the ventricles. They are involved in the production of CSF and the cilia on the ependymal surface help to filter and circulate the CSF throughout the CNS.
- Microglia. Microglia are the smallest and rarest neuroglia in the CNS. They are phagocytic, white blood cells that have migrated across the capillary walls in the CNS and provide protective functions, similar to those of white blood cells.

PNS glial cells

- Schwann cells. Schwann cells produce the myelin sheath around peripheral and cranial nerves.

Further information for health professionals and the public

Crossman AR and Neary D (2005) *Neuroanatomy: an illustrated colour text.* Edinburgh: Churchill Livingstone.

Action potentials

The action potential sequence is essential for communication between the sensory, integrative and motor functions of the nervous system. In response to stimuli, the cell membrane of a nerve cell goes through a sequence of depolarization from its resting state followed by repolarization back to its original state.

Depolarization

- A stimulus is received by the dendrites of a nerve cell
- Voltage-gated channels open and sodium (Na^+) ions enter the cytoplasm.
- If the stimulus is sufficient, more Na^+ channels open and the potential increases from –70 mV up to +30 mV.
- The channels then close, ensuring that the inner membrane contains more positive than negative ions, a process called depolarization.

Repolarization

- Once the Na^+ channels are closed, potassium (K^+) channels open to allow K^+ to move out of the cell and the membrane begins to repolarize back towards its resting potential.
- Since the K^+ channels function more slowly, the depolarization has time to be completed.
- To allow both Na^+ and K^+ channels to open simultaneously would prevent the generation of a further action potential.
- As the membrane repolarizes to –70mV and the K+ channels close, the membrane potential returns to its normal resting levels. The membrane is now in its pre-stimulation state and the action potential is complete.

Refractory period

A refractory period prevents the neuron from receiving other stimuli until it has returned to its resting state.

All-or-nothing principle

- A small stimulus either in amplitude or duration will cause no change in membrane potential.
- Progressively larger stimuli eventually reach a stimulus level that can evoke an action potential (*threshold* stimulus).
- A stimulus greater than the threshold level will elicit an action potential of the same magnitude each time; either the stimulus is sufficient to generate an action potential or it is not.

Continuous conduction

Impulses are transmitted at 1m/s along unmyelinated fibres. At the peak of an action potential the inside of a cell has an excess of positive ions, which spread along the inner surface of the membrane. This leads to the threshold being triggered further along the axon and in turn moves the action potential along the axon.

Saltatory conduction

Impulses are transmitted at 50m/s in myelinated fibres and depolarization can only occur at the Nodes of Ranvier, where the axon is exposed.
Speed of transmission is determined by:
- Temperature
- Presence or absence of myelin
- Fibre diameter

Factors affecting conduction

- Toxic substances—drugs, virus, infections
- Demyelination
- Fatigue
- Critical illness

Further information for health professionals and the public

Martini, F. and Bartholomew, F. (1999). *Essentials of anatomy and physiology*, 2nd edn. New Jersey: Prentice-Hall.
Tortora, G. and Derrickson, B. (2006). *Principles of anatomy and physiology*, 11th edn. London: Wiley.

Neurotransmission

A neuron propagates an action potential along its axon and transmits this impulse across a gap (synapse) between two neurons or between a neuron and an effector cell by releasing neurotransmitters. These chemical transmitters trigger a reaction in the post-synaptic neuron or effector cell, e.g. muscle cells, glands or endocrine cells.

The impulse may stimulate or inhibit the receiving cell, depending on the neurotransmitter and receptor involved.

- A synapse functions in one direction only
- Neurotransmission involves the transfer of information across the synaptic cleft and occurs through the release of chemicals called neurotransmitters
- A typical neuron will receive input from thousands of synapses

Neurotransmitters

The most common neurotransmitters are:
- Acetylcholine (ACh) in cholinergic synapses within the bulbospinal motor neurons, autonomic preganglionic fibres, postganglionic cholinergic fibres, and many neurons in the CNS.
  - It is rapidly broken down by the enzyme acetylcholinesterase.
- Noradrenaline (norepinephrine [NE])
- Dopamine
- Gamma-aminobutyric acid (GABA)
- Serotonin.

There are known to be over 100 neurotransmitters whose effects are still being researched.

Name	Effect	Action
Serotonin	Modulates hunger sensations, controls behaviour, sleep and affects neuro-endocrine control	Inhibitory
Dopamine	Involved with fine motor movement from the basal ganglia.	Inhibitory
Norepinephrine	Major transmitter in parts of the autonomic nervous system.	Excitatory and inhibitory
Gamma-aminobutyric acid (GABA) and glycine	Affects the synapses in the spinal cord, cerebellum, basal ganglia and some higher centre in the brain.	Excitatory

The process of neurotransmission

- Depolarization of the terminal membrane causes voltage channels to open, allowing calcium ions (Ca^{2+}) to enter the cytoplasm and trigger the release of the neurotransmitters into the synaptic cleft.
- Neurotransmitters diffuse across the cleft and bind to receptors on the post-synaptic membrane. Chemically regulated Na^+ channels in the post-synaptic cell are then stimulated producing a graded depolarization.

- The post-synaptic receptor is inactivated almost immediately to allow repeated stimulation of receptors and the neurotransmitter is promptly recycled back into the presynaptic nerve terminals or destroyed.
- The synaptic vesicles contain several thousand molecules of neurotransmitters. On stimulation they release these chemicals into the cleft.

Further information for health professionals and the public

Tortora, G. and Derrickson, B. (2006) *Principles of anatomy and physiology*, 11th edn. London: Wiley.

Neurotransmitters in health and illness

Impaired impulse transmission is the primary cause of many neurological and psychiatric disorders.

Environmental, physiological or psychological factors may also adversely affect the function of neurotransmitters, generating illness or disease processes.

Neurological disorders and neurotransmitters

- Alzheimer's disease and epilepsy—↓ levels of GABA
- Botulinum toxin inhibits the release of acetylcholine preventing muscle contraction
- Myasthenia gravis results from antibodies that damage acetylcholine receptors causing generalized neuromuscular weakness
- Parkinson's disease—insufficient dopaminergic neurons in the basal ganglia and substantia nigra
- Serotonin is implicated in onset of migraine

Neurotransmitters and drugs

- Schizophrenia—neuroleptic drugs help to block dopamine receptors
- Depression and anxiety disorders respond to benzodiazepines that affect the release of GABA
- Mood disorders—tricyclic drugs such as fluoxetine affect serotonin levels
- Anaesthetic agents—e.g. neostigmine, physostigmine, diisopropyl fluorophosphates gas, atracurium (curare-based drugs), inhibit the function of the neurotransmitters.

Functional areas of the brain

Frontal lobe

Functions

- Largely responsible for contralateral control
- Motor cortex is located in the precentral gyrus
- Language—Broca's area controls motor production of speech
- Personality
- Initiative, appropriateness, inhibitions—facilitation/suppression
- Cortical inhibition of bladder and bowel voiding

Parietal lobe

Functions

- Sensory cortex is located within the post-central gyrus
- Appreciation of posture, touch, passive movement, temperature
- Lower visual fields
- Auditory and visual aspects of comprehension
- Concept of body image
- Awareness of environment
- Visuospatial awareness and ability to construct shapes

Temporal lobe

Functions

- Auditory cortex
- Language interpretation (Wernicke's area)
- Learning and memory—recent and remote
- Area of the limbic lobe
- Upper visual pathways

Dominant hemisphere

- Important in the hearing of language

Non-dominant hemisphere

- Important in the hearing of sounds, rhythm and music

Occipital lobe

Functions

- Perception of vision
- Connection with other lobes for interpretation, memory, etc.

The cerebellum

- An automatic processing centre with two primary functions:
  - Adjustment of the postural muscles and programming and fine-tuning of movements controlled at the conscious and subconscious level
  - Balance and coordination of voluntary movement

Brainstem

- Midbrain, pons, medulla oblongata (autonomic nuclei)
- Cardiovascular centres—heart rate, strength of muscular contractions, and flow of blood

- Respiratory centre—rate and rhythm
- Cranial nerve nuclei—VIII, IX, X. XI and XII
- Relay stations—decussation of tracts to opposite side of the brain
- Reticular formation—consciousness

Limbic system

A functional grouping rather than an anatomical one.
- Establishing emotional states
- Links the conscious intellectual functions of cerebral cortex with the unconscious and autonomic functions of the brainstem
- Facilitates memory storage and retrieval

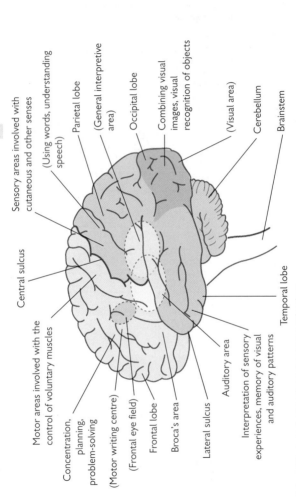

Fig. 2.3 Lateral view of the brain, functional area descriptions in brackets.
Reproduced from Fitzgerald O'Connor I., Urdang M. (2008) *Handbook for Surgical Cross-Cover*, with the permission of Oxford University Press.

Spinal pathways

Motor neurons that carry impulses from the cerebral cortex to the cranial nerve nuclei or the spinal cord are called upper motor neurons (UMN).

A lower motor neuron (LMN) extends from the spinal cord to skeletal muscle.

Damage to an LMN will result in a flaccid paresis of the muscle due to the lack of innervation. Injury to a UMN will produce some degree of spasticity caused by persistent stimulation and contraction of the muscle.

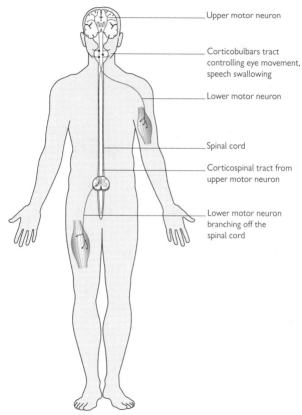

Upper motor neuron

Corticobulbars tract controlling eye movement, speech swallowing

Lower motor neuron

Spinal cord

Corticospinal tract from upper motor neuron

Lower motor neuron branching off the spinal cord

Fig. 2.4 An example of a motor neuron.

Autonomic nervous system

The autonomic nervous system (ANS) controls all the body's 'automatic' functions, i.e. those outside voluntary control. ANS neurons span both the CNS and PNS and control homeostasis.

Main functions/systems controlled by the ANS

- Cardiovascular system
- Respiration
- Digestion
- Excretion
- Thermoregulation

The ANS is divided into two main subdivisions: sympathetic and parasympathetic. These normally work in tandem and there is a balance between the effects of the two divisions.

Sympathetic division

The sympathetic division predominates during stress and is responsible for the 'fight or flight' response.

Parasympathetic division

The parasympathetic division predominates during rest and digestion, is responsible for emptying the bladder and bowel, and generally produces effects that are the opposite of sympathetic stimulation.

Table 2.1 Main sympathetic and parasympathetic effects

Target organ/function	Sympathetic response	Parasympathetic response
Pupil	Dilatation	Constriction
Heart rate	Increased	Decreased
Blood flow to heart and skeletal muscles	Increased	Decreased
Blood pressure	Increased	Decreased
Airways	Dilatation	Constriction
Respiratory rate	Increased	Decreased
Gut peristalsis	Decreased	Increased
Saliva production	Reduced	Increased
Gut secretions	Reduced	Increased
Bladder muscle	Relaxation	Constriction
Urethral sphincter	Contraction	Relaxation
Sweat production	Increased	
Body hair	Erect—goose bumps	
Adrenal glands	Secrete adrenaline and noradrenaline	

Cranial nerves

There are 12 pairs of cranial nerves that arise from nuclei within the brainstem. Some are purely sensory, some are mixed, i.e. motor and sensory, and some carry the autonomic i.e. sympathetic and parasympathetic innervations to internal glands or organs like the heart and lungs.

	Cranial nerve	Action	Innervation and function
I	Olfactory	Sensory	Transmits the sense of smell. Starts from olfactory mucosa in the nose and ends in the olfactory bulbs. They may be damaged in head injury, base of skull fractures, frontal lobe tumours or some forms of epilepsy.
II	Optic	Sensory	Carries visual information from the eyes. The optic nerves start at the retina and intersect at the optic chiasma before terminating at the lateral geniculate nuclei at the thalamus.
III	Oculomotor	Motor	Involved in eye movements and parasympathetic control of pupil size. From the midbrain, innervates four of the six muscles that control movement of the eyeball (superior, medial, inferior rectus and inferior oblique muscles).
			Controls autonomic (parasympathetic), supply of the shape of the lens and amount of light entering the eyes. III nerve lesions cause ptosis, loss of pupil constriction, squint and double vision.
IV	Trochlear	Motor	Controls eye movements by innervating the superior oblique muscle. Damage results in double vision.
V	Trigeminal	Mixed	Transmits sensory information from the head, face and motor control of the muscles for mastication. Three branches: ophthalmic (eye, nasal cavity, sinuses forehead and nose; maxillary (lower eye lid, lip, cheek and nose; and mandibular (temples, lower gums and teeth).
VI	Abducens	Motor	Controls the movements of the eye by innervating lateral rectus muscle. Paralysis causes convergent squint.

(Continued)

	Cranial nerve	Action	Innervation and function
VII	Facial	Mixed	Controls muscles of facial expression and transmits the sensation of taste from the anterior $^2/_3$ of the tongue. Also conveys parasympathetic supply to lacrimal, submandibular and sublingual glands.
VIII	Vestibularcochlear (acoustic)	Sensory	Sensation of hearing (cochlear portion) and balance and position (vestibular portion).
IX	Glossopharyngeal	Mixed	Controls movement of muscles in the throat, parasympathetic control of the parotid glands, sensation of taste from posterior $^1/_3$ of the tongue, and is involved in the detection of blood pressure changes in the aorta.
X	Vagus	Mixed	The motor portion controls the muscles in the pharynx, larynx and palate, essential for swallowing, and visceral organs in the thoracic and abdominal cavity. Also responsible for parasympathetic control of the heart, lungs, and abdominal organs.
XI	Spinal accessory	Motor	The cranial root supplies palate, pharynx and larynx along with the vagus nerve. The spinal root controls the muscles in the neck and shoulders.
XII	Hypoglossal	Motor	Controls movement of the tongue. Separate branches supply three of the four extrinsic muscles and all intrinsic muscles of the tongue.

The blood–brain barrier

The blood–brain barrier (BBB) provides protection for the delicate brain by governing substance movement between the blood and the brain. It performs this task by strictly regulating nutrient entry and inhibiting noxious substances including endogenous metabolic waste and therapeutically used xenobiotic substances across the brain capillary wall.

Although primarily made up of the endothelial cells that form brain capillaries, other cells interact with brain capillary endothelium to form the BBB including:

- Astrocytes
- Preicytes
- Neurons
- Other glial cells

The BBB is formed by the unity of these cells and interaction of the cells causes structural and functional changes in the brain capillary endothelial that confers BBB properties (Fig. 2.5).

Structural differences

Tight junctions

As a result of the above cell interactions, extremely effective and occlusive 'tight junctions' occur at cell–cell joint interfaces.

Reduced fenestrations and membrane surface area

The brain capillary endothelia posses very few fenestrations, which limits substance movement across the capillary wall. In addition, the luminal membrane of brain capillary endothelium is relatively devoid of folds which reduces its surface area available for substance diffusion.

Together these structural changes virtually eliminate the passage of water-soluble substances from the blood to the brain. Water-soluble substances like electrolytes, glucose and water-soluble amino acids have to be transported across the membrane through other means.

Fat-soluble substances are able to diffuse across the blood–brain barrier, but the BBB possesses a number of mechanisms that limit the diffusion of potential toxins across the capillaries into the brain. These mechanisms constitute the chemical differences found in brain capillaries compared with peripheral capillaries.

Chemical differences

Increased number of mitochondria

Brain capillary endothelium possesses a high number of mitochondria, which generate energy adenosine triphosphate (ATP) to drive the metabolic activities of the endothelium.

Drug efflux proteins

The BBB contains a number of membrane-bound and intracellular proteins that recognize a large number of fat-soluble substances. Drug efflux proteins are found in the luminal membrane of the endothelial cell and are thought to eject lipidic substances that are diffusing from the blood to the brain. These proteins eject substances against their concentration gradient, i.e. from membrane (low concentration) to the bloodstream (high concentration), to do this they utilize a large amount of energy in the form of ATP. There are different drug efflux proteins these include:

- P-glycoprotein (Pgp)
- Breast cancer resistance protein (BCRP)
- Multidrug resistance-related protein (MRP)

Of these drug efflux proteins, Pgp may play a significant role in limiting the entry of drugs into the brain, limiting their effect in CNS pathologies.

In addition to drug efflux, these proteins may play a role in transport of hormones and other homeostatic mediators from the brain to the bloodstream.

Drug metabolizing enzymes in the BBB

A large number of metabolic enzymes are expressed in the brain. Apart from a possible role in metabolizing medication, they play a role in oxidative processes in the brain.

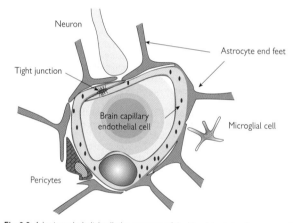

Fig. 2.5 A brain endothelial cell: the structure of the blood–brain barrier.

Cerebral haemodynamics

Intracranial contents

There are three main components within the skull:
- Brain and intracellular fluid (85%)
- Cerebrospinal fluid (7–10%)
- Blood (7–10%)

These three constituents are incompressible, i.e. they cannot be squashed into a smaller space, but they are interchangeable.

The Monroe Kelly doctrine

As the intracranial volume is fixed, changes in the volume of any of the components within the skull will necessitate a compensatory change in volume of one or more of the other components if intracranial pressure (ICP) is to remain constant.

Neurophysiology

- Cerebral blood volume (CBV) refers to the amount of circulating blood in the brain and is controlled by autoregulatory systems in the brain stem.
- CBV is affected by the systemic blood pressure (BP), cardiac function, blood viscosity, chemical and metabolic factors (Ph, CO_2 and O_2 values).
- Hypotension—mean arterial pressure (MAP) < 60mmHg—following severe brain injury is associated with increased disability and mortality.
- Normal ICP = 0–10mmHg.
- Cerebral perfusion pressure (CPP) represents the driving force behind maintaining a blood pressure gradient to the brain. 60–70mmHg is recognized as the critical threshold.
- CPP can only be calculated once ICP is recorded as the difference between the systemic MAP and the cerebral ICP.

$$CPP = MAP{-}ICP$$

- Cerebral compliance represents the brain's ability to adjust and maintain normal equilibrium against changing or increasing volumes.
- The degree of compliance is affected by the amount of additional volume, the amount of free space in the skull and the time available to accommodate any of the changes, e.g. slow-growing tumour compared to an acute extradural haematoma.
- When the volume of one or more of the contents begins to increase, the brain can initially compensate to maintain a normal CPP and ICP.
- Ultimately small increases in intracranial volume will dramatically increase ICP and reduce CPP.
- Once all compensatory mechanisms have been depleted, ICP will rise.

Compensation mechanisms

Reduction in CSF volume

CSF volume may be reduced through:
- Increased reabsorption
- Reduced production
- Diplacement to lumbar theca

Reduction in blood volume

Cerebral veins become compressed and blood is forced into the dural sinus, returning to the venous circulation.

Brain shift and herniation

Brain tissue moves into any available space until it begins to be compressed through the foramen magnum, known as cerebral herniation or coning.

Further information for health professionals and the public

Woodward, S. and Mestecky, A.-M. (2009) *Evidence-based neuroscience nursing.* Oxford: Wiley-Blackwell.

Cerebrospinal fluid circulation

CSF is a clear, colourless fluid that cushions and protects the brain and spinal cord from injury.

500ml of CSF is produced daily (25ml/hr) by the choroid plexus in the lateral, third and fourth ventricles and by the ependymal cells lining the ventricles.

The amount of CSF circulating through the ventricular system is only 120–150ml at any one time, indicating the degree to which it is being continuously produced and reabsorbed.

Composition
- Water
- Protein
- Electrolytes:
  - Sodium
  - Potassium
  - Chloride
  - Glucose
- Lymphocytes

CSF pressure and ICP

Normal CSF pressure is:
- Lying—60–180 mm H_2O
- Sitting—200–350 mm H_2O

ICP is directly affected by changes in the volume of CSF within the brain. These changes in volume may be the result of:
- Change in the rate of production of CSF.
- Obstruction to CSF flow.
- Changes in the rate of reabsorption of CSF.

Abnormalities in over-production, circulation, or reabsorption of CSF can result in hydrocephalus and may be an indication for insertion of an external ventricular drain.

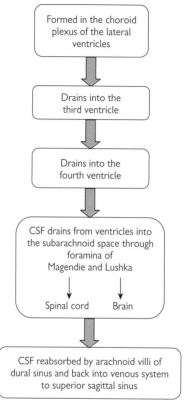

Fig. 2.6 The flow of cerebrospinal fluid.

Cerebral blood circulation

Arterial circulation (📖 see inside front cover)

A significant number of neurological disorders and secondary complications are related to cerebral circulation dysfunction. The brain demands 20% of the total cardiac output to maintain its normal function and autoregulation ensures that cerebral blood flow remains relatively constant by responding to changes in the diameter of the cerebral blood vessels.

The brain is unable to store oxygen or glucose, which leaves it particularly vulnerable to any interruption in its blood supply. Irreversible brain damage can occur within 2 minutes of oxygen (O_2) deprivation.

• The anterior communicating artery connects the right side of the brain to the left.
• The posterior communicating artery provides collateral circulation, joining the posterior circulation to the anterior circulation.

Venous circulation

The venous circulation drains deoxygenated blood from the superficial surface of the cerebral hemispheres and the internal structures within the brain. The superficial drainage flows into various dural sinuses positioned over the cerebrum. The largest is the superior saggittal sinus, which lies over the midline of the cerebrum from front to back.

Venous blood from the deeper cerebral structures drains into large veins that feed into the large vein of Galen, merging with the inferior saggittal sinus and flowing into the straight sinus then into the jugular veins.

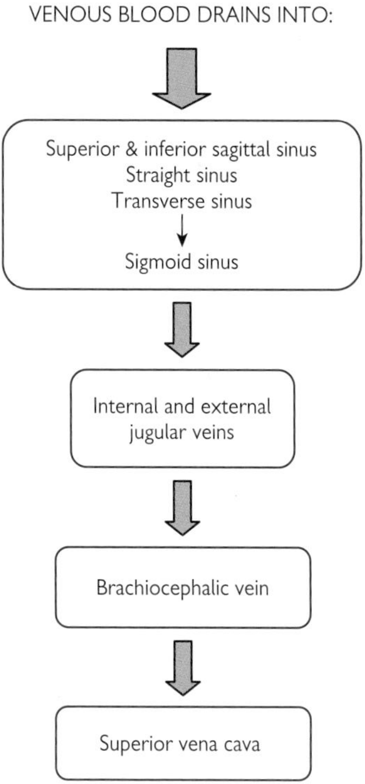

VENOUS BLOOD DRAINS INTO:

Superior & inferior sagittal sinus
Straight sinus
Transverse sinus
↓
Sigmoid sinus

Internal and external
jugular veins

Brachiocephalic vein

Superior vena cava

Fig. 2.7 Drainage of venous blood.

Neurological assessment

Assessment of level of consciousness

Consciousness is defined as a general awareness of oneself and the environment with the ability to respond appropriately to external stimulus. It is sensitive to and frequently the first indicator of neurological damage. Any deterioration can occur rapidly over minutes or very slowly over hours or weeks, depending on the cause.

Consciousness spans a broad continuum from fully aware and awake to deeply unresponsive to almost all external stimulation.

There are two mechanisms that influence level of consciousness (LOC):

1. Arousal—damage to the reticular activating system in the brain stem will affect the LOC.
2. Awareness—diffuse damage across the cerebral hemispheres will adversely affect cognitive functions.

Aetiology of altered LOC

- Metabolic—hypoglycaemia, hyperglycaemia, renal, pancreas and liver
- Electrolyte imbalance
- Neurolological—epilepsy, tumours, stroke, transient ischeamic attacks
- Hypoxic–ischaemic injury—head injury, carbon monoxide poisoning
- Infective—meningitis, encephalitis
- Cardiovascular—vasovagal response, arrhythmias
- Environmental—overdose, toxins, allergies
- Psychiatric disorders and psychotropic drugs (amphetamines, tricyclic antidepressants).

Diagnosis and investigations

Identification of the cause of altered LOC begins with taking a detailed past medical history (from the patient, relatives or carers), history of the presenting complaint and drug history (including prescribed medication and history of drug abuse).

Initial examination includes:

- Complete neurological assessment (including GCS)
- Vital signs—temperature, BP and pulse, oxygen saturation
- Assessment of changing respiratory pattern
- Assessment of breath odour (e.g. smell of alcohol, pear drop smell may indicate ketones)
- Limb assessment—assess tone, posture, reflexes
- Check for signs and symptoms of meningism (indicative of subarachnoid haemorrhage (SAH), meningitis, or infection)
- Evidence or a history of seizure activity
- Examination for skin lesions, e.g. rashes, bruising, pigmentation
- Fundoscopy—signs of: papilloedema, subhyaloid haemorrhages, infection retinopathy diabetes, hypertension)
- Otoscopy—evidence of bleeding or CSF leakage from the ear

Initial investigations may include:

- Urinalysis—for presence of glucose
- Full blood screen—including blood glucose, urea and electrolytes, liver function levels, full blood count, toxicology (blood or urine).
- CT scan or MRI

- Arterial blood gas analysis
- Electroencephalogram (EEG)
- Lumbar puncture

Defining coma

A patient is assessed as being in a state of 'coma' when the GCS is eight or below i.e.:
- Eyes open to pain E2
- Weak flexion to a central painful stimulus M4
- Incomprehensible sounds V2

Prognosis

The longer the period of unconsciousness, the greater the chance of disability.

Younger patients have the greatest chance of making a better recovery following their initial injury.

Long-term prognosis is affected by the premorbid state of the patient.

Glasgow Coma Scale

This 15-point scale was developed by Jennett and Teasdale (1974) and assesses the patient's level of consciousness by evaluating three behavioral responses directly corresponding to a region in the brain:

- Eye opening
- Verbal response
- Motor response

The scale allows the practitioner to make rapid, repeated evaluations of the patient's neurological status in response to a stimulus.

Each response carries a numerical value that correlates with the patient's best level of responsiveness or degree of deficit. The highest possible score is 15, the lowest possible score is 3 indicating:

- No eye opening (E1)
- No verbal response (V1)
- No movement in response to painful stimuli (M1)

Eye-opening response

Eye opening evaluates the patient's level of wakefulness thereby assessing the integrity of the ascending reticular activating system (📖 see Chapter 2, p 45).

Scoring eye-opening response	
Score 4	Eyes open spontaneously as the practitioner approaches patient
Score 3	The eyes open in response to speech
Score 2	The eyes open in response to a peripheral pain e.g. side of the fingernail distal to the last interphalangeal joint,(applied with graduating intensity for 10–15 seconds)
Score 1	No response to verbal or painful stimulus

'C' is recorded if the patient is unable to open their eyes due to peri-orbital swelling.

Verbal response

Verbal response assesses the Wernicke's speech centre (language centre) and Broca's speech centre, (coordinating expressive speech) in the temporal/frontal lobes respectively.

❶ Establish hearing acuity prior to assessment.

Scoring verbal response	
Score 5	Orientation to time, place and person. The patient should be able to state who they are (personal details), where they are (city or hospital), and the month and year
Score 4	Confusion. The patient gives inaccurate responses but is still able to talk in sentences
Score 3	Inappropriate words. The patient responds to questions but words are random or muddled and do not form complete sentences
Score 2	Incomprehensible sounds. The patient answers but with no clear discernable words, frequently moans or cries
Score 1	No response from patient to voice or any painful stimuli

'T' is recorded if the patient has an endotracheal tube or tracheostomy tube.

Motor response

Motor response evaluates the integrity of the motor strip in the cerebral cortex as well as ability to understand language and simple commands.

Scoring motor response	
Score 6	Patient obeys at least two commands or instructions ensuring that it isn't a mere reflex action, e..g. lift up arms, stick out tongue, display teeth, stick up thumb
Score 5	Patient localizes towards a central painful stimulus in an attempt to remove the pain, e.g. supra-orbital pressure, trapezium squeeze. Arm moves across the midline towards the level of the chin
Score 4	Normal flexion occurs when the patient flexes their arm at the elbow towards the source of the pain
Score 3	Abnormal flexion, known as decorticate movement. The patient bends their arm at the elbow and rotates wrist in a primitive posture
Score 2	Extension to pain, known as a decerebrate response when the patient extends their arms away from the source of the pain
Score 1	No response from arms to a central painful stimulus

Best practice guidance

- The **best** response from the arms is recorded.
- Even small changes can be significant and must be actioned.
- All sections of the chart must be completed as appropriate to the patient's condition. Any omissions or deviations in neurological status must be explained in the patient's records.
- Dots (•), not lines or ticks, must be used to fill out the GCS chart.

- Individual documentation of responses provides the clearest indication of cerebral function, i.e. E4, V5, M6—do not sum the scores.
- On commencement of shift handover one set of observations must be performed together (assessment must include the form of painful stimuli used and the specific questions used to assess orientation).
- A complete set of observations is carried out by the same person and wherever possible, continuity of observations should be maintained by the same person throughout the shift.
- Patients and relatives have the opportunity to discuss the results of the GCS assessment and its relevance to their individual needs.
- Student nurses should always complete GCS observations under direct supervision of a qualified practitioner.
- ❶ If in doubt—check your results with another nurse. Do not assume that you have got it wrong—the patient's condition may have changed.
- ❶ Report any deterioration immediately to the nurse in charge/medical staff and consider increasing the frequency of the observations.
- Serial assessments are more important than a one-off assessment of GCS

Reference

Jennett, B. and Teasdale, J. (1974) Assessment of coma and impaired consciousness: a practical scale. *Lancet*, 2: 81–4.

Further information for health professionals and the public

NNBG (2007) National Neuroscience Benchmarking Group. British Association of Neuroscience Nurses http://bann.org.uk.

Woodward, S. (1997) Practical procedures for nurses. No 5.1 Neurological observations. Glasgow Coma Scale. *Nursing Times*, 93(45 Suppl.): 1–2.

Woodward, S. and Mestecky, A.-M. (2009) *Evidence-based neuroscience nursing*. Oxford: Wiley-Blackwell.

Pupillary assessment

Pupil assessment forms an important part of the neurological assessment of the patient. Changes in the size, shape or speed of reaction of the pupil is frequently a **late** sign of increasing intracranial pressure.

Regular, repeated comparison with previous assessments is useful to identify subtle signs of change.

Normal
- Shape—should be round. Oval or irregular shape may indicate cerebral damage or compression of the cranial nerve.
- Pupils should be equal in size (25% of population have unequal pupils—aniscoria—with no known aetiology or pathological consequence).
- Size is 3–5 mm in diameter **prior to** shining a light into the eyes.
- They react briskly to light.
- Both pupils constrict to a light stimulus consensually (simultaneously).

Prerequisites to note
- Any pre-existing irregularities in pupil shape due to ophthalmic procedures e.g. trauma, cataracts, false eye, other disease processes or base of skull surgery causing local nerve damage.
- Medication that might cause the pupil to constrict, e.g. narcotics or topical beta blockers.
- Medication that might cause the pupil to dilate, e.g. atropine, tricyclic antidepressants.

Pupil examination
- Examination should be performed in a semi-darkened room, using a bright pen-torch.
- Ask the patient to look at a distant object when testing reaction (prevents accommodation and convergence reflex interfering with assessment).
- Accommodation reflex is observed by asking the patient to re-focus their vision from a distant object to a near object.
- Observe both eyes to confirm the responses are equal and symmetrical.
- It is important to assess both direct and consensual reflexes.
- ❶ The use of an ophthalmoscope is contraindicated as the light isn't strong enough to provoke a good response, similarly a large torch should not be used as the beam of light is too broad.
- Reaction should be recorded as: + pupil reacting, – no reaction, SL sluggish or slight reaction.
- Promptly report any changes from the patient's baseline to medical staff.

Assessment of reaction to light
Direct light response—move the beam of light from the outer aspect of the eye towards the pupil. The pupil should react briskly and return to its original size immediately after it is removed. Repeat the procedure for each eye, noting any differences.

Consensual reaction—both pupils should constrict when a light source is applied to one eye.
❶ Do not move the torch from one eye to the other across the bridge of the nose when assessing.

Abnormal pupil reactions

- A unilateral, unreactive pupil may be caused by an expanding mass (e.g. tumour, blood clot, or abscess) causing herniation of part of the temporal lobe through the tentorium cerebelli (a fold of dura) and compressing the 3rd cranial nerve.
- Bilateral, fixed dilated pupils may be an indication of herniation of the medial temporal lobe and is regarded as a terminal sign.
- Bilateral pinpoint pupils are invariably difficult to assess as reacting, but may be indicative of pontine heameorrhage or opiate overdose.
- Hippus reaction occurs when the pupil dilates and constricts. This 'twinkling' effect can be observed when there is increasing pressure on the 3rd cranial nerve.

Assessment of limb movements

The evaluation of limb movements forms an important part of the patient's neurological assessment and provides a baseline for future assessments and comparisons.

Any inexplicable change in limb movements may be an indication of brain injury and may help to determine the extent and position of the damage.

The results of this assessment are to be recorded alongside pupil reactions and GCS on a neurological assessment chart.

Prerequisites to note

- Pre-existing medical history may preclude normal limb movement, e.g. stroke, musculoskeletal or spinal disorders.
- Any acute orthopaedic injuries must also be taken into consideration.
- It is important to assess the patient's level of comprehension prior to the assessment, a patient with some degree of dysphasia or aphasia may not be able to understand the commands.
- The type of movement (involuntary or spontaneous), should be observed as well as comparing the strength of the limbs on both sides of the body.

Assessing limb movement

Limb movement is assessed initially by direct instruction.

Direct instruction—ask the patient to lift their limbs against gravity or move their limbs against a slight resistance. Power in all four limbs is assessed individually as:

- **Normal**—movements within the patients' normal power and strength.
- **Mild weakness**—cannot fully lift limbs against gravity and finds it difficult to move against resistance.
- **Severe weakness**—is able to move limbs laterally but cannot move against gravity or resistance.

For those patients that are unable to obey commands testing how the limbs react when a painful stimulus is applied should be observed.

Response to pain—the patient's response to central painful stimulus (e.g. trapezium squeeze) and their attempts to remove it is assessed. These reactions can present as:

- Normal flexion or withdrawal:
  - Rapid movement
  - The arm is drawn away from the trunk of the body
  - The elbow flexes
  - No muscle stiffness
- Abnormal flexion:
  - Slow movement
  - Forearms and hands are held against the body and the limbs have a hemiplegic position
  - The elbow will be flexed
  - Muscle stiffness is present

- Extension:
  - Limbs straighten, stretch, and extend
  - External rotation of the shoulders and forearms
  - Muscle stiffness is present
- No motor response (after application of maximum pain stimulus).

Swallowing assessment

Many patients with neurological problems experience dysphagia (swallowing difficulties). These patients are at risk of aspiration and developing chest infections and aspiration pneumonia. It is not always obvious when a patient aspirates, as they do not always cough and splutter. This is a problem known as silent aspiration.

Swallowing assessment is vital to ensure that patients are safe and that those patients who are at risk of aspiration do not develop problems. One of the first signs of a swallowing problem may be respiratory distress.

⚠ If in doubt—keep the patient nil-by-mouth (NBM) and refer to the speech and language therapist (SLT) for assessment. It is better to be safe than sorry.

Nursing bedside swallowing assessment

Some Trusts permit nursing bedside assessment of swallowing, while others do not. Local guidelines and policies should be followed at all times.

❶ Presence of a 'gag reflex' is **NOT** an indication of a safe swallow.

Patients should be assessed sitting up and with their head upright. Patients who are not sufficiently conscious to stay in this position and maintain attention should not be assessed further.

Assess general factors that contribute to safe swallow:
• Lip movements and ability to seal lips
• Tongue movement
• Ability to cough voluntarily
• Voice quality (a 'wet'-sounding voice may indicate aspiration e.g. of the patient's own saliva)

Assess ability to swallow a teaspoon of water:
• Observe the patient swallow and check for upward movement of the larynx during swallow
• Observe for any delay in swallowing more than a couple of seconds after the water has been put into the patient's mouth
• Observe for delayed cough up to 1 minute after swallowing
• Observe for pooling of liquid in the cheeks
• Check voice quality again for 'wet' or 'gurgly' voice which may indicate that the water is sitting around the laryngeal opening and has not been swallowed
• Observe for obvious signs of aspiration, e.g. coughing, choking or respiratory difficulty

If any of the above signs are present then the patient's swallow should be regarded as unsafe and necessary precautions taken as described above.

SLT assessment of swallowing

SLTs are able to undertake much more detailed assessment of swallowing function. Bedside assessment is performed, but videofluoroscopy may be indicated at a later date to identify specific problems.

Videofluoroscopy

Videofluoroscopy involves the patient swallowing radio-opaque liquids and solids of varying consistency while a real-time X-ray video is taken. This is then analysed by the SLT and radiologist.

No specific patient preparation is required.

Further information for health professionals and the public

Woodward, S. and Mestecky, A.-M. (2009) *Evidence-based neuroscience nursing*. Oxford: Wiley-Blackwell.

Pain assessment

Pain is a subjective experience, and can only be accurately described and assessed by the person experiencing it. Nurses can often allow their judgement and other factors to get in the way. Some procedures we would think of as minor and not particularly painful may often cause more pain than major neurosurgery. Don't make any assumptions about patients' pain—use a pain assessment tool.

Pain assessment tools

An appropriate assessment tool to the setting and patient's cognitive function should be chosen. Detailed assessment tools (e.g. the McGill pain questionnaire) would be no help for critically ill or confused patients, but may be good for chronic pain assessment.

Three key elements of pain need to be assessed:
- Quality
- Quantity
- Site

As well as duration + any exacerbating/relieving factors.

Examples of tools suitable for acute setting
- Numerical rating scale (e.g. the patient rates pain on scale between 0–3 or 0–10).
- Visual analogue scale (VAS)—the patient is asked to put a mark on 10cm line with no other markings than 0 and 10 to provide anchors at either end.
- Pain ruler (vertical scale showing markings from 0–10).
- Wong Baker faces scale. A series of pictures of faces showing different facial expression—especially useful for non-English speakers and children.

Examples of tools suitable for chronic pain assessment
- Oxford Pain Score
- McGill Pain Questionnaire

Factors that influence nurses' decision-making
- Personal experience of pain
- Personal background, culture, and ethnicity of the nurse
- Patient behaviour—patients laughing and joking are often not believed to be in pain, but may be using distraction to take their mind off the pain or be putting on brave face in front of visitors
- Patient age (older patients are more likely to be believed but less likely to be given analgesia due to fears of sedation and respiratory depression)
- Systemic obs: nurses look to elevated pulse (P) and BP to confirm patient reports of pain, but within 24hrs of acute pain, the body physiologically adapts and observations normalize
- Patient gender and lifestyle

Nursing interventions
- ⚠ Golden Rule: Believe what the patient is telling you and document their rating of pain, not what you think
- Use an appropriate pain assessment tool
- Re-check pain score after giving analgesia

Neuropathic pain assessment

Neuropathic pain is caused by damage to or a disturbance of either the central or peripheral nervous system. It may be acute or chronic.

Common conditions that may produce neuropathic pain include:
- Shingles
- Diabetic neuropathy
- Guillain–Barré syndrome (during the recovery phase)
- Trigeminal neuralgia
- MS
- Post-stroke
- Phantom limb pain following amputation

Neuropathic pain is different from other acute and chronic pain. It is often described as a constant burning or throbbing sensation, and patients may experience parasthesia and a constant sensation of 'pins and needles'. Patients should be assessed by a neurologist and undergo detailed neurological examination, with special attention being paid to sensory testing and assessment.

Neuropathic pain assessment tools

There are a number of specific neuropathic pain assessment tools available and guidelines for the assessment of neuropathic pain have been produced following a systematic review of the evidence by the European Federation of Neurological Societies (Cruccu et al., 2004).

The quality and intensity of the pain should be assessed and recorded separately, as with any pain assessment.

A simple pain assessment tool, e.g. a VAS, may be sufficient to assess neuropathic pain, but tools such as the McGill pain questionnaire are not recommended.

Further information for health professionals and the public

Cruccu, G., Anand, P., Attal, N. et al. (2004) EFNS guidelines on neuropathic pain assessment. Eur J Neurol, 11(3): 153–62.

White, S. (2007) in Woodward, S. (ed.) Neuroscience nursing: assessment and patient management, chapter 3, pp 29–40. London: Quay Books.

Assessment of sedation

The monitoring and assessment of levels of sedation is essential in the management of the critically ill patient.

Over or under-sedation is associated with longer lengths of stay, and increased levels of morbidity and mortality.

Aim of sedation

- Facilitate nursing care interventions
- Reduce anxiety, stress, and provide amnesia
- Promote sleep and hypnosis, reducing the incidence of post-traumatic stress disorder
- Control pain and enable the patient to tolerate unpleasant procedures or therapies
- Reduce the risk of accidental self-extubation or removal of invasive lines and catheters
- Reduce the use of neuromuscular blocking agents for patients requiring mechanical ventilation support
- May reduce the period of time spent on mechanical ventilation, leading to early discharge from the intensive care unit
- Depresses autonomic responses, reducing oxygen consumption and improving ventilator synchrony
- Facilitate a level of patient comfort that enables cooperation, communication and participation in care

Over-sedation

- May increase the period of time that the patient is ventilated, with corresponding increase in the cost of care
- Respiratory depression—prolonging the weaning process
- In the non-ventilated patient, resulting in severe hypercarbia, hypoxia and respiratory arrest

Under-sedation

- Increases blood pressure, pulse rate and oxygen consumption
- Inadvertent removal of essential tubes and catheters
- May precipitate development of a post-traumatic stress disorder following discharge
- Patients receiving neuromuscular blocking agents can be more at risk of under sedation

Sedation scoring systems

- Each individual response to sedation is variable; monitoring ensures the correct dose is administered.
- Sedatives may be administered intermittently or continuously depending on the duration of the therapy.
- Effective pain control reduces secondary complications, improves patient compliance and hastens recovery. Adequate analgesia reduces the necessity for other sedative therapy.
- There are several validated scoring tools available:
  - Linear analogue scales—allow various components of sedation to be measured independently.

- The Ramsay Sedation Scale is one example that uses six different levels or scores, according to how rousable the patient is. It is suitable for use in both intensive therapy unit (ITU) settings and general areas where narcotic or sedative drugs are administered.
- Unlike the Glasgow Coma Scale, the stimulus applied should not be painful or cause discomfort; rather, the assessment should be more observational and must not overly disturb the patient's sleep pattern.
- Assessment may be further augmented by the use of a bispectral monitor. An index score below 60 Bispectral Index (BIS), correlates with a Ramsey score of VI.

Ramsay Sedation Scale

I. Patient is anxious, agitated and restless
II. Patient is cooperative, oriented, and tranquil
III. Patient responds to commands only
IV. Patient exhibits brisk response to light stimulation
V. Patient responds sluggishly to stimulation
VI. Patient exhibits no response

Further information for health professionals and the public

DeJonghe B., Cook D., Appere-de-Vecchi C., Guyatt G., Meade M., & Outin H. (2000). Using and understanding sedation scoring systems: a systematic review. *Intensive Care Medicine* 342: 1471–1477.

Assessment of cognition

Cognition describes mental processes such as thinking, perception and memory. Cognition involves a number of different elements, all of which need to be assessed:
• Orientation
• Memory
• Attention and concentration
• Ability to evaluate
• Affect/mood
• Abstract reasoning
• Insight

Simple bedside assessment

Ask the patient to read a newspaper headline or short article and then have a conversation with them about what they have read. For those who have problems with English language or dysphasia—use the pictures. For example, can they recognize famous faces, or can they recognize and appreciate the differences between a range of facial expressions?

By asking the patient to read the paper you will be able to assess all of the above at the bedside:
• Does the patient understand what you have asked them to do and have they followed the instruction?
• Are they able to hold their attention on the paper long enough to carry out the task?
• Can they remember what they have just read?
• Can they discuss the story and draw conclusions about future implications of what they have read?

Mini Mental State Examination (MMSE)

This is the most commonly used bedside screening tool to identify levels of cognitive impairment and has been shown to be a valid and reliable tool since it was published (Folstein et al., 1975), although it cannot be used with patients who do not speak English or who have aphasia.

This tool is easy to use at the bedside and will identify whether a patient has cognitive impairment, but will not tell you why. It takes only a few minutes to administer.

The MMSE assesses the following cognitive elements:
• Orientation to time and place
• Registration (initial memory) and short-term memory (lasts seconds to minutes
• Language ability
• Calculation ability

A score out of 30 is given and scores between 24–30 are considered within normal limits.

Specific cognitive assessment

For some patients more detailed cognitive assessment is required and these patients would require referral to a clinical neuropsychologist.

References

Folstein, M.F., Folstein, S.E., McHugh, P.R. (1975) 'Mini-mental state'. A practical method for grading the cognitive state of patients for the clinician. *J Psychiatr Res*, 12(3): 189–98.

Further information for health professionals and the public

Woodward, S. and Mestecky, A.-M. (2009) *Evidence-based neuroscience nursing*. Oxford: Wiley-Blackwell.

Functional assessment—Barthel Index

Functional assessment is primarily used within rehabilitation settings to determine functional outcomes from rehabilitation.

There are a variety of tools available to assess functional outcomes, with the most commonly used being the Barthel Index and functional independence meaure (FIM)/functional assessment measure (FAM).

These tools aim to provide clinicians and researchers with an objective and reliable assessment of disability and function. They can also be used to evaluate the effectiveness of rehabilitation service provision.

Barthel Index

The Barthel Index (Mahoney and Barthel, 1965) is a widely used scale for assessing functional outcomes in rehabilitation settings.

While this is primarily used by allied health professionals, nurses may also find it a simple and useful tool to assess functional outcomes for their patients.

Scoring

Score the patient for each item and the sum will give a total score out of 20.

Difficulties

The tool is very subjective and open to interpretation. For many items there is no indication as to the level of assistance required, so the Barthel Index may not be very sensitive to changes in the patient's ability over time, compared to other functional assessment tools.

Item	Scores
Bowels	0 = dependent on intervention 1 = some episodes of faecal incontinence/soiling 2 = continent
Bladder	0 = dependent on intervention 1 = some episodes of urinary incontinence 2 = continent
Grooming	0 = dependent 1 = independent
Toileting	0 = dependent 1 = assistance required 2 = independent
Feeding	0 = dependent 1 = assistance required 2 = independent
Transfer	0 = dependent 1 = maximal assistance 2 = minimal assistance 3 = independent
Mobility	0 = dependent 1 = independent using wheelchair 2 = assistance from one person to walk 3 = independent
Dressing	0 = dependent 1 = assistance required 2 = independent
Stairs	0 = dependent 1 = assistance required 2 = independent
Bathing	0 = dependent 1 = independent

Mahoney and Barthel (1965).

Further information for health professionals and the public

Mahoney, F.I. and Barthel, D.W. (1965) Functional evaluation: the Barthel index. *Maryland State Medical Journal*, 14: 61–5.

Functional assessment

Functional independence measure (FIM)

The FIM was produced by Granger *et al.* in 1986 and practitioners need to be trained in its use and scoring, to ensure reliable and consistent results are obtained.

While most nurses will not be required to use this tool themselves, they may be part of the assessment process through case conferences and will need to be able to comment on the patient's abilities detailed below.

It is a widely used functional assessment scale and can be completed in approximately 20 minutes, either at a case conference, by observing the patient or by telephone interview. It consists of 18 items and is designed to assess change in the patient's function and independence over time during the course of rehabilitation treatment. Each item is scored against the patient's level of dependence/independence from 0 (complete dependence) to 7 (independence).

This is a valid and reliable tool, but does have limitations for use with certain neurological conditions as it does not assess many functions related to cognition or communication. FIM has a wider scoring scale and therefore is often more sensitive to change than the Barthel index.

Items covered by FIM are:
- Self-care:
  - Feeding
  - Grooming
  - Bathing
  - Dressing upper body
  - Dressing lower body
  - Toileting
- Sphincter control:
  - Bladder
  - Bowel
- Mobility:
  - Transferring to bed, chair or wheelchair
  - Transferring to toilet
  - Transferring to bath and shower
- Locomotion:
  - Ambulation
  - Stairs
- Communication:
  - Comprehension
  - Expression
- Social cognition:
  - Social interaction
  - Problem-solving
  - Memory

Functional assessment measure (FAM)

This tool was developed to complement the FIM. A further 12 items were identified which could be added to the initial 18 identified in FIM to create a 30-item scale.

The main areas addressed by FAM are those that were less well covered by FIM, i.e. cognition, communication, behaviour and ability to function in the community, which are often the issues identified as being most important to the patients.

A UK version of FIM+FAM has been developed.

Additional items covered by FAM include:

- Self-care:
  - Swallowing
- Mobility:
  - Transfer to car
- Locomotion:
  - Community mobility
- Communication:
  - Reading
  - Writing
  - Speech intelligibility
- Psychological adjustment:
  - Emotional status
  - Adjustment to limitation
  - Employability
- Cognitive function:
  - Orientation
  - Attention
  - Safety judgement

Reference

Granger, C.V., Hamilton, B.B. and Sherwin, F.S. (1986) *Guide for the use of the uniform data set for medical rehabilitation*. Buffalo, New York: Uniform Data System for Medical Rehabilitation Project Office.

Further information for health professionals and the public

Hall, K.M., Hamilton, B.B., Gordon, W.A., *et al.* (1993) Characteristics and comparisons of functional assessment indices: disability rating scale, functional independence measure, and functional assessment measure. *J Head Trauma Rehabil*, 8: 60–74.

Hawley, C.A., Taylor, R., Hellawell, D.J. and Pentland, B. (1999) Use of the functional assessment measure (FIM+FAM) in head injury rehabilitation: a psychometric analysis. *J Neurol Neurosurg Psychiatry*, 67: 749–54.

Nutritional assessment

It has long been known that hospitalized patients are at risk of malnutrition. This is a particular problem for patients with neurological problems affecting both patients with long-term conditions and those who are acutely or critically ill for a variety of reasons.

Some patients may develop problems with nutrition due to difficulty feeding themselves or swallowing, while others develop malnutrition due to the hypermetabolic state and catabolism that occur following severe trauma.

⚠ Nutritional assessment of neurological patients is vital and falls very squarely in the lap of nursing staff.

A valid and reliable tool should be used for nutrition assessment. Many nutrition assessment tools are available and there may be one that has been specifically developed for use within a local Trust. Other care areas may use a nationally recognized tool such as the Malnutrition Universal Screening Tool (MUST) (BAPEN, 2003). Other guidelines and screening tools are recommended by the European Society for Clinical Nutrition and Metabolism (ESPEN).

BAPEN questions

The British Association of Parenteral and Enteral Nutrition (BAPEN) has set out four questions that every patient must be asked on admission to hospital:
• Have you unintentionally lost weight recently?
• Have you been eating less than normal?
• What is your normal weight?
• How tall are you?
This is the bare minimum assessment required. All patients should be weighed and have their height recorded.

Malnutrition Universal Screening Tool

The MUST has been developed by BAPEN for use in either acute or community settings. The tool is designed to identify those patients who have or are at risk of malnutrition, or who are obese. It is available from the BAPEN website.

Body Mass Index

Body mass index (BMI) is a measure of height to weight ratio. It is calculated using the following formula:

$$\frac{\text{Weight (Kg)}}{\text{Height}^2 \text{ (m}^2)}$$

❶ As this calculation uses actual body weight it may not give an accurate indication of nutritional status in a patient who is fluid overloaded and should be used with caution.

Anthropometric assessment

Anthropometric nutritional assessments give a measure of lean body mass (muscle mass) and body fat, which are often better indicators of nutritional status than BMI.

Nurses do not usually perform these assessments, but they may be carried out by a dietitian.

These measurements include:
- Skinfold thickness (assesses body fat) can be measured at various sites e.g. triceps, biceps.
- Mid-arm circumference (assesses muscle and bone + subcutaneous fat).
- Mid-arm muscle circumference is calculated from the above two measurements and gives an indication of protein-energy malnutrition.

Biochemical and laboratory assessment

Some patients who are critically ill require a more exact measure of nutritional status and data from which to calculate nutritional requirements.

An example may be the use of nitrogen balance to calculate the protein requirements of the patient. This is done by measuring the nitrogen content from urea in the patient's urine over 24 hours. If nitrogen is being eliminated then the patient is said to be in a positive nitrogen balance and they are receiving sufficient protein intake. If no nitrogen is eliminated the opposite is true.

While these tests are carried out by a dietitian the nurse must:
- Record all food intake during the 24-hour period.
- Collect all the patient's urine for 24 hours after the first void on the morning of the test.

Further information for health professionals and the public

British Association for Parenteral and Enteral Nutrition http://www.bapen.org.uk/
British Association for Parenteral and Enteral Nutrition (2003) *Malnutrition Universal Screening Tool: 'MUST'*. Redditch: BAPEN.
European Society for Clinical Nutrition and Metabolism http://www.espenblog.com/

Assessment of bladder function

Continence and bladder problems are common in neurological disorders. Continence assessment is a nursing role and detailed assessment is often required.

All patients should be asked a trigger question to identify whether they are likely to have a bladder problem. Some Trusts have developed lists of trigger questions which will alert the nurse to the likelihood of a problem.

Examples of trigger questions:

- How many times do you need to empty your bladder during the day? (Normal 6–7 times).
- How many times do you have to get up to empty your bladder at night? (Normal 0–1 time).
- Do you ever have to rush to a toilet urgently to empty your bladder?
- Do you ever feel that you do not empty your bladder fully?

If a bladder/continence problem is suspected from the trigger questions, a detailed continence assessment must be performed.

Continence assessment checklists

The use of an assessment checklist/continence assessment tool is advised as this will:

- Act as an aide memoir and make sure nothing is omitted.
- Make sure a logical sequence to assessment is followed.
- Provide a means of documenting data.
- Act as a baseline for evaluating interventions.

A valid and reliable tool should be used, but not many have been validated in practice (Woodward, 2006).

Detailed continence assessment

Detailed assessment of bladder problems must include the following:

General history

- Past medical, surgical and obstetric history (don't assume that the continence problem is due to the neurological condition)
- Drug history (check the medications to see if there are any side-effects that affect the bladder)
- Mobility and manual dexterity
- History of how the problem is currently managed

Urinary symptoms

- Frequency (more than 6–7 times per day)
- Nocturia (more than once at night)
- Urgency
- Hesitancy (difficulty getting going)
- Straining to void
- Post-micturition dribbling
- Nocturnal enuresis (bedwetting)
- Leak on exertion (small amount of urine lost on coughing, sneezing, laughing, etc.)
- Dysuria (burning sensation on passing urine)

Physical examination
- Observe patients perineal skin condition for signs of excoriation and wetness
- Per rectum (PR) examination to assess for constipation
- Observe for signs of uterine prolapse

Investigation
- Urinalysis—especially for nitrites and leucocytes (indicates infection)
- Post-void residual measurement (preferably using a bladder scan as this is non-invasive, but if not available an in–out catheterization may be performed)
- Consider referral for urodynamics

Further information for health professionals and the public

Woodward, S. (2006) Development of a valid and reliable tool for assessment of urinary incontinence in people with neurological problems. *British Journal of Neuroscience Nursing*, 2(5): 247–55.

Association for Continence Advice http://www.aca.uk.com

The Bladder and Bowel Foundation http://www.bladderandbowelfoundation.org

Assessment of bowel function

Faecal incontinence and other bowel problems are common in neurological disorders. Bowel assessment is a nursing role and detailed assessment is often required.

As with bladder assessment, all patients should be asked a trigger question to identify whether they are likely to have a bowel problem. Some Trusts have developed lists of trigger questions which will alert the nurse to the likelihood of a problem.

Examples of trigger questions:

- How often do you have a bowel motion? (Normal not more than 3 times per day and not less than once every three days).
- Do you ever have to rush to a toilet urgently to empty your bowel?
- Do you ever feel that you do not empty your bowel fully?
- Do you have to strain to empty your bowel?

If a bowel/faecal incontinence problem is suspected from the trigger questions, a detailed bowel assessment must be performed.

Bowel assessment checklists

The use of a bowel or faecal incontinence assessment checklist is advised as this will:

- Act as an aide memoir and make sure nothing is omitted
- Make sure a logical sequence to assessment is followed
- Provide a means of documenting data
- Act as a baseline for evaluating interventions

Examples of such tools can be found in Norton and Chelvanayagam (2004).

Detailed bowel assessment

Detailed assessment of bowel problems must include the following:

General history

- Past medical, surgical and obstetric history (don't assume that the bowel problem is due to the neurological condition)
- Drug history (check the medications to see if there are any side-effects that affect bowel)
- Diet and fluid intake
- Mobility and manual dexterity
- History of how the problem is currently managed
- Effect of bowel problem on lifestyle and relationships

Bowel symptoms

- The most bothersome symptoms/main problem for the patient
- Usual bowel habit/frequency (any deviation from normal limits should be noted)
- Consistency of stool (Use the Bristol Stool Form Scale—copies are available from Norgine Ltd)
- Urgency or lack of urge
- Bleeding PR (on wiping or in toilet—blood loss in the toilet is a red flag symptom and should be investigated further)
- Mucus passed
- Straining

- Feeling of incomplete evacuation
- Soiling or faecal incontinence
- Pain associated with bowel motions, either before or during defecation (site of pain—rectal/abdominal; is it relieved on defecation?)
- Digitation (using a finger in rectum or vagina to assist bowel to empty)

Physical examination
- Observe patient's perineal skin condition for signs of excoriation and soiling, scars and anal fissure/hemorrhoids/rectal prolapse, etc.
- PR examination to assess for constipation

Investigation
The patient may need referral for more detailed investigations, e.g.
- Anorectal physiology (testing of anal sphincter function and reflexes)
- Colonic transit studies (plain abdominal x-ray after ingestion of radio-opaque markers) to diagnose slow transit

Reference

Norton, C. and Chelvanayagam, S. (2004) *Bowel continence nursing*. Beaconsfield: Beaconsfield Publishers Ltd.

Further information for health professionals and the public

Norton, C. et al. (2008) *Oxford Handbook of Gastrointestinal Nursing*. Oxford: Oxford University Press

Association for Continence Advice http://www.aca.uk.com

The Bladder and Bowel Foundation http://www.bladderandbowelfoundation.org

Neurological investigations

Computerized tomography scan

A computerized tomography (CT) scan is a specific X-ray procedure in which a computer is used to summate and reconstruct images obtained in multiple planes. Several X-rays are passed through the area of the body being scanned from different directions simultaneously.

The X-rays are detected having passed through the tissues and their relative strength is measured. X-rays that passed through less dense tissue such as CSF or brain tissue will be stronger than X-rays that have passed through denser tissue such as bone.

The relative density of the tissues is then calculated by a computer and an image displayed, with very-low-density areas (e.g. air in the sinuses or CSF within the ventricles) showing up as black and high-density areas (e.g. skull bones) showing up as white. Brain tissue density lies between these two extremes and appears as shades of grey.

Contrast media may be injected to show areas of enhancement. Where the blood–brain barrier has been disrupted, e.g. around a tumour or cerebral abscess, contrast is able to pass through into the brain tissue and will be evident on the image.

Patient preparation

- A CT scan may be performed as an outpatient procedure and requires minimal preparation.
- Patients are normally asked to remove contact lenses or glasses, hair clips and hearing aids prior to the scan.
- Very young patients, non-compliant patients or patients with severe movement disorders will usually require sedation to ensure that they remain still for the duration of the scan.

Post-procedure care

- No specific post-procedure care is required, but the patient should be observed until fully alert if sedation has been used.

Safety features

The potential risk associated with a CT scan are very similar to conventional X-rays due to the use of ionizing radiation that may increase the risk to a foetus or increase the risk of developing a malignancy.

Occupational exposure is monitored and staff must attend yearly updates to comply with health and safety regulations.

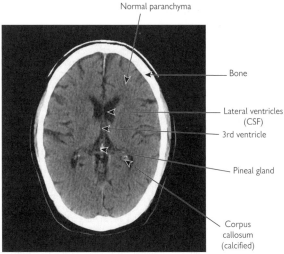

Normal paranchyma

Bone

Lateral ventricles
(CSF)

3rd ventricle

Pineal gland

Corpus
callosum
(calcified)

Fig. 4.1 CT scans use ionizing radiation to generate two-dimensional cross-sections of structures. They are used to determine the extent of bone destruction or calcification. Dense structures such as bone appear as white, other soft tissues appear in varying shades of grey, black represents air spaces. Images can be further enhanced with intravenous radio-opaque contrast medium. CT is particularly useful in detecting haemorrhage, hydrocephalus, large tumours, cerebral atrophy, and in imaging the bones of the skull base.

Magnetic resonance imaging

Magnetic resonance imaging (MRI) is a relatively new imaging technique that produces very detailed images of internal organs and tissues. Patients lie inside a large cylindrical magnet, while radio waves many thousands of times stronger than the earth's magnetic field are passed through the patient's body. This forces the nuclei of the body's atoms into a different alignment, and then when the signal is stopped and the atoms realign in their normal position, they send out radio waves which are picked up by the scanner and converted into an image.

MRI is non-invasive and does not involve X-rays, but the magnet is incompatible with many implantable devices or metal prosthesis.

Patient preparation
- Identify any contraindications. If the patient is unconscious a close relative must be approached for the information.
- Warn the patient about the claustrophobic effects of entering the scanner and that they will be able to communicate with staff.
- Assist the patient to change into a gown and remove watches, jewellery and hair clips. Mobile phones and credit cards must not be taken into a scan room as the magnetic information stored within them will be erased.
- ⚠ Anyone moving into the vicinity of the scanner must not take any ferromagnetic objects into the room to avoid 'missile effect' objects flying into the scanner causing damage or injury.

⚠ Cautions
- Pregnancy—injection of contrast medium and scans during the first trimester should be avoided.
- Noise—vibrations produce a loud noise that patients can find very disturbing. Ear protection is provided that plays music requested by the patient and allows staff to communicate with the patient.
- Claustrophobia—panic attacks may occur. Some patients will require sedation or anaesthetic.

❶ Absolute contraindications
- Cardiac pacemakers, vagal nerve stimulators, internal defibrillators, cochlear implants and deep brain stimulators, insulin or baclofen pumps, shell fragments, older aneurysm clips and metal fragment in the eyes associated with people involved with metal working.
- Titanium alloy materials are normally MRI compatible. Patients are asked for detailed information relating to the prosthesis including insertion date and model number to clarify compatibility.

Post-procedure care
No specific post-procedure care is required.

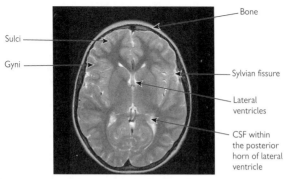

Fig. 4.2 MRI scans can be used to complement the results from CT scans. It is a non-invasive medical imaging investigation that uses magnetic fields and non-ionizing radio-frequency signals. The intensity of the signal describes the brightness and clarity of the various tissues that are described as hyperintense or 'bright', iso-intense 'grey' or hypointense, 'dark' and this is used to compare possible abnormalities against the appearance of normal tissues. Interpretation of the scans will depend on the type of image recorded and the use of contrast medium. T1 images—CSF is shown as 'black'. T2 images CSF will be 'white'.

Functional MRI

Functional MRI (fMRI) is a form of MRI scanning that has been used since the early 1990s to examine functional activity within the brain.

It is now the most common form of imaging used to map the functional activity of the brain due to its low risk profile and wide availability. It is more commonly used than either positron emission tomography (PET) or single photon emission computerized tomography (SPECT) scanning, which are generally only used for research.

Functional MRI shows the metabolism of oxygen, based on the assumption that this correlates with neuronal activity.

Brain neurons cannot store oxygen or glucose and when an area of brain is active, more oxygen is required so the blood flow to this area of brain increases. This can be measured, as oxygenated blood gives off a different MRI signal to deoxygenated blood.

While in the scanner patients may be asked to undertake a series of cognitive tests or other tasks/activities, depending on the functional area of brain being assessed.

Patient preparation

The patient completes a comprehensive questionnaire, as for routine MRI scanning; if the patient is unconscious a close relative is approached for the information.

Other preparation would be the same as for MRI (📖 see Magnetic resonance imaging, p 94).

Post-procedure care

As for MRI, no specific post-procedure care is required.

MR and CT angiography and venography

MR and CT angiography are non-invasive and therefore are much less risky than conventional angiography.

MR angiography

MR angiography (MRA) is used to visualize blood vessels within the brain and neck using the MRI scanner rather than X-rays and CT scanning.

It may be performed with or without contrast media and as no X-rays are used does not carry the same risks as conventional angiography.

MR angiography can also be performed without the need for injecting contrast media directly into the femoral or other major artery, thereby eliminating the risk of haemorrhage.

If contrast media are used they will be injected intravenously via a peripheral cannula.

Patient preparation

The patient completes a comprehensive questionnaire; if the patient is unconscious a close relative is approached for the information.

Post-procedure care

As for MRI, no specific post-procedure care is required.

CT angiography

CT angiography (CTA) is particularly useful for imaging cerebral vessels to:
- determine suitability for thrombolysis
- detect atherosclerosis which may lead to ischaemia
- detect small aneurysms or arteriovenous malformations (AVM)
- examine in detail the blood supply to a tumour prior to surgery

Patient preparation

- Assist the patient to change into a gown for the procedure if necessary
- The patient should remove any jewellery, glasses, hearing aids and dentures
- ⚠ Check any allergies, especially to contrast media on previous occasions
- The patient may need to be NBM for a period before the scan if contrast is to be used
- Warn the patient that they will need to remain still for the duration of the scan

Post-procedure care

No specific post-procedure care is required

MR and CT venography

Cerebral venous circulation may also be a source of problems and these vessels can also be imaged by MR or CT venography.

Positron emission tomography scanning

What is a PET scan?

Positron emission tomography (PET) scans are not widely available and are often used for research purposes.

It is one of a number of investigations carried out within nuclear medicine departments and is one form of functional neuroimaging, showing metabolic activity within the nervous system, rather than structure per se.

PET scans use an injection of a positron emitting radioactive form of glucose or a similar inhaled form of oxygen. Following the injection these travel to areas of high glucose or oxygen metabolism, e.g. in the brain, and these areas therefore become visible on the scan. Positrons are emitted as the radioactive substance breaks down and 3D, colour images are produced.

Some cells, e.g. malignant cells, divide rapidly and have increased metabolic activity. If they are present, injected radio nuclides become trapped and the PET scan detects this. PET can also be used to diagnose conditions such as epilepsy or Alzheimer's disease.

Patient preparation

- Patients should not drink caffeine-based drinks or alcohol and should not smoke for 24 hours prior to the scan—this can affect cell metabolism
- ⚠ Do not administer glucose infusions to patient prior to PET scanning.
- Patients may be required to have nothing to eat or drink for anything between 4–12 hours prior to the scan depending on the scan being performed—check detailed instructions with the department
- Patient education is important. Warn the patient that they will need to:
  - Rest for approx 1 hour in the department after the injection to allow the radioactive glucose to be distributed throughout the brain tissue—may take a book with them if well enough or may like to take a personal stereo/MP3 player to alleviate boredom
  - Undergo the scanning process for approx 1 hour—need to lie still during the scanning
  - Alert the staff in the scanning department if they feel unwell during the scan
  - May be asked to undertake some cognitive assessments while being scanned, e.g. mental arithmetic, answering questions

Post-procedure care

- Encourage patient to drink plenty to flush radioactive substances from the body—they decay quickly, but this will help
- No other specific nursing care is required, but the patient should not have contact with babies or pregnant women for between 6–24 hours post-scan—check specific timings with the department that carried out the scan.

Further information for health professionals and the public

NHS Direct http://www.nhsdirect.nhs.uk

Single photon emission computed tomography scanning

SPECT is another non-invasive imaging technique that involves the scanning of gamma rays and, like PET, enables assessment of brain function.

SPECT differs from PET in that the radioisotopes injected are helped to cross the blood–brain barrier and are taken up in the areas of the brain that have the highest blood flow through them. These radioisotopes are detected by a gamma camera and images are available immediately following the injection.

SPECT was initially used to measure cerebral blood flow and can detect alteration in blood flow due to a number of neurological conditions that disrupt this, e.g.

- stroke
- head injury not visible using other imaging techniques
- partial seizures
- seizure origin when evaluating patients for epilepsy surgery
- spinal stress fractures

Patient preparation

- Patient education is important. Warn the patient that they will need to:
  - Undergo the scanning process for between 20 minutes and approx 1 hour—need to lie still during the scanning
  - Alert the staff in the scanning department if they feel unwell during the scan
  - Rest for approx. 10–20 minutes following the injection
- ⚠ Patients may experience an allergic reaction to the radioisotope injection. Ensure that adrenaline is prescribed for use as required before the patient goes to the scan room
- During the procedure observe the patient for reactions to the injection, e.g. itching, shortness of breath

Post-procedure care

- Encourage patient to drink plenty of fluids to flush radioactive substances from the body.

Cerebral angiography

Cerebral angiography involves imaging of cerebral blood vessels to detect aneurysm or AVM. It may be invasive or non-invasive (MR angiography). Invasive angiography carries a risk of about 1% of stroke and therefore is normally avoided unless absolutely necessary. Angiography can be conducted as a day case.

Invasive angiography is carried out under sedation or rarely general anaesthetic (GA), usually via a puncture in the femoral artery and catheter fed up through the vascular system to the carotids to inject radio-opaque dye.

X-ray images of the skull are taken before and after injection of dye, then the computer subtracts the plain image from the other to leave a view of just the blood vessels containing the dye.

Pre-procedure care

- Ensure the patient is given a full explanation of the procedure and consent is obtained
- Good patient hygiene ↓risk of infection: patients should take a bath or shower on the day and wear a clean gown
- It is not necessary to shave the groin and this may increase risk of infection if skin is cut
- The patient may need to be NBM for few hours beforehand if GA is to be administered
- Inpatients should be accompanied to imaging and handed over to nursing staff

Nursing role during procedure and in imaging dept

- Reassure the patient throughout and explain the need to lie still
- Check consent and patient preparation
- Scrub to assist during the procedure
- IV cannulation and administration of sedation
- Post-procedure recovery—systemic obs and check site
- Nurse-led discharge may be possible if day cases are carried out in the department

Post-procedure care

- Regular systemic obs (temperature, pulse, respirations (TPR) and BP)) + neuro obs (minimum half hourly)
- Check puncture site for haemorrhage and haematoma
- Bedrest for 4 hours
- Oral fluids and diet once sedation effects have worn off and swallowing is safe
- ▶▶If bleeding occurs apply pressure and call doctor immediately
- ❶If a haematoma occurs apply a pressure dressing and inform doctor

Possible complications
- Haemorrhage
- Haematoma formation
- Puncture site infection
- Cerebral vasospasm
- Stroke

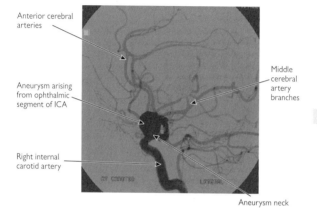

Fig. 4.3 A cerebral angiogram showing position of an aneurysm on the anterior cerebral blood supply.

Electroencephalography

Electroencephalography (EEG) is the non-invasive study of small, constantly changing electrical potentials from the brain, which can be recorded from the scalp. Voltage differences from various parts of the brain are measured. The resulting traces represent summation of post-synaptic potentials generated by interconnecting neurons.

Clinical use of EEG
- To classify epilepsy syndrome and therefore optimize treatment
- To confirm the diagnosis of non-convulsive status
- To monitor depth of anaesthesia, particularly in the treatment of status epilepticus
- To distinguish between encephalopathies and primary psychiatric syndromes
- In certain circumstances to distinguish epileptic seizures from other disorders, such as non-epileptic attacks, syncope and movement disorders
- In a child who shows unexplained regression or loss of speech and language
- To monitor the EEG response to treatment in certain epileptic syndromes e.g. childhood absence epilepsy
- To investigate the appearance of new seizure types in subjects with known epilepsy, e.g. infantile spasms
- Unexplained altered consciousness such as semi-comatose or comatose states

Method of recording
- 21 electrodes are attached to the scalp with collodion glue or adhesive paste
- Electrode positions are measured using the 'International 10/20 system' of electrode placement
- Routine recordings are taken in the waking state predominantly with subject's eyes closed. Brief periods of eye opening are also recorded
- Simultaneous electrocardiogram (ECG) recorded
- Additional electrodes can be added to record specific areas of interest

Patient preparation
Other than an explanation of the procedure, no specific patient preparation is required.

Peri-procedural activation techniques
- Hyperventilation: undertaken vigorously for 3–5 minutes can activate generalized epileptiform discharges. Useful in childhood absence epilepsy where a failure to evoke epileptiform changes makes the diagnosis unlikely
- Photic stimulation: a strobe light is placed 30cm from the subject. Frequencies from 1–60 Hz are presented during eye opening and closure. Production of self-sustaining, generalized epileptiform abnormalities seen in photosensitivity

- Sleep deprivation: subject usually stays awake for 24 hours. Increased yield of abnormalities, particularly epileptiform
- Natural or drug-induced sleep: may increase the yield of epileptiform abnormalities and certain seizure types are seen more often in sleep

Post-procedure care
- No specific post-procedure care is required
- Assist the patient to wash their hair to remove the glue if required

Interpreting EEG
Normal activity
- Alpha activity: frequency range 8–13 Hz. Seen over the posterior regions of the brain. Can be higher amplitude on the dominant side. It is seen during eye closure
- Beta activity: frequency range >13 Hz. Seen symmetrically over both hemispheres, maximal frontally. Dominant frequency in subjects with eyes open or who are anxious
- Theta activity: frequency range 4–<8 Hz. Normally seen in young children. Also seen in drowsiness.
- Delta activity: frequency <4 Hz. Normally seen in slow wave sleep in adults. Also seen in babies

Abnormal activity
Epileptiform
- Focal: discharges manifest as sharp waves or spikes. Localization can be made from recordings using the 10–20 system, but supplementary electrodes are often useful. The temporal area is the most common location of focal epileptiform activity and of interictal discharges
- Generalized: discharges usually take the form of spike-wave or polyspike-wave complexes. Often having an anterior predominance particularly in the primary generalized epilepsies

Non-epileptiform
- Focal: seen over areas of the brain where there is focal damage to the cortex. Usually seen as an increase in slow activity or at times as a decrease in amplitude of EEG signals
- Generalized: diffuse abnormal slow rhythms seen in encephalopathies (usually metabolic), hydrocephalus and post-ictal states. Most commonly seen frontally. Can also manifest as symmetrical, bilateral slowing of normal background rhythms

Electromyography

Electromyography (EMG) records the electrical activity within muscles.

EMG can be used to differentiate between muscle weakness due to primary disease in the muscle itself and weakness caused by neurological problems.

Needle electrodes are placed directly into the muscle through the skin to record the activity within the body of the muscle.

Activity in the muscle is measured when the patient is at rest, but sometimes they may be asked to voluntarily contract the muscle during recordings. Action potentials generated during this contraction will be recorded and assessed.

Patient preparation

• Patient education is important and they should be informed that:
  • Small needle electrodes will be placed into the muscles being tested and that this may feel similar to having an intramuscular (IM) injection
  • The muscles may feel bruised for a short time/few days following the investigation
  • No other specific patient preparation is required

Post-procedure care

No specific post-procedure care is required, but the patient may require some mild analgesia.

Evoked potentials

Evoked potentials assess the conduction velocity along a nerve pathway. Damage to the myelin sheath will delay conduction velocities.

A number of different evoked potentials can be measured:

- Auditory evoked potentials (AEP) measure conduction velocity along the auditory pathway from the ear to the auditory cortex in the temporal lobe
- Visual evoked potentials (VEP) measure conduction velocity along the visual pathway from the back of the eye to the visual cortex in the occipital lobe
- Somato-sensory evoked potentials (SSEP) measure conduction velocity along sensory pathways from periphery to sensory cortex in parietal lobe

With all evoked potentials a stimulus is applied and then the time taken for this to be recorded in the brain is measured. This conduction velocity is then compared with normal values in milliseconds to determine if it is reduced.

Each test normally lasts approx 30 minutes.

AEPs

These are sometimes known as brainstem auditory evoked potentials (BAEPs).

The patient wears headphones and a series of clicks are generated by a computer and played through the headphones. The recordings are taken from scalp electrodes placed on the scalp over the auditory cortex. Electrodes are attached in the same way as for EEG.

White noise is played into the opposite ear, to ensure that the AEP is being recorded from one side at a time.

Patients need to rest in a relaxed position during the test and may rarely be sedated.

VEPs

The patient is asked to sit in front of a chequerboard display on a screen or to look at a flash of light. The light is flashed on and off at predetermined intervals, or more commonly the black and white squares on the chequerboard are alternated. Recordings are taken from scalp electrodes placed over the occipital lobe.

SSEPs

The patient is asked to sit relaxed in a chair or lie on a couch. As with AEPs it is important that the patient remains relaxed throughout and mild sedation may be administered.

Skin electrodes are placed over a large nerve in an arm or leg and a small electrical current is applied intermittently. This should not be painful, but patients might feel a sensation of slight tapping on the skin.

Patient preparation
- Patient education is important and they should have the procedure explained to them
- If the patient is having VEPs make sure they take their usual glasses for distance/reading with them—they will need to wear these during the test

Post-procedure care
No specific post-procedure care is required, but the patient should be observed until fully alert if sedation has been used.

Lumbar puncture

Lumbar puncture (LP) involves placing a fine bore-needle into the spinal canal at the level of the cauda equina to obtain a specimen of CSF for analysis.

This is usually carried out at the patient's bedside and a nurse is required during the procedure to both assist the doctor performing the LP and support and reassure the patient throughout.

LP should never be performed on a patient with raised ICP and mass lesions inside the cranium as this may lead to brain herniation and coning.

Pre-procedure preparation

- Position the patient lying on their left side, curled up with knees drawn up to their chest (fetal position)—this helps to open up the spaces between the vertebrae for insertion of the needle. Rarely, if it is not possible for the patient to lie flat or the LP cannot be performed successfully, the patient may sit up on the side of their bed, leaning over a bed table and supported on pillows.
- The nurse may be asked to assist in preparation of the trolley/ equipment for the LP.
- The patient should wear a gown or loose clothing that will allow access to the spine and allow bony landmarks (e.g. iliac crest) to be located easily.
- △ Check for allergies to skin prep solutions, e.g. iodine-based preparations.
- Patient must consent to the procedure and must have been informed of risks by person taking consent.

During the procedure

- Reassure the patient throughout the procedure.
- Local anaesthetic is injected into the skin and dura surrounding the spinal canal—warn the patient that this may sting.
- The spinal needle (trochar and cannula) is then introduced into the spinal canal through the disc space usually at L4–L5 or L5–S1 once the local anaesthetic has taken effect. It is vital to ensure the patient remains still throughout.
- Once *in situ* the trochar is removed and CSF will flow through the hollow spinal needle.
- CSF pressure may be recorded at this point by attaching a manometer.
- Nurse may be asked to assist in collection of specimens—hold a universal container just below the spinal needle where the CSF is dripping slowly. Do not touch the needle with the specimen container. Remember that CSF is a body fluid so gloves should be worn. Ensure containers are labeled in the order in which they are collected—it is usual to collect 3.
- Once the procedure has been completed and needle removed, apply pressure for a short time to the puncture site and then dress with a small plaster.

Post-procedure care

- Encourage patient to rest for a short period of time before mobilizing
- Encourage patient to drink plenty of fluids
- Check puncture site for CSF leak
- Record systemic observations on completion of the procedure

Potential complications

Post-LP headache

This will occur in approx. 1 in 4 patients. There is no evidence that prolonged flat bedrest (e.g. 4–6 hours) post-procedure will reduce this risk.

This is thought to be due to low CSF pressure, possibly from a dural tear following the procedure and most will resolve within a few days/one week. Risk can be reduced by using smaller needles and good technique.

If headache occurs this is worsened by sitting up—encourage patient to lie flat, stay in bed and drink lots of fluids. Administer simple analgesia, e.g. paracetamol, as prescribed.

CSF leak

- Check puncture site for clear, straw-coloured fluid. If this occurs CSF leak can be confirmed by testing the fluid for the presence of glucose.
- Apply pressure to site and inform medical staff.
- Observe patient for post-LP headache

Change in level of consciousness

In rare cases a patient may deteriorate neurologically. This is a medical emergency. If this occurs, record neurological assessment every 15 minutes and inform medical staff immediately.

Infection and meningitis

Rarely a patient may deteriorate some time after the procedure. There is a risk that infection may be introduced and cause meningitis. Advise patients to report symptoms of nausea and vomiting, worsening headache and neck stiffness and any occurrence of pyrexia.

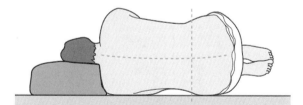

Fig. 4.4 The correct patient positioning in preparation for lumbar puncture.

Reproduced from *Medicine*, volume 32, M. Sharief, Lumbar puncture and CSF examination, pages 44–46 with permission from Elsevier.

Muscle biopsy

Needle muscle biopsies are most commonly performed and may be carried out under local anaesthetic in a ward area.

If a larger piece of muscle tissue is required, then the procedure is carried out in theatre through a small incision in the skin (open biopsy), under local anaesthetic.

Muscle biopsy will obtain a sample of tissue to be used to differentially diagnose muscle and nervous disorders.

Pre-procedure preparation

- Consent must be obtained from the patient and risks of the procedure must be explained by the person taking that consent.
- ⚠ Check for allergies to skin prep solutions, e.g. iodine-based preparations.
- Ensure the patient is wearing a gown or has removed relevant articles of clothing.
- Position the patient semi-recumbent or in a comfortable position in bed.
- Biopsies are usually taken from the top of the thigh—place an incontinence sheet under the patient's leg to prevent skin prep solutions from running onto the bed.

During the procedure

- Assist the medical staff as required and reassure the patient throughout the procedure.
- Explain to the patient that the local anaesthetic may sting, but that they should not feel any pain. Explain that they may feel some pulling or pressure.

Post-procedure care

- Apply a dressing to the wound site and observe half-hourly for bleeding and haematoma formation
- Record a set of systemic observations following the procedure
- Administer analgesia as required, as prescribed—the site may feel sore for a few days following the biopsy

Sleep studies

Sleep studies are carried out to assess respiratory function during sleep and to identify problematic sleep apnoea syndromes.

Sleep apnoea

Resp. rate fluctuates throughout the night and brief periods of apnoea are normal during rapid eye movement (REM) sleep.

Sleep apnoea can be problematic when these episodes become prolonged and may be caused by:

- Brainstem infarct
- Mechanical problems/obstruction:
  - Obesity
  - Myxoedema
  - Acromegaly

Patients with sleep apnoea often experience snoring, sleepiness during the day and early morning headaches.

Sleep studies

These involve the patient being admitted for overnight monitoring of oxygen saturation, sometimes with video recording.

Further assessment and sleep studies may be performed with the patient receiving nasal continuous positive airway pressure (CPAP).

Patient preparation

Patient may be admitted late in the evening and discharged the following morning once they are awake.

Ensure patients bring an overnight bag, toiletries and a change of clothes for the following day.

- Warn the patient that you will be going into their room on an hourly basis to check their oxygen saturation levels, but will not need to wake them.
- Apply O_2 saturation probe to a finger and secure with tape. Ensure this is comfortable.
- Patient may go to sleep whenever they feel ready.

Post-procedure care

No specific post-procedure care is required and the patient is usually free to leave after breakfast, unless they need to wait and see a technician.

Offer the patient breakfast.

Common drugs and treatments

Neurotransmitters

Naturally occurring neurotransmitters are chemicals that relay signals from the pre-synaptic nerve terminal across the synapse to a receptor in the post-synaptic neuron. They are released as a calcium-dependent process and synthesized and terminated within the neuron they are released from. Synthetic neurotransmitter must mimic the effect of the natural neurotransmitter, when applied exogenously.

Neurotransmitters and drugs

- Drugs can alter the stages of neurotransmission to treat neurological and non-neurological disorders.
- Fig. 5.1 shows how drugs may affect neurotransmission.

Neurotransmitter receptors

- Neurotransmitters exert their effects on target cells by binding to receptors which are proteins on neuron membranes.
- Binding of the neurotransmitter to the receptor causes a chemical or electrical change in the target cell; different receptors cause different changes.
- Receptors are neurotransmitter-specific, e.g. dopamine receptors specifically bind dopamine.
- Neurotransmitters are able to exert a range of effects by binding to a range of specific receptors at different locations within the CNS—these receptor subtypes exert different effects on target cells.

Drugs and receptors

Drugs that bind to receptors can be classified in two ways:

- *Agonists*—drugs that bind to the receptor and mimic the effect of the neurotransmitter, e.g. dopamine agonists bind to dopamine receptors in the striatum.
- *Antagonists*—drugs that bind to receptors but have no effect, i.e. blocking the effect of the neurotransmitters. Antipsychotic drugs exert their effects by blocking dopamine receptors.

As well as binding to the intended receptor to exert a therapeutic effect, drugs may bind to other receptors, either as agonists or antagonists, and may cause side effects. Tricyclic antidepressants, for example, such as amitriptyline, often used for neuropathic pain, block muscarinic acetylcholine receptors producing 'anti-cholinergic' side effects of blurred vision, dry, mouth, urinary retention etc.

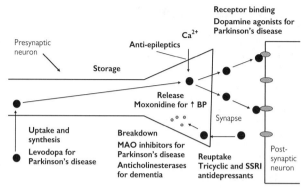

Fig. 5.1 Drug treatments targeted for neurological disorders.

Intravenous immunoglobulin

Immunoglobulins are pooled normal human immunoglobulins (concentrated antibodies), extracted from human plasma from healthy individual donations and must be treated and administered with the same level of caution and respect as any other blood product.

General notes

- Initial indications for intravenous immunoglobulin (IVIg) were immunodeficiency disorders; at higher doses IVIg alters immune response by mechanisms not yet fully understood and is used to treat various autoimmune disorders
- Common neurological indications:
  - Guillain–Barré syndrome
  - Acute exacerbation of myasthenia gravis
  - CIDP (acute and chronic inflammatory demyelinating polyneuropathy)
  - Multifocal motor neuropathy
- Usual starting dose is 2g/kg given over 2–5 days (e.g. 0.4g/kg for 5 days):
  - Doses are rounded down to nearest bottle size

Important notes

With the exception of Guillain–Barré syndrome all neurological indications for IVIg are unlicensed ones. Further details of efficacy, guidance on the use of IVIg and safety aspects related to administration can be found within the Association of British Neurologists Guidelines, and the Department of Health (2008) National Patient Safety Agency.

IVIg is a blood product with a risk of viral transmission although this risk is now very low. The risk of variant CJD transmission is as yet unknown.

Potential side effects

Infusion-related; often subside with reducing or temporarily stopping infusion rate.

- Headache
- Chills
- Fever
- Backache
- Anaphylaxis (rare)—stop infusion immediately and treat as per local anaphylaxis guidelines

Other side effects:

- Mild, reversible neutropaenia/lymphopaenia
- Renal damage, particularly from formulations with high sucrose content
- Plasma hyperviscosity—rare reports of cerebral and myocardial infarction
- Aseptic meningitis
- Skin rashes

Administration details

- Adhere to the summary of product characteristics and/or local guidelines.
- Infusion rates are product-specific but first dose infusions are started slowly to minimize the risk of adverse effects; the infusion rate is increased according to patient tolerance.
- Although the active ingredient in IVIg is the same from brand to brand, there are differences in the manufacturing processes which means that the products should not be used interchangeably.
- IVIg can be administered via a peripheral cannula or a butterfly device (21 or 23 gauge). A giving set with an in-built airway and a 15-micron filter should be used as albumin can occasionally precipitate out of solution.
- Subsequent infusion and treatment courses repeated within 6 weeks can be commenced at the previously tolerated infusion rate without titration.
- Due to potential risk of anaphylaxis, the patient should be closely monitored initially.
- All batch numbers and adverse effects should be recorded in the patient records as per local guidance.
- The Department of Health plans to maintain a national database of IVIg usage to monitor indications for IVIg and collect other long-term data.

Monitoring

Prior to commencement of infusion, baseline observations must be recorded.

Observations must be repeated at each change of infusion rate and 4-hourly thereafter.

Observations of the patient must be continued for one hour after completion of the first infusion and then 20 minutes after subsequent infusions in line with manufacturer's instructions.

Further reading

Association of British Neurologists Guidelines http://www.theabn.org/documents/IVIg-Guidelines-2008.pdf

Department of Health (2008) *Clinical guidelines for immunoglobulin use*, 2nd edn. London: Department of Health.

Steroids

General notes

- Corticosteroids exist naturally in the body as aldosterone, hydrocortisone, and corticosterone, and are produced in the adrenal cortex.
- Corticosteroids affect carbohydrate and protein metabolism (glucocorticoid activity), and water and electrolyte balance (mineralocorticoid activity).
- Corticosteroids are crucial for survival—they are synthesized in the adrenal cortex in response to the body being placed in stressful situations (e.g. illness, surgery).
- Hydrocortisone (glucocorticoid activity) and fludrocortisone (mineralocorticoid activity) are used in replacement therapy in patients with adrenal failure (e.g. Addison's disease).

Anti-inflammatory actions

- The main therapeutic application of glucocorticoids are their potent anti-inflammatory and immunosuppressive actions.
- Steroids have intracellular actions, acting at the cell nucleus to reduce production of inflammatory mediators and increase production of anti-inflammatory mediators; they also reduce vasodilation.
- Commonly used steroid drugs include:
  - Hydrocortisone
  - Prednisolone
  - Methylprednisolone
  - Dexamethasone
- The drugs do not have equal anti-inflammatory potency, i.e. they are not equivalent on a milligram to milligram basis.

  750 micrograms dexamethasone ≡ 5mg prednisolone ≡ 4mg methylprednisolone ≡ 20mg hydrocortisone

i.e. Dexamethasone is most potent and hydrocortisone is least potent. Corticosteroids are used for numerous conditions with an underlying inflammatory or auto-immune pathology. The list of clinical indications are endless but common indications include:

- Clinically disabling relapses of multiple sclerosis
- Reduction of cerebral oedema associated with brain tumour, neurosurgery or traumatic head injury
- Myasthenia gravis (used carefully—rapid dose titration can exacerbate condition)
- CIDP
- Vasculitis
- Adjunctive treatment to drug therapies which carry a risk of anaphylaxis, e.g. some monoclonal antibodies

Side effects

- Metabolic side effects:
  - Cushing's syndrome—excessively high levels of cortisone due to numerous causes including pituitary adenoma, adrenal gland

disease, small cell lung neoplasms or steroid use, produces a range of symptoms:
- 'Moon face' and increased abdominal fat
- Skin thinning
- Hypertension
- Poor wound healing
- Muscle wasting
- Cataracts
- Osteoporosis
- Hyperglycaemia
- Weight gain
- Suppressed response to infection and a greater risk of opportunistic infection
- Dyspepsia/indigestion
- Alteration of mood
- Suppression of endogenous corticosteroid synthesis—rapid or abrupt withdrawal of corticosteroids after prolonged treatment can lead to potentially fatal acute adrenal insufficiency.

Notes on side effects

- Inflammatory conditions should be treated using the lowest dose possible to minimize side effects; steroid-sparing agents are often added to achieve this (🕮 see Immunosuppressants, p 120).
- The incidence of side effects is related to the dose and duration of treatment—metabolic side effects, except transient hyperglycaemia from high dose treatment, are unlikely from a short-course, i.e. less than 2 weeks.
- Patients should be always be given a steroid card and the duration of treatment or date for review should be confirmed.
- Oral corticosteroids are usually taken in the morning to coincide with when the body maximally produces endogenous steroids.
- Side effects can be reduced by prescribing on alternate days or pulsed regimes.
- Patients likely to require long-term steroid treatment (e.g. myasthenia gravis, vasculitis) should be prescribed appropriate prophylaxis against steroid-induced osteoporosis as bone-thinning effects of steroids are greatest during initial treatment.
  - Bisphosphonates, calcitriol and hormone replacement are therapeutic options.
  - Bisphosphonates are commonly prescribed.
  - Calcium and vitamin D supplements may be prescribed for patients with poor dietary vitamin D intake but should be given at least 2 hours either side of a bisphosphonate as the absorption of the latter is greatly reduced by concomitant administration.

Immunosuppressants

General notes

Immunosuppressants are commonly co-prescribed with steroids as 'steroid-sparing agents' to reduce steroid requirements and long-term side effects. The therapeutic goal is to completely withdraw steroids or maintain the patient on the lowest dose of steroids possible.

Immunosuppressants are less toxic than steroids but do carry a risk of significant side effects (Table 5.1)—the risks and benefits should be discussed with the patient prior to commencing treatment.

Mode of action

Cyclophosphamide, methotrexate and azathioprine are cytotoxic agents developed initially as anti-cancer treatments.

Their anti-proliferative action produces broad immunosuppression by suppressing the production of rapidly dividing cells of the immune system, including lymphocytes.

- All three drugs can cause bone-marrow suppression therefore patients should be aware to immediately report unusual bleeding and bruising as well as infection.
- Full blood count monitoring (FBC) is also recommended.

The immunosuppressant action of ciclosporin is thought to be due to inhibition of T lymphoctes as well as inhibiting production of interleukin 2 and interferon gamma.

Mycophenolate blocks the proliferation of lymphocytes via a more selective mechanism than the broad anti-proliferative agents such as azathioprine.

Long-term immunosuppression

- Patients receiving long-term immunosuppression have a higher risk of developing opportunistic infections.
- Patients treated with immunosuppressants have a higher risk of developing cancer.

Table 5.1 Commonly used immunosuppressant agents and indications in neurological disease

Drug	Indications	Dose range[1]	Adverse effects[1]
Azathioprine	CIDP, multifocal motor neuropathy, myasthenia gravis, multiple sclerosis, polymyositis, vasculitis	2–3mg/kg/day[2]	Gastrointestinal side effects, bone marrow suppression, rash, hepatotoxicity
Ciclosporin	Behçet's syndrome, myasthenia gravis, polymyositis, sarcoidosis		Gastrointestinal side effects, headache, tremor, parasthesias, electrolyte and lipid abnormalities, hypertension, renal dysfunction
Cyclophosphamide	Induction and maintenance of remission in vasculitis	Pulsed regimes of 10–15mg/kg PO/IV or continuous regimes of 1–2mg/kg/day	Nausea, alopecia, bone marrow suppression, haemorrhagic cystitis,[3] bladder cancer
Methotrexate	Vasculitis, dermatomyositis	2.5–25mg weekly PO	Bone marrow suppression, mouth ulcers/stomatitis, pulmonary fibrosis, hepatotoxicity[4]
Mycophenolate	Myasthenia gravis, vasculitis	500-1500mg BD	Diarrhoea, leucopenia, progressive multifocal leukoencephalopathy

1. For full guidance on each drug please consult local guidelines and individual summary of product characteristics (SPC) http://www.emc.medicines.org.uk/ although please note that indications and doses may be outside of the drug company recommendations.
2. Patients may be measured for thiopurine methyl transferase activity. TMPT is one of the enzymes that metabolizes azathioprine; lower levels may increase the risk of adverse effects. Patients with low TMPT activity should be cautiously initiated on treatment.
3. Haemorrhagic cystitis results from a highly reactive metabolite, acrolein, passing through the bladder. The patient should be encouraged to drink plenty of fluid to flush acrolein out of the body. Mesna neutralizes acrolein and can be considered for patients at risk of haemorrhagic cystitis; it is generally not required for cyclophosphamide doses <1.5g.
4. Adverse reactions can be minimized by co-prescribing folic acid 5mg. Various regimes are prescribed including 5mg taken weekly 2 days after methotrexate or 5mg daily except on the day of methotrexate.

Analgesia

General notes

Analgesics may be used for a variety of reasons in neuroscience, to relieve mild discomfort such as a headache, the severe pain of acute conditions such as subarachnoid haemorrhage or to optimise sedation in the ventilated patient, It may also be used to control the neuropathic pain that is caused by damage to nerve fibres.

Paracetamol

- Mode of action not fully understood but use is widespread.
- Side effects are very rare but hepatotoxic in overdose which can be fatal.
- Adult dose is 0.5–1g every 4–6 hours; not more than 4g in 24 hours
- Available in combination with opioid analgesics
  - Co-codamol
  - Co-dydramol
- Contained within many over-the-counter analgesics and cough and cold remedies—check drug charts and drug histories carefully to avoid accidental overdose.

Non-steroidal anti-inflammatory drugs (NSAIDs)

- E.g. ibuprofen, diclofenac, naproxen, indometacin
- Have analgesic, anti-inflammatory and anti-pyretic properties
- Inhibit production of inflammatory prostaglandins
- Particularly good for inflammatory pain
- Possible side effects include:
  - Indigestion/dyspepsia, peptic ulceration
  - Renal impairment, particularly when given with other nephrotoxic drugs such as ACE inhibitors and Angiotensin II receptor antagonists
  - Increased bleeding risk—use cautiously with warfarin
  - Exacerbation of asthma in some patients
- Indometacin is used specifically in hemicrania

Opioids

- Modulate pain pathways by acting at opioid receptors within the brain and spinal cord.
- Potent analgesic agents that can be used in acute and chronic pain, including neuropathic pain.
- Opioids have varying potencies and are not equivalent dose for dose, e.g. fentanyl is 100–150 times more potent than morphine; a 25mcg/hr patch is equivalent to up to 90mg per day of oral morphine.

Weak opioids	**Strong opioids**
Codeine (oral, injection)	Morphine (oral, injection)
Dihydrocodeine (oral, injection)	Oxycodone (oral, injection)
	Fentanyl (patch and lozenge)

Side effects from opioids include:
- Nausea and vomiting
- Constipation
- Respiratory depression
- Drowsiness
- Itching (from morphine)
- Confusion and hallucinations
- Dependence and abuse potential

With the exception of constipation, patients develop tolerance to side effects with chronic treatment.

Where appropriate, simple analgesia such as paracetamol or NSAIDs should initially be used and then stepped up to the weak opioids such as codeine and dihydrocodeine, and then the stronger opioids.

Neuropathic pain

Causes include:
- Demyelination (multiple sclerosis and Guillain-Barré syndrome)
- Diabetic neuropathy
- Herpes simplex virus (post-herpetic neuralgia)
- Amputation (phantom limb pain)
- Stroke
  Drug treatments include:
- Opioids. e.g. morphine, tramadol
- Antidepressants. e.g. amitriptyline, imipramine, duloxetine
- Anticonvulsants. e.g. gabapentin, pregabalin, carbamazepine, lamotrigine
- Local anaesthetics. e.g. lidocaine patches
- Cannabinoids. e.g. nabilone (unlicensed indication)

Levodopa and drugs for Parkinson's disease

General notes
- The motor symptoms of Parkinson's disease (PD) are attributable to the death of dopamine-producing neurons in the basal ganglia.
- Drug treatments for the motor symptoms of PD augment or mimic dopamine function in the brain.
- Not all forms of Parkinson's disease (e.g. vascular Parkinsonism) respond well to drug treatment.
- **Correct timing of drug administration is very important for optimal symptom control.**
- Drug treatments are symptomatic only.
- Treatment of symptoms become more difficult with disease progression.
- Long-term treatment, especially with levodopa, is associated with the development of motor fluctuations which include:
  - Dyskinesias
  - End of dose wearing off effect (off)
  - Rapid and sometimes unpredictable on–off switches

Drug treatments
L-dopa (levodopa)
This is the biological precursor of dopamine and is converted to dopamine within the brain.

Combination with peripheral decarboxylase inhibitors, benserazide (co-beneldopa) and carbidopa (co-careldopa) greatly reduce side effects.

Dopamine agonists
These mimic the effects of dopamine by activating dopamine-specific receptors in the basal ganglia—they can be classified chemically as ergot-derived and non-derived (see adverse reactions).

Ergot derived	**Non-derived**
Bromocriptine	Pramipexole
Cabergoline	Ropinirole
Pergolide	Rotigotine (a 24 hour patch)

Monoamine oxidase B (MAO-B) inhibitors and catechol-o-methlytransferase (COMT) inhibitors
These increase dopamine action by blocking the enzymes that normally break down dopamine.

MAO-B inhibitors	**COMT inhibitors**
Selegiline	Entacapone
Rasagiline	Tolcapone

- *Amantadine* may increase dopamine action possibly by inhibiting the reuptake of dopamine by dopamine neurons.

- *Apomorphine* is a very potent dopamine agonist administered by subcutaneous injection with a rapid onset and short duration of action.

Treatment options—early disease
- Levodopa, dopamine agonists, MAO-B inhibitors.
- Levodopa is the gold standard treatment but is associated with long-term motor complications.
- Dopamine agonists and MAO-B inhibitors may be considered in younger patients.

Treatment options—PD with motor complications
- Modified-release levodopa preparations have slightly more prolonged effect, reducing off time, and reduced peak concentrations which are associated with dyskinesia.
  - Modified-release preparation must be swallowed whole.
  - ⚠ Please take care: modified-release preparations look and sound very similar to standard release preparations.
- COMT inhibitors prolong the duration of levodopa but can cause dyskinesia by increasing peak concentrations.
- Amantadine can relieve dyskinesia.
- Apomorphine for off episodes; continuous infusion for people experiencing frequent and/or unpredictable off episodes.
- Disadvantages of apomorphine are:
  - High cost
  - Issues of administration (needs to be injected)
  - Cutaneous irritation from long-term use—apomorphine should always be diluted with sodium chloride 0.9% for infusion

Side effects common to all treatments
- Nausea and vomiting:
  - May be reduced by taking tablets with food
  - Domperidone is treatment of choice
  - Centrally acting dopamine antagonists e.g. metoclopramide, prochlorperazine, worsen motor symptoms and should be avoided
- Postural hypotension
- Neuropsychiatric side effects—hallucinations (visual), paranoid ideation, pathological gambling, hypersexuality
  - More common with dopamine agonists

Side effects that are drug-specific
- Coloured urine—from entacapone (reddish-brown colour)
- Hepatotoxicity—associated with tolcapone; regular LFT monitoring required
- Fibrotic reactions—pulmonary, cardiac and retroperitoneal fibrosis reported with ergot derived dopamine agonists

Disease-modifying therapies for multiple sclerosis

The aims of disease-modifying therapies (with the exclusion of methylprednisolone) are to reduce relapses and disease progression which in clinical trials is often measured by the expanded disability status scale (EDSS). Available treatments include:

- Beta-interferons—interferon beta-1a (Rebif® and Avonex®) and interferon beta-1b (Betaferon®).
- Glatiramer acetate.
- Mitoxantrone.
- Plasma exchange
- Natalizumab
- High-dose methylprednisolone for clinically disabling relapses

General notes

Beta-interferons are indicated for relapsing–remitting multiple sclerosis. Their expense has led to the development of criteria for their use.

Active disease defined as one or more of:

- Two clinically significant relapses in the last two years.
- One disabling relapse in the last year.
- Active MRI scan containing new or gadolinium-enhancing lesions that have developed in the last year.

Mitoxantrone and plasma exchange may be considered for highly active MS that does not respond to disease-modifying therapy.

Due to its expense, natalizumab has been approved by NICE for rapidly evolving relapsing remitting multiple sclerosis which is defined by two or more disabling relapses within one year, and one or more gadolinium-enhancing lesions on MRI or significant increase in lesion load compared with a previous MRI.

Beta-interferons

- Interferons are produced naturally in response to viral infection; the exact mechanism in MS is not yet fully understood.
- The route of administration varies from product to product:
  - Avonex® is administered by intramuscular injection
  - Rebif® and Betaferon® are administered by subcutaneous injection
- Common side effects include:
  - Injection site reactions (rotate injection sites)
  - Flu-like symptoms
  - Headache
  - Blood disorders—neutropaenia, lymphopaenia etc. (monitoring required)
  - Increases in liver enzymes
  - Depression

Glatiramer acetate

- The mechanism of action is not fully understood.
- Common side effects include:
  - Injection site reactions (rotate injection sites)
  - Flu-like symptoms

- Headache
- Chest pain and palpitations
- Anxiety and depression
- Gastrointestinal side effects—nausea, vomiting, constipation

Mitoxantrone

Is a cytotoxic agent: great care should be taken with administration.
Potential side effects include:
- Bone marrow suppression
- Blue discoloration of urine and sclera
- Hepatotoxicity
- Cardiotoxicity—cumulative effect which limits prolonged use
- Nausea and vomiting
- Extremely irritant in the event of extravasation—refer to local guidelines

Plasmapheresis

See p 130.

Natalizumab

- Monoclonal antibody against α4 integrin:
  - Inhibits transfer of T cell lymphocytes into the CNS
- Administered by intravenous infusion every 4 weeks
- Infusion related side effects include:
  - Dizziness
  - Nausea
  - Urticaria
  - Rigors
  - Hypersensitivity, including anaphylaxis (<1% patients)
- Progressive multifocal leukoencephalopathy (PML) has been reported in several patients taking natalizumab in combination with beta-interferon

Anti-epileptic drugs

General notes

Anti-epileptic drugs (AEDs) are frequently prescribed for the control and management of patients with epileptic disorders, however, they may also be useful in pain management, particularly for trigeminal neuralgia and post-hepatic neuralgia. AEDs are frequently used prophylactically to prevent seizures, in the management of patients following head injury, neurosurgical procedures, and brain tumours.

Principles of drug treatment for epilepsy

AEDs reduce electrical excitability of neurons by various mechanisms. Some agents (e.g. lamotrigine) have several actions giving them a broad spectrum of action producing efficacy against different seizure types. Many AEDs can cause CNS side effects in a dose-related manner, e.g.

- Drowsiness
- Somnolence
- Ataxia
- Nystagmus
- Cognitive impairment

With the exception of status epilepticus drug therapy is normally initiated at a low dose and titrated according to seizure control and side effects.

Modified-release carbamazepine

- Cause less fluctuation in plasma levels, often improving seizure control and reducing CNS side effects from peak plasma concentrations.
- Prescriptions should be checked carefully and clarified with the medical or pharmacy staff if there is any discrepancy.
- Modified-release formulations should not be crushed or chewed.

Phenytoin suspension administration via enteral feeding tubes

- The chemical form of phenytoin in suspension formulation is different to the capsule and injection formulation; the dose needs to be altered if a patient is changed to phenytoin suspension.
- Enteral feeding: concomitant administration with enteral feed significantly reduces phenytoin absorption—enteral feeding should be withheld 2 hours either side of phenytoin administration via feeding tubes.

Phenytoin sodium dose (capsule or IV form)	Phenytoin suspension equivalent dose
100mg	90mg
200mg	180mg
250mg	225mg
300mg	270mg
350mg	315mg

Drug treatment for convulsive status epilepticus

Check local treatment protocols which should include treatments for reversible causes e.g. hypoglycaemia. Drug treatments include:

Benzodiazepines

- Lorazepam (IV)
- Diazepam (IV/PR)
- Midazolam (buccal / nasal)

Often first line treatment in status protocols. Possible side effects are:

- Respiratory depression
- Hypotension
- Cardio-respiratory collapse

Careful patient monitoring of pulse and respiratory rate, blood pressure and oxygen saturation essential—side effects may be prolonged, especially with diazepam.

Phenytoin

IV loading doses can be given (15–20mg/kg in adults) to rapidly achieve therapeutic levels. Side effects from infusion can be:

- Cardiac arrhythmia*
- Hypotension*
- Thrombophlebitis and tissue damage with extravasation

* ⚠ Rate-related reactions: infusion rates should not exceed 50mg/min; consider reducing rate in elderly patients. Cardiac monitoring advised.

Phenytoin injection may precipitate after dilution—administration of neat injection is recommended.

If diluted, mix with sodium chloride 0.9% only and include 0.2 micron in-line filter; monitor solution for cloudiness (precipitation)—do not leave solution standing.

Phenobarbital

IV loading doses can be given, (10mg/kg in adults), to rapidly achieve therapeutic levels. Rapid infusion can cause:

- Hypotension
- Respiratory depression

Infusion rate should not exceed 100mg/min in adults. Close patient monitoring advised.

Failure to control status epilepticus may necessitate the use of anaesthetic agents, including propofol and thiopental. Such agents will be used in a critical care environment with appropriate monitoring.

Therapeutic plasma exchange

General notes

Plasma exchange (plasmapheresis), involves the removal and separation of plasma from blood cells and replacement of albumin (commonly a mixture of human albumin and sodium chloride 0.9%). The procedure is largely indicated for autoimmune diseases, It works by removing inflammatory mediators and autoantibodies in conditions such as:

- Guillain–Barré syndrome
- Myasthenia gravis
- CIDP
- Plasma exchange is usually considered after treatment with IVIgs has been ineffective. IVIgs are more frequently used due to their comparable efficacy with plasma exchange and the ready availability and relative ease of administration
  Possible adverse effects of both these treatments include:
- Hypotension
- Hypersensitivity reactions to plasma substitute
- Thrombosis
- Hypocalcaemia resulting in tingling and parasthesia
- Citrate is used as an anticoagulant and causes hypocalcaemia

Plasma exchange and drugs

- Drugs highly bound to protein may be removed by plasma exchange.
- Where possible, doses should be delayed until after the plasma exchange procedure, but individual patients should be discussed with medical staff.

Neurological emergencies

Rising intracranial pressure and coning

Physiology

As the intracranial volume is fixed, changes in the volume of any of the components demands a compensatory change in the volume in one or more of the other components if intracranial pressure is to remain constant, known as the Monroe–Kelly hypothesis (📖 see p 54, Cerebral haemodynamics).
The skull contains:

- Cerebrospinal fluid: 7–10%
- Brain and intracellular fluid: 85%
- Blood: 7–10%
- As pressure increases the brain tries to compensate by:
  - Reduction in CSF volume:
    (a) through reabsorption
    (b) fall in production
    (c) displacement to lumbar theca
  - Blood volume displacement—cerebral veins are compressed and blood drains into the venous circulation.
  - Brain displacement—the brain is displaced from one intracranial compartment to another, until it finally becomes compressed through the foramen magnum.
- An increase of intracranial pressure above 40–50 mm Hg will obstruct cerebral blood flow resulting in diffuse, generalized ischemia.
- The skull of a baby can adjust to small changes in pressure. Once the sutures close, the skull becomes rigid.

Contributory factors

- Space-occupying lesions—tumour, haemorrhage, abscess
- Cerebral oedema—head injury, inflammation, infections
- Hydrocephalus—subarachnoid hemorrhage, infection
- Hypoxia and hypercapnia

Coning or cerebral herniation

As the brain becomes increasingly compressed, it begins to move from one area of the skull to another. There are three types of herniation:

- Supratentorial herniation—displacement of the cingulate gyrus compressing the pericallosal arteries resulting in ischaemia and infarction.
- Trans-tentorial herniation—the uncus of the temporal lobe is pushed between the midbrain and the tentorium, compressing the ipsilateral oculomotor nerve, observed as a fixed, dilated pupil.
- Cerebellar tonsillar herniation—pressure on the posterior fossa compresses the pons and displaces the cerebellar tonsils into the foramen magnum. Affects the pneumotaxic centres in the brainstem resulting in cardiac and respiratory arrest.

Status epilepticus

Status epilepticus (SE) is a prolonged seizure of any form or repeated seizures without regaining consciousness, lasting for 30 minutes or more. Status epilepticus is categorized as follows:

- Convulsive tonic–clonic SE:
  - Common in children, persons with learning disabilities and those with structural cerebral pathology
  - Presents with generalized tonic–clonic seizures, which give the clinical diagnosis
- Non-convulsive SE should be considered in patients with undiagnosed alteration of mental state. Diagnosis is heavily dependent on EEG.

Causes

- Acute infection, especially in children
- Stroke
- Hypoxia
- Metabolic derangements
- Alcohol intoxication or withdrawal
- Progression of underlying pathology
- Withdrawal of anti-epileptic drugs (AEDs) in patients with epilepsy

Stages of status epilepticus

- Prestatus:
  - A stage of increasing seizures lasting hrs to days which usually precede status epilepticus. Treatments shown below may avert progression to status epilepticus
- Early status:
  - The first 30 minutes of continuous convulsive seizure activity matched by continuous EEG seizure activity
- Established status:
  - Occurs 30–60 minutes when homeostatic mechanisms become inadequate and there is unmet demand. After 60 minutes decompensation occurs with significant changes in vital parameters
- Refractory status:
  - Lasts more than one hour and continues despite first line treatment
  - ↑ risk of brain injury—hypoglycaemia, hypoxia–ischaemic damage
- Subtle:
  - May emerge if seizures continue for hours. Clinically obvious convulsive activity slowly declines in amplitude and extent
  - Coma deepens and any motor activity may be limited to twitches around the eyes or mouth. EEG monitoring vital.
  - Mortality in subtle status is 65% compared to 27% in overt status in adults.

Management of convulsive status epilepticus

Management depends on several factors which include:

- The stage of status epilepticus.
- Whether it is the first presentation of epilepsy.
- Previous anti-epileptic medication taken and/or recent changes.
- Other potential causes such as psychogenic non-epileptic seizures.

Aims of care
- Control seizures
- Prevent physiological compromise
- Restore treatment for patients known to have epilepsy

Management
Prestatus
- If patient is alert between seizures, oral benzodiazepines such as clobazam 10mg may stop the flurry of seizures.
- If drowsy between seizures give diazepam 10–20mg rectally repeated once after 10 minutes if seizure continues **or**
- Midazolam 10mg buccally repeated after 10min if seizure continues.

Stopping status epilepticus
- Lorazepam i.v. usually 4mg bolus. Repeated after 10–20 minutes if the seizures continue.
- If seizures continue 30 minutes after first injection, administer:
  - Phenytoin infusion 15–18mg/kg at a rate of 50mg/min **or**
  - Fosphenytoin infusion 15–20mg PE/kg – 150mg PE/min
  - **and/or** phenobarbital bolus 10mg/kg at a rate of 100mg/min

Refractory status
- If measures fail to control the seizures, the patient should be transferred to ITU for treatment with barbiturate therapy.
- Propofol may also be beneficial in status epilepticus.
- Elective ventilation is often continued for 12–24 hours after last clinical or EEG evident seizure and then weaned off.
- Upon recovery consider long-term management with AEDs.

Monitoring and other management
- Resuscitate where necessary and maintain cardiorespiratory function
- Secure airway and administer oxygen, hypoxia is often severe
- Establish cause of seizures
- Check neurological observations, vital signs, ECG, routine blood levels
- Give prescribed treatment accordingly for any derangements
- Intensive monitoring including EEG
- Thiamine for any history of alcoholism

Non-epileptic attacks
The diagnosis of non-epileptic attacks should be considered if the seizures appear atypical and do not respond to initial treatment.

Epidemiology and prognosis
- Convulsive tonic–clonic status epilepticus incidence of 18–28 per 100,000 persons (9000–14,000 new cases in the UK).
- Accounts for 3.5% of admissions to neurological intensive care.
- Mortality is about 20%, and depends primarily on the cause
- The prognosis of status is mainly determined by the cause;
- Permanent neurological and mental decline may result especially in children
- Risk of morbidity increases with duration of the episodes.

Neuromuscular respiratory failure

Many neurological conditions can result in respiratory failure. Some may cause a rapid deterioration in respiratory function requiring careful monitoring and sometimes emergency intervention e.g.:
- Myasthenia gravis
- Guillain–Barré syndrome

Other conditions will cause respiratory failure more slowly and this should be managed in a controlled and planned way e.g.:
- Motor neurone disease
- Chronic neuropathies
- Chronic myopathies

Monitoring respiratory function

Assessment is vital and some aspects of respiratory assessment are more useful than others. The following should be monitored regularly:
- Respiratory rate.
- Observe for use of accessory muscles for breathing, shallow breathing, nasal flaring.
- Forced vital capacity (FVC)—this measures the amount of air the respiratory muscles are able to move, i.e. the largest volume exhaled slowly after a maximum inspiratory breath, and will be reduced in neuromuscular respiratory failure.
- Oxygen saturation.
- Arterial blood gas analysis.

⚠ Peak flow is NOT useful in these patients as this is a measure of airway resistance and their airways are not usually narrowed.

Forced vital capacity

- Measure using a spirometer.
- Don't get the patient to blow hard—this may damage the spirometer
- Ensure a good lip seal or use a face mask if good lip seal is not possible
- Ask the patient to blow as long as they can and encourage them to keep going.

If you do not have a spirometer a crude assessment of vital capacity can be made by asking the patient to take a deep breath and then count out loud for as long as they can without taking another breath.

FVC is measured against normal values for the individual compared with age, height and sex matched norms and should be approx 70–75 ml/kg.

FVC <20 ml/kg or a 30% drop requires emergency intervention, but as a general rule:

⚠ If a patient's FVC falls towards 1.5L, refer for an urgent medical assessment.

Patients will often be electively ventilated before their VC falls too low, but between 1.5–1.0L emergency ventilation may be required.

Nursing management

- Maintain regular observations of respiratory function, especially FVC
- If respiratory function deteriorates as above:
  - Call doctors urgently to review patient
  - Sit patient up to minimize pressure on the diaphragm and allow maximal ventilation
  - Administer oxygen as prescribed
  - Ensure crash trolley is at hand, but keep just outside the patient's room so as not to cause alarm
  - Reassure patient and stay with them
  - Assist doctors in assessing patient
  - Fast bleep anaesthetist if required and prepare patient for transfer to a critical care unit

Further information for health professionals and the public

Garner, A. and Amin, Y. (2006) The management of neuromuscular respiratory failure: a review. *British Journal of Neuroscience Nursing*, 2(8): 394–8.

Aspiration

Patients may cough during aspiration or it may be silent, i.e. without coughing and choking.

Common causes of aspiration

- Aspiration of gastric contents during induction of anaesthesia or intubation/vomiting or if the patient is unconscious for other reasons and their airway is unprotected.
- Neurological problems, e.g:
  - Stroke
  - Motor neurone disease
  - Parkinson's disease
  - Head injury
  - Multiple sclerosis
  - Other neurological conditions that cause dysphagia

Consequences of aspiration

- Chest infection and pneumonia
- Reduced oxygenation
- Death

Patient assessment

- Assess patient swallow (📖 see Swallowing problems (dysphagia) p 164)).
- Assess respiratory function:
  - Rate and depth
  - Oxygen saturation
  - Auscultation for crackles and reduced air entry
- Record temperature regularly.

Nursing care if aspiration is suspected

- Sit patient up if condition allows
- Keep nil-by-mouth
- Stop nasogastric (NG) feed and check position of tube if applicable
- Check oxygen saturation and administer oxygen as prescribed
- Perform tracheal suctioning if the patient is intubated
- Seek urgent medical review

Acute cord compression

Contributory causes
- Spondylosis (particularly in the elderly)
- Acute disc prolapse
- Spinal metastases
- Primary spinal tumours (ependymoma, meningioma)
- Direct trauma (☐ see Spinal cord injury, p 332).

Presenting symptoms
- Following complete cord compression there will be complete loss of function (motor, sensory, and autonomic reflexes) below the level of the lesion.
- Incomplete spinal compression can present with varying symptoms that make diagnosis difficult.
- Sensory loss.
- Acute back pain.
- Urinary urgency or painless retention.
- Constipation or faecal incontinence.

Diagnosis
- Medical history—presenting signs and symptoms
- Full neurological examination
- Radiology—MRI scan, plain spinal X-rays
- Chest X-ray
- Routine bloods, clotting, erythrocyte sedimentation rate (ESR), calcium, vitamin B12

Complications
- Temporary or permanent neurological deficits—particularly motor signs
- Spinal shock
- Cauda equina syndrome—damage to the lumbosacral nerve roots affecting the legs, bladder and bowels

Management
- Surgical decompression
- Radiotherapy
- Steroid theapy
- Conservative management—immmobilization

Autonomic dysreflexia

Autonomic dysreflexia is characterized by acute and rapid onset of hypertension in patients who have a spinal cord injury, usually above mid-thoracic level (T6 and above). It is triggered by painful or noxious stimuli below the level of the injury.

The hypertension is caused by over-stimulation of the sympathetic nervous system. The spinal lesion prevents upward ascension of pain messages and causes a mass reflex stimulation of the sympathetic nerves below the lesion along with marked vasospasm. Attempts by the body to respond to this inappropriate stimulation of the sympathetic nervous system fail because descending nerve tracts are blocked, further perpetuating the hypertension.

Autonomic dysreflexia needs to be treated early and appropriately as the rapid rise in blood pressure can lead to seizures, cerebral haemorrhage, myocardial infarction and death. It is only seen after recovery from spinal shock when reflex activity has returned.

Presentation

Symptoms are diverse but include:
- Severe hypertension
- Bradycardia
- Bilateral pounding headache
- Sweating and flushed, blotchy skin above the level of injury
- Goose flesh below the level of injury
- Nasal congestion
- Shivering
- Anxiety
- Nausea

Aims of care

Autonomic dysreflexia should be treated as a medical emergency. Care is initially directed at control of blood pressure and identification and removal of cause of pain/noxious stimuli. The following treatment should be administered:
- Sit the patient upright.
- Loosen any tight clothing.
- Monitor BP every 2–5 minutes during episode.
- Aim to find cause and remove noxious stimuli.
- Rapid survey of possible triggering factors.
- Check bladder and perform catheterization if required.
- Check for faecal impaction/constipation.
- Exclude other causes of pain/noxious stimuli.
- If elevated BP does not decline after 1 minute or cause can not be found then medical treatment is essential.

Triggering factors

The most common cause of autonomic dysreflexia is distended bladder either due to catheter blockage or other form of outlet blockage.
Other causes include:
- Distended bowel/constipation
- Pressure sore

- Sunburn
- Urinary tract infection (UTI)
- Bladder spasm
- Visceral pain/visceral trauma
- Ingrown toenail
- Deep vein thrombosis (DVT)
- Pregnancy/labour
- Severe anxiety

Medical treatment

- Immediate blood pressure reduction using antihypertensive drugs.
- Usual treatment with rapid action/short duration drugs, e.g. nitrates.
- If oral nitrates do not work consider intravenous medication.
- Patient should be monitored for any signs of hypotension post medication.

Prevention

Patient education is essential to prevent recurrent episodes. This should include counselling in relation to bladder, bowel and skin management.

Further information for health professionals and the public

Spinal Injuries Association http://www.spinal.co.uk

Neurogenic shock

Neurogenic or vasogenic shock is caused by the sudden loss of control of the sympathetic portion of the autonomic innervation system, controlling the contractibility of the smooth muscle in the arterioles, venules and small veins. It is characterised by a sudden decrease in vascular tone and resistance, as the vessels dilate fluid volume is increased in the circulatory system triggering a corresponding fall in blood pressure. It occurs more frequently in lesions or injuries occurring above T6 spinal level.

It is important to differentiate from other types of shock (anaphylactic, septic or hypovalaemic shock) that may co-exist in various situations.

Contributing factors

- Acute trauma/damage to the spinal cord
- Severe fluid loss
- Drugs
- Genral anaesthetic
- Neurological disorders

Signs and symptoms

Clinical signs include:
- Bradycardia with strong amplitude—less than 50–70bpm.
- Hypotension caused by effects of peripheral vaso-dilation.
- Neurological deficits
- Reduced skin temperature below level of lesion affected by environmental temperature.
- Inability to sweat normally below level of lesion.

Management

- Avoid administering large amounts of intravenous fluid to correct hypotension unless BP < 80mmHg systolic.
- Treat bradycardia <50bpm with bolus doses of atropine.
- Perform pharyngeal and tracheal suctioning with care—may induce bradycardia and asystole.
- Use of suxamethonium is contra-indicated in acute cord compression—may precipitate cardiac arrest.

Further reading

Spinal Injuries Association http://www.spinal.co.uk

Post-operative deterioration

Neurosurgical post-operative deterioration is a consequence of complex surgery to the brain and spinal cord.

Failure to detect and promptly intervene and manage the episode can have devastating consequences for the patient.

Complications can follow any routine surgical procedure, particularly when they involve a general anaesthetic.

General management

- Record vital signs—respiratory pattern and rate, pulse and BP.
- Prevention of hypovaleamia—central venous pressure (CVP) and blood pressure recording.
- Apply prophylactic anti-thrombosis measures—compression stockings, flowtron boots.
- Provide analgesia without over-sedating or compromising the level of consciousness.
- Pain is aggravated by anxiety, fear and communication difficulties—patients will need continued reassurance and explanation.
- Control hyperpyrexia—paracetamol, active cooling measures.
- Monitoring of blood electrolytes, clotting, ESR, haemoglobin.
- Observe wound for signs of haematoma, CSF leakage.
- Observe for signs of infection.
- Change position to avoid pressure effect problems.
- Manage any pre-existing disease or disability.
- Ensure the family are kept informed of treatment, progress and prognosis.
- Work with multidisciplinary team in preparation for discharge/transfer.

Respiratory support

- Blood gas analysis—signs of hypoxia and hypercapnia.
- Monitor respiratory rate and oxygen saturation.
- Observe for signs of retained secretions. Damage to the cranial nerves, particularly the hypoglossal and glossopharyngeal nerves, may depress normal airway protective mechanisms, leading to aspiration of oral secretions.
- Chest physiotherapy.

Circulatory management

- Maintain an accurate fluid balance.
- Maintain normovolaemia—normal levels of potassium and sodium.
- Give colloids to maintain CVP and cerebral perfusion pressure (CPP).
- Administer vaso-active drugs to maintain CPP.
- Initiate oral feeding as soon as clinical condition allows.
- Commence enteral feeding if swallow reflex assessed as unsafe.
- Record urine output hourly and monitor specific gravity of urine (signs of diabetes insipidus).

Neurosurgical management
- Glasgow Coma Scale observations—observing for changes from baseline.
- Assess limb movements, sensation and power.
- Monitor cranial nerve function and integrity.
- Record at least hourly pupil reactions
- Observe for signs of seizure activity
- Maintain head elevation to 15–30°.

Following cranial surgery

There are numerous problems and complications that can develop following craniotomy. Early diagnosis and prompt interventions can prevent neurological deterioration.

Contributory causes

- Hypoxia and hypercapnia
- Extradural, subdural, intracerebral haematoma formation
- Diffuse brain swelling
- Seizures
- Infection
- Infarction
- Hydrocephalus

Immediate/acute complications

- Ineffective airway or breathing problems
- Inadequate blood gases
- Inadequate cough or gag reflex—aspiration of secretions
- Wound haemeorrhage or haematoma
- Focal neurological deficits—sensory and motor changes
- Altered level of consciousness—raised intracranial pressure—↓GCS, ↓conscious level, changes in behaviour, motor deficits, headache, changes in pupil response
- Vital signs—Cushing's triad; ↑BP, ↓Pulse, changing respiratory pattern, widening pulse pressures
- Electrolyte imbalance—fluid loss, diabetes insipidus
- Pyrexia
- General post-operative complications (paralytic ileus, DVT, nausea, vomiting, pain)

Short-term complications

- Infection—wound, meningitis
- Cerebral abscess
- Cerebrospinal fluid leak (otorrhoea, rhinorrhoea), aerocoele
- Hydrocephalus
- Cognitive impairment—agitation and confusion
- Altered bladder function, sensory or motor dysfunction
- Altered bowel function—altered diet, NG feeding, drug therapy

Long-term complications

- Osteomyelitis
- Epilepsy
- Carotid cavernous fistula
- Skull defects
- Hydrocephalus
- Diffuse brain damage
- Focal brain damage
- Personality changes
- Poor memory (short-term)
- Speech and language problems

Medical and nursing management

- Assess airway, breathing and circulation and active resuscitation measures.
- Check arterial blood gases—elective mechanical ventilation.
- Check blood urea and electrolytes, glucose, blood cultures, FBC, and ECG.
- Perform a baseline neurological examination:
  - Level of consciousness
  - Pupil reactions—equal, size, shape
  - Eye movements—III, IV, VI cranial nerves
  - Motor responses—abnormal flexion, extension, flaccid
- Arrange CT/MRI scan.
- Control raised Intracranial pressure:
  - External ventricular drain to reduce CSF pressure
  - Cerebral diuretics (mannitol)
  - ICP bolt to measure ICP
  - Fluid management/vaso-active drugs to maintain CPP
- Maintain normothermia.
- Anticonvulsant therapy to control seizure activity.
- Maintain patient safety—protect invasive lines, raise cot rails, consider use of restraints for extreme cases (📖 see p 152).
- Swallow assessment, particularly for posterior fossa craniotomies.
- Pain control.
- Accurate fluid balance.
- Monitor urine and serum osmolarity for signs of diabetes insipidus or syndrome of inappropriate anti-diuretic hormone secretion (SIADH).
- Liaise with members of multidisciplinary team.
- Refer to specialist agencies—early discharge planning.

Following spinal surgery

New neurological deficit following spinal surgery is rare but requires urgent diagnosis and prompt interventions to prevent permanent neurological disability.

Contributory causes

- Large vessel damage during surgery
- Extradural haematoma—in the cervical region may cause weakness or significant disability
- Local damage to nerve roots
- Oedema and swelling

Immediate/acute complications

- Acute airway or respiratory problems.
- Hypovolemic shock (tachycardia, ↓BP, ↑resps, ↓urine output).
- General post-operative complications associated with anaesthetic.
- Sensory or motor deficits.
- Bladder and bowel disturbance.
- Cauda equina syndrome (weakness, sensory loss, urinary incontinence or retention, pain).
- Wound haemorrhage or haematoma.

Short-term complications

- Infection.
- Epidural abscess—compresses the spinal cord causing myelopathy, ischaemia and infarction.
- Dural tear—cerebrospinal fluid leakage from the lumbar thecal space into the surrounding tissue.
  - Can occur in a small number of patients.
  - In severe cases a pseudo-meningocele may form below the incision site.

Long-term complications

- Spinal instability—an increased risk with multilevel laminectomy. Can lead to development of kyphosis, subluxation and increasing deficits.
- Inflamation and fibrosis—recurrence of symptoms due to compression of local blood supply to the nerve roots. Long-term damage may lead to ischemia and infarction.
- Spinal stenosis may intensify original symptoms.
- Sexual dysfunction.
- Persistent pain and symptoms that are unresolved following surgery.

Management

- Assess airway, breathing and circulation and resuscitate if necessary
- Check blood urea and electrolytes, glucose, blood cultures, ESR/CRP (C-reactive protein), FBC and ECG.
- Spinal observations and neurological examination.
- CT/MRI scan.

- Some patients following a cervical laminectomy may require a swallow assessment by a trained practitioner or speech and language therapist if the laryngeal nerve has been damaged.
- A lumbar drain will help to reduce the pressure of CSF over the dural tear and promote healing.
- Bed rest for short periods to allow the leak to heal.
- A small number may require surgical intervention to repair the torn dura.

Following neuroradiological interventions

Complications following invasive neuroradiological interventions for diagnosis or treatment are less common than those following surgical intervention. Early recognition, diagnosis and intervention can prevent and reduce neurological deterioration.

Typical interventions

- Myelography
- Cisternogram
- Lumbar puncture

Normally, catheter angiography approaches are via the femoral artery:

- Cerebral, spinal angiography (including stenting)
- Coiling, embolization
- Endarterectomy

Possible catheter angiography complications

Puncture site

- Haematoma (usually femoral), large vessel dissection,
- Psuedoaneurysm and ruptured vessels.
- A-V fistula—following multiple puncture attempts.
- ⚠ Important to check clotting status prior to procedure.

Cerebral

- Vasospasm
- Stroke
- Vasovagal reactions

Spinal

- Spinal cord ischaemia

Other general complications

- Headache
- Infection
- Siezures
- Ischaemia and infarction—hemiparesis/plegia
- Pulmonary emboli
- Dysphasia/aphasia
- Visual field defects

Related to contrast media

- Allergic reactions
- Vomiting
- Urticarial rashes
- Anaphylaxis
- Seizures

Post-procedural care

- Cardiovascualr observations
- GCS observations
- Bed rest as clinical condition demands
- 📖 See also Chapter 4, p 100

Acute behavioural disturbance and use of restraint

Patients with neurological problems may exhibit disturbed behaviour for a variety of reasons. Often this is due to the inability of the brain to process information correctly and can be caused simply by sensory overload or deprivation as well as a host of neurological metabolic and other causes. (For causes of confusion see 📖 Chapter 7, pp 155–178).

Consequences of neurological disturbance

Behaviour that is identified as challenging is often a consequence of pain, fear, frustration or confusion. This is frequently manifest by physical or psychological symptoms.

Cognitive

Memory impairment, attention deficits, perceptual and visual–spatial problems, language difficulties.

Emotional difficulties

Frustration, rapid mood swings, emotional flattening or lability, apathy, disinhibition, anxiety, depression, obsessional behaviour.

Physical

Paralysis or reduced mobility, ataxia, visual difficulties, loss of smell and taste, epilepsy, fatigue headaches, sexual arousal.

Priority of care

Maintain the safety of both the patient and others.

- Some patients may be at risk to themselves due to wandering away from the safe environment of the ward or pulling out tracheostomy tubes or invasive arterial and central lines.
- Other patients may become aggressive or violent and present a risk to staff, other patients and visitors.

Restraint

The use of restraint is a controversial issue and is subject to considerable legislation to prevent inappropriate or excessive use. There are many physical and psychological complications that may results from using restraints:

Skin breakdown and trauma	Loss of dignity
Compromised circulation	Depression
Aspiration pneumonia	Apathy
Incontinence	↑ Anxiety and dependency
↓Cardiac function	↑ Fear, panic anger
↓Nerve conduction	↑ Agitation

However, in acute neuroscience and critical care areas there is still a clinical indication for restraint if: according to the Mental Capacity Act:
- The person lacks capacity and it will be in the person's best interest.
- It is firmly believed that restraint is necessary to prevent the patient from harming themselves.
- The restraint is a proportionate response to the likelihood of the person suffering harm and seriousness of that harm.

Additional considerations
- Use of restraint must not be an alternative to inadequate human or environmental resources.
- Restraint should always be a last resort when all other less intrusive methods of managing the problem have failed to achieve the desired outcome.
- The patient and their family should be engaged in discussions to inform them of the reason and choice of restraint.
- If an alternative to a proposed restraint is identified, and yet the restraint continues, the use of the restraint will be seen as an abusive act.

Management of patients with behavioral disturbance
- Speak calmly and slowly.
- Give simple instructions.
- Do not shout.
- Orientate the patient to their environment.
- Do not grab the patient to try and restrain them—this may make them more confused and aggressive.
- Encourage family and friends to sit with the patient—a familiar presence may reassure them and calm the situation.
- If the patient is mobile and is being aggressive or violent—ensure you have a clear exit from their room.
- Monitoring behaviour to identify triggers for their behaviour, i.e. observing for antecedents, noting type of behaviour and its consequences (ABC charts).
- Try to remove 'bothersome' interventions—catheters, lines.

Risk assessment
When restraints are employed in the clinical area a comprehensive risk assessment must be completed that clarifies:
- Why the restraint is necessary.
- What restraint is to be used?
- When the restraint is to be used.
- Details of who approved the restraint.
- When the restraint should stop/time limits for the restraint—visual observation to be made every 30 mins.
- The patient must be released from the restraint every hour.
- Commercially produced restrainers should be consistently used.

Common problems and symptoms

Change in level of consciousness

Consciousness is defined as a state of awareness of oneself and the environment. There are many causes of an altered state of consciousness, such as those summarized below:

Intracranial causes	Extracranial causes
Most of the intracranial causes of altered consciousness result in either raised intracranial pressure or cerebral hypoxaemia, e.g:	Metabolic causes:
	Hypoxia
	Hypercapnia
	Uraemia
Trauma	Hepatic encephalopathy
Tumours	Endocrine causes:
Infection: meningitis, encephalitis	Hypo/hyperglycaemia
Oedema	Other causes:
Stroke	Poisoning
Subarachnoid haemorrhage	Drug/alcohol intoxication
Dementia	

The next two topics deal with management of common altered states of consciousness, confusion and coma.

Caring for a confused patient

Patients may appear confused for a variety of reasons and this altered state of consciousness may be due to acute confusional disorders or may be a chronic problem. Confusion may be transient or cognitive function may progressively decline. Priorities of care are to:

- Assess the level of consciousness and confusion (📖 see Chapter 3, p 62)
- Maintain the safety of the patient and others
- Maintain patient dignity
- Promote quality of life
- Promote self-care and independence with activities of living as far as possible
- Provide emotional support for patient and family
- Provide practical advice and support for family and carers
  Caring for such patients requires an interdisciplinary approach

Caring for an acutely confused patient

The care of an acutely confused patient is considered in Chapter 6.

Caring for a patient with cognitive decline

- Assess cognitive function (📖 see Chapter 3, p 78).
- Assist patient to remain independent with activities of living and give clear, simple instructions at all times.
- Orientate to time and place:
  - Place a clock in the patient's room where it can be clearly seen.
  - Remind them of the date and time.
  - Patients may experience a disturbed sleep–wake cycle and night-time waking with daytime somnolence is common.
- Administer medication and monitor side effects—it is unlikely that patients will be able to do this independently.
- Observe patient and maintain safety if they are wandering—this can be a common problem—follow at a safe distance and do not try to grab the patient and pull them in another direction. Instead, gently guide them back towards the ward.
- Assist patient and family to develop strategies to maintain social activities. Social isolation can become a problem and depression may occur.
- Provide families and carers with contact information for voluntary organizations and support groups.
- Make arrangements for respite care for patient to enable carers to have a break from time to time.

Caring for an unconscious patient

Patients who are unconscious are completely dependent on nursing care to maintain their safety and activities of living. Patients may be unconscious for a variety of reasons, and the loss of consciousness may be sudden and acute or may have developed progressively over a period of time. For some patients the loss of consciousness is expected to resolve, while for others it may not.

Care should be planned to ensure all activities of living are maintained:

- Maintaining a safe environment:
  - Ensure patient is nursed safely in bed
  - Use bed rails with care to ensure patient does not fall out of bed, but these should not be used if the patient is confused and may climb over them, falling and injuring themselves
- Breathing:
  - Ensure airway is maintained
  - Administer humidified oxygen as prescribed if required
  - Assess respiratory function—rate, depth, oxygen saturation etc.
  - Care for endotracheal/tracheostomy tubes if required
  - Suction patient according to Trust guidelines
- Communicating:
  - Speak to patient at all times and explain all procedures—the patient may still be able to hear
  - Encourage family and friends to sit with patient and talk to them
  - Use non-verbal communication, e.g. touch
  - Observe for non-verbal signs of pain e.g. agitation and restlessness, grimacing
- Eating and drinking:
  - Unconscious patients should be NBM as they will be unable to protect their airway
  - Patient is at risk of aspiration (🕮 see Chapter 6, p 138)
  - Maintain IV infusion as prescribed & check IV site for phlebitis (redness/swelling)—patient will be unable to tell you if this is painful
  - Administer NG/percutaneous endoscopic gastrostomy (PEG) feeds as prescribed if required—taking care to check position of NG tube before use and observe PEG site for inflammation
- Eliminating:
  - Monitor urine output and bowel function (🕮 see Chapter 3, pp 86–89)
  - Catheterize patient if accurate hourly urine output is needed, otherwise use sheaths, pads and pants and other aids/appliances to contain urine lost
  - Ensure the patient does not become constipated or strain—this can elevate ICP
- Personal cleansing and dressing:
  - Bed-bath unconscious patient and change sheets daily or more frequently if sweating profusely
  - Pay particular attention to eye care: patients that have lost blink reflex and cornea may become dry and damaged
  - Ensure mouth-care is provided regularly

- Controlling body temperature:
  - Check temperature regularly
  - Remove coverings if patient becomes pyrexial
- Mobilizing:
  - Conduct risk assessment for moving and handling and pressure areas
  - Turn the patient and adjust position 2 hourly to reduce risk of pressure sores developing
  - Provide pressure-relieving equipment and beds as required
  - Carry out passive limb exercises
  - Position the patient to reduce spasticity and risk of contractures
- Working and playing:
  - Discuss employment with the patient's family
  - Provide an in-patient certificate for an employer if required
  - Refer to social worker for support with financial circumstances and benefits if required
  - Ask the family if the patient enjoys listening to particular music and encourage family to bring in MP3 player/personal stereo. Use intermittently and monitor patient response
- Expressing sexuality:
  - Ensure the patient's dignity is maintained
  - Nurse in single sex ward/bay if possible
  - Encourage partners to visit and spend time with the patient
- Sleeping:
  - Assess for discomfort and administer analgesia as prescribed if required
  - Assess level of consciousness
- Dying
  - Discuss prognosis and provide emotional support to family
  - Discuss preferred place of care for end of life as appropriate with family

Further information for health professionals and the public

Hickey, J.V. (2003) *The clinical practice of neurological and neurosurgical nursing*, 5th edn. Philadelphia: Lippincott

Woodward, S. and Mestecky, A.-M. (2009) *Evidence-based neuroscience nursing*. Oxford: Wiley-Blackwell.

Seizures

Seizures are transient episodes of altered neurological function, during which a person may or may not experience alteration of awareness or loss of consciousness and can manifest with one or more of the following phenomena; sensory; motor or psychic.

Causes
- Epilepsy
- Acute symptomatic seizures:
  - Alcohol, drugs-therapeutic or recreational
  - Metabolic disorders e.g. renal failure
  - Cerebral hypoxia
  - Pre eclampsia
- Hyperpyrexia-febrile convulsions

Epidemiology
- Incidence of single seizure in Britain is 20/100,000
- Incidence of febrile convulsion in Britain is 50/100,000
- Lifetime prevalence (cases who have ever had a seizure) 20/1000
- Seizures remit in 70% of cases on treatment

Presentation
Manifestations include some of the following symptoms:
- Motor manifestations—jerking (clonus), spasms or posturing, focal or generalized convulsions, head or eye version (turning).
- Speech arrest, choking sensations.
- Loss of consciousness.
- Sensory manifestations such as numbness, tingling, flashing lights, sensation of epigastric rising.
- Autonomic changes, e.g. blood pressure, heart rate, skin colour etc.
- Psychic manifestations, e.g. disturbance in memory, dream-like states, alteration of awareness.
- Automatisms—involuntary motor actions in a state of impaired awareness, e.g. chewing, fiddling movements of hands, aimless walking etc.

Nursing care in a clinical setting
Management of seizure
- Safety:
  - Loosen any tight clothing around patient's neck.
  - Protect patient from injury (remove sharp or hard objects from the vicinity; or guide patient away from danger.
  - Cushion patient's head if they fall down.
  - Once the seizure has finished, aid breathing by gently placing patient in recovery position.
  - If respirations are compromised, provide oxygen as prescribed
  - Stay with patient until fully recovered.
- Ensure treatment is administered as prescribed, e.g. IV diazepam, buccal midazolam.

Documentation and observation of seizure activity

It is vital that nurses make accurate records of seizure activity including:

- Date time and duration.
- Did the patient cry out?
- Did the patient have an aura?
- In which part of the body did the twitching begin and did it progress?
- Did the patient lose consciousness?
- What colour was the patient's skin during the seizure?
- Did the patient turn their head to one side at the start of the seizure?
- What activity did the eyes have? Did the pupils react to light?
- Was the patient incontinent of urine or faeces?
- Did the patient bite their tongue?
- Was any injury sustained? If so what?
- Did the patient hyperventilate?
- Did the patient complain of any after effects?
- Was the patient confused?
- Baseline observations intra and post 'ictally'.
- Record GCS, BP, pulse and O_2 sats, ECG.

Nursing care in a primary care setting

Ambulance support may be required in a community setting. Send for an ambulance if:

- It is a first seizure
- The seizure lasts more than 5 minutes before use of emergency medication
- Seizures continue 10 minutes after administering emergency medication where prescribed
- There is evidence of respiratory compromise and injury

Further information for health professionals and the public

National Society for Epilepsy (NSE) http://www.epilepsynse.org.uk
Epilepsy Action (EA) http://www.epilepsy.org.uk
International League Against Epilepsy (ILAE) http://www.ilae-epilepsy.org
NICE (2004) *The epilepsies: the diagnosis and management of the epilepsies in adults and children in primary and secondary care.* London: National Institute for Health and Clinical Excellence.

Pain

Pain is a subjective experience and defined by the person experiencing it. Pain is commonly experienced by patients with neurological problems although it may be related to an underlying problem and not related to their neurological condition.

Pain may be related to:
• Headache (discussed further in ☐ Chapter 8, p 216)
• Spasticity
• Muscle cramps
• Poor positioning and posture
• Dystonia
• Paraesthesia and neuropathic pain
• Emotional distress
• Underlying co-morbidity, e.g. arthritis

A thorough and detailed pain assessment is vital to determine the cause and nature of the pain. Give patients time to tell you about their symptoms, especially if they have difficulty communicating.

Pain management

Pain is often under-reported and under-treated, especially amongst older patients. Pain related to neurosurgery may also be underestimated. More extensive surgery is often less painful than anticipated and procedures that might be considered more minor often result in more pain. Patients are also often given less analgesia than required due to fears of masking neurological signs and there is sometimes a reluctance to use opioid analgesia post-operatively.

Patients' reports of pain should be believed, documented, acted upon and then reassessed.

The mainstay of pain management remains analgesia—starting with simple analgesia and increasing. Nurses should always administer analgesia as prescribed and assess the effectiveness.

Different analgesics are used for different types of pain, e.g:
• Simple analgesia (paracetamol) for headaches.
• As above + codeine or tramadol, moving up to morphine for post-op neurosurgical patients.
• Anticonvulsants (e.g. carbamazepine, gabapentin) are useful for neuropathic pain.
• Muscle relaxants, antispasmodics and botox may be prescribed for muscle spasm and spasticity.

Non-pharmacological methods of pain relief

The following may also be helpful in alleviating patients' pain and should be offered where appropriate. Nurses will not be able to instigate all of the following interventions, but may be able to discuss alternatives with medical staff and allied health professionals.
• Distraction, e.g. watching TV, listening to music
• Careful positioning and repositioning
• Physiotherapy and passive movements
• Application of heat/cold

- Transcutaneous electronic nerve stimulation (TENS)
- Massage
- Acupuncture

Chronic/complex pain management

Some patients' pain is difficult to alleviate and a referral to pain management teams or specialist palliative care services may be required.

Palliative care should not only be considered for patients who are terminally ill and specialist palliative care practitioners have a lot of expertise in symptom control.

Pain may not just be a physical problem and may be due to emotional distress or spiritual pain. Multidisciplinary team involvement in pain management is vital.

Nurses need to be the patient's advocate in pain management.

Further information for health professionals and the public

Woodward, S. and Mestecky, A.-M. (2009) *Evidence-based neuroscience nursing*. Oxford: Wiley-Blackwell.

Swallowing problems (dysphagia)

Dysphagia, or difficulty swallowing, is a common problem seen in patients with neurological disorders and may be due to a variety of conditions:

- Altered consciousness
- Spasticity of muscles of face and pharynx
- Flaccidity and paralysis of muscles of face and pharynx
- Cognitive problems
- Affect and mood (e.g. depression)
- Dyspraxia—uncoordinated voluntary movement

Consequences of dysphagia

- Aspiration, leading to chest infection and possibly death
- Malnutrition
- Dehydration
- Increased infection risk
- Increased length of stay
- Poor wound healing
- Psychological distress

Nursing patients with dysphagia

- Patient safety is paramount—aim of care is to prevent aspiration and maintain adequate nutrition and fluid intake
- Assess swallowing early (📖 see Chapter 3, p 61) and refer to SLT for further assessment
- ❶ If swallow is unsafe—keep patient nil-by-mouth
- Liaise with SLT to identify individualized swallowing programme/ techniques, which may include:
  - Always supervise patients while taking food or fluid orally
  - Ensure staff members are trained in feeding techniques if patients are unable to feed themselves
  - Protect mealtimes and ensure sufficient staffing
  - Alter consistency of food and fluid—thickened fluids and puréed diet may be recommended
  - Alter temperature of food and fluids. For some patients cold fluids are easier to swallow as they cause more sensory stimulation
  - Always ensure patient sits upright
  - Some patients may be recommended to tuck their chin down towards their chest when swallowing, which helps to protect airway
  - Some patients may be recommended to swallow twice after each mouthful
  - Check patient is not pooling food in the cheek pocket and that the mouth is empty before taking the next mouthful
  - Feed patients slowly and with small mouthfuls, ensuring they have time to trigger a swallow
  - Do not use straws for patients to drink through or 'wash food down' by following a mouthful with water
  - ⚠Observe for signs of aspiration during feeding, e.g. wet voice, coughing and choking

- Observe for signs of silent aspiration (in which the patient does not cough etc), e.g. pyrexia, altered respiratory function, productive cough

Further information for health professionals and the public

Woodward, S. and Mestecky, A.-M. (2009) *Evidence-based neuroscience nursing*. Oxford: Wiley-Blackwell.

Communication problems

Communication problems are common in patients with neurological disorders. The most commonly encountered problems fall into two main categories:

• Dysphasia/aphasia—this is a language problem, whereby the patient may or may not understand what is being said to them (receptive dysphasia) or may be unable to find the right words to express what they want to say (expressive dysphasia). It is unlikely that a patient has purely expressive dysphasia and will usually have an element of receptive dysphasia as well.

• Dysarthria—this is a problem with the motor production of speech often due to difficulty coordinating movement of the face, lips, tongue and muscles of the pharynx and breathing in order to produce speech. These patients understand everything that is being said to them and know what they want to say, but just can't get the words out, with speech often being slurred.

• Dyspraxia—this is a problem with motor programming of speech. Voluntary coordination of speech production is lost, but the patient may be able to respond with automatic gestures and words, e.g. say hello, wave, smile appropriately. These patients know what they want to say, but are unable to produce sounds in the correct order.

Communicating with patients with speech and language problems

• Assess speech deficit and refer to SLT for an early detailed assessment.
• Liaise with SLT to identify effective communication methods for the individual patient. This may include use of:
  • Picture boards
  • Pen and paper to enable patient to write
  • Light writer and other electronic communication aids
• Do not shout at the patient—they are not deaf and this can lead to frustration.
• Use active listening at all times.
• Allow time for the patient to express what they want to say.
• Do not finish their sentences for them. Again this can be frustrating and is often incorrect.
• Do not avoid spending time communicating with patients who have difficulty—this has been shown to increase social isolation and depression.
• Always speak slowly and clearly.
• Ensure that you face the patient when communicating and maintain eye contact. It is important that the patient is able to see your facial expression when you are speaking to them.
• If a patient has any element of receptive dysphasia, always use short sentences and simple instructions.
• Confirm that you have understood what the patient wanted to say by using yes and no.
• Don't pretend you have understood if you haven't.

- Encourage the patient to have a go—any attempt at communication should be encouraged.
- Minimize environmental distractions and background noise.

Further information for health professionals and the public

Woodward, S. and Mestecky, A.-M. (2009) *Evidence-based neuroscience nursing*. Oxford: Wiley-Blackwell.

Spasticity

Spasticity is a disorder of the tonic stretch reflex and results in increased muscle tone, stiffness and often painful muscle spasms. It is a common feature of central nervous system problems such as:
- Traumatic brain injuries
- Multiple sclerosis
- Stroke

Left untreated patients with increased tone will develop contractures, pressure sores and difficulty with activities of living and socializing. Patients often develop a pattern of extensor spasm with the head tipped back and legs extended—this is not a good functional position and makes swallowing and communication difficult as well as independent mobilizing. This position can also lead to patients sliding out of a chair.

Prevention of spasticity

- Position patient in an anti-spastic posture—liaise with physiotherapist as to the best position for the patient from day 1.
- ⚠ Avoid noxious stimuli—these will often trigger spasm in a patient prone to spasticity and will make existing spasticity worse:
  - Full bladder
  - Blocked catheter
  - Constipation and faecal impaction
  - Tight clothing/leg-bag straps round the legs
  - Pain
  - Stress
  - Anxiety
  - Pressure sores
- Lie the patient supported on their side in bed before getting them up—this will help to reduce tone and severe extensor spasm.
- Do not pull quickly on affected limbs—spasticity is velocity driven and the quicker a force is applied the more spasticity will result. Instead, when dressing patients etc, move the limb slowly with firm, gentle forces. The spasticity will often suddenly 'give' and the limb will relax and move. This is known as 'clasp-knife'—like opening a stiff penknife.
- Reposition the patient regularly and ensure they are comfortable with all extremities supported.
- Administer medication as prescribed to reduce spasticity e.g:
  - Anti-spasmodics (baclofen, dantrolene).
  - Muscle-relaxants (diazepam)
  - Anticonvulsants (e.g. gabapentin, carbamazepine)—reduce muscle spasm and pain.
- Some patients may be prescribed botox for specific muscle groups or have intrathecal pumps inserted for administration of baclofen directly into the spinal canal.

Prevention of secondary complications

- Check pressure areas regularly and ensure pressure-relieving aids are used appropriately.

- Ensure hands are positioned supported on a pillow with the fingers outstretched. Do not give the patient something to hold or a ball to squeeze as this will only encourage the fingers to curl in flexor spasm. Long-term the patient will not be able to uncurl the fingers as the soft tissues will shorten and contract into this position.
- Ensure good personal hygiene, especially inside the palm of the hand, which often becomes enclosed, sweaty and offensive smelling.
- Put limbs and muscles through a range of normal movement—passive exercises—liaise with the physiotherapist to prevent contractures.
- Liaise with OT and physio re splinting and orthotic supports.

In severe cases, if a patient has developed contractures due to spasticity, surgery may be indicated to allow the limbs to be positioned in a more functional position, but prevention is always better than cure!

Flaccidity

Flaccidity or loss of muscle tone is a common feature of neurological conditions affecting the lower motor neuron. If a muscle loses its nerve supply and no impulses are therefore transmitted to it, the muscle will lose tone, becoming flaccid, and may waste.

Flaccidity can be seen in a range of neurological conditions e.g.

- Guillain-Barré syndrome
- Peripheral neuropathies or injuries
- Motor neuron disease
- Spinal cord injury (depending on level of injury)

Caring for patients with flaccidity

- Support affected limbs and joints at all times in a good functional position.—e.g. feet at 90° at the ankle, otherwise the foot will drop and the patient will not be able to walk in the long term
- Liaise with physiotherapist and OT re positioning and splinting
- If orthotic splints are provided, ensure these are removed at least once per day and pressure areas are inspected
- Ensure limbs are put through a range of movements and passive exercises every day—liaise with physiotherapists re: exercises to be performed and frequency
- Ensure joints are supported and not able to hyperextend, e.g. knees. Muscles help to provide support around a joint and hyperextension injuries can result. Use profiling bed to help support patient in a good functional position
- Ensure analgesia is administered as prescribed—joints may become painful.
- Ensure DVT prophylaxis is instigated as prescribed when indicated, e.g. thrombo-embolus deterrent (TED) stockings, anti-coagulation according to NICE guidelines. Patients with muscle flaccidity are particularly at risk of DVT as the deep veins have lost the support of the muscles that they lie within, which can cause endovascular damage, not just because of reduced mobility.

Further information for health professionals and the public

NICE (2009) *Reducing the risk of venous thromboembolism (deep vein thrombosis and pulmonary embolism) in patients admitted to hospital.* London: National Institute for Health and Clinical Excellence.

Following burr hole surgery and craniotomy

Craniotomy is a general term that describes an operation to open the skull (cranium) in order to access the brain for surgical repair.

Brain surgery is generally the first line of treatment for brain injuries and conditions and may be performed as:

1. An emergency procedure following head injury, brain haemorrhage, infections, abscess, oedema.
2. A planned procedure to remove a tumour or to clip an aneurysm.

Burr holes

- Can be performed under a local or general anaesthetic.
- The hair is shaved around the burr hole site.
- Head movement is minimized by positioning on a shaped headrest that is usually clamped using a frame fixed to a table.
- Following a skin incision, one or more small burr holes are made in the skull with a drill into the exposed skull.
- Stereotactic frames, image-guided computer systems, or endoscopes are used to guide instruments through the burr holes.
- Burr holes may be used for minimally invasive procedures:
  • Insertion of a ventricular shunt to manage hydrocephalus.
  • Insertion of a deep brain stimulator to treat PD.
  • Insertion of an intracranial pressure (ICP) monitor.
  • Obtaining a biopsy for histology.
  • To drain a chronic subdural haematoma (CSDH).

Craniotomy

- A general anaesthetic is usually required.
- After the scalp is prepared with antiseptic, a skin incision is made, usually behind the hairline. Sometimes a hair-sparing technique can be used that requires a small shaved area around the incision.
- Craniotomies are named according to the area of skull removed.
- A craniotomy may be small or large depending on the underlying problem.
- Complex craniotomies are often used to perform skull base surgery. They involve the removal of part of the skull that supports the base of the brain, cranial nerves and blood vessels. Extensive reconstruction is frequently required.
- Craniotomies may be used to:
  • Remove or treat large brain tumors, aneurysms, or AVMs
  • Treat the brain following a skull fracture or injury (e.g., gunshot wound)
  • Remove tumours that have invaded the skull
  • A craniotomy is used to connect the burr holes to create a removable bone flap that is stored until replaced at the end of the procedure or at a later date. If the bone flap is not replaced, the procedure is called a craniectomy.

- Following the surgery, if the bone flap is replaced it is secured with stitches or wire, the dura, muscle and skin are sutured and a drain may be inserted to remove residual blood.
- Stitches or staples are usually removed 7–10 days following surgery.

Potential complications

Actual risk depends on the complexity of the operation.

No surgery is without risks. General complications include haemorrhage, DVT, reactions to anesthesia, chest infection.

Specific complications related to a craniotomy may include:
- Wound or bone flap infection
- Intrinsic damage to the brain during surgery
- Meningitis
- Seizures—anticonvulsants are not routinely prescribed.
- Cerebral oedema—bone flap may be removed, sterilized, and stored carefully until it is required
- Local damage—facial muscle, sinuses, cranial nerves
- CSF leak—may require repair

Operations involving the temporal lobe frequently damage the muscles controlling jaw opening, leaving the mandible stiff and painful to open wide. Recovery is aided by chewing gum.

Post-operative nursing care

- Perform a baseline neurological examination:
  - Level of consciousness
  - Pupil reactions—equal, size, shape
  - Motor responses—abnormal flexion, extension, flaccidity
- Maintain normothermia.
- Administer anticonvulsant therapy to control seizure activity as prescribed.
- Maintain patient safety—protect invasive lines, raise cot rails, consider use of restraints for extreme cases.
- Swallow assessment, particularly for posterior fossa craniotomies.
- Administer analgesia as prescribed for pain control.
- Maintain accurate fluid balance.
- Liaise with members of the multidisciplinary team.
- Refer to specialist agencies—early discharge planning.
- See also care of the unconscious patient.

Specific issues to consider

The patient will need to inform the Driver and Vehicle Licensing Authority (DVLA) of their surgery and their driving licence may be suspended due to a risk of seizures. For the latest guidelines refer to the DVLA website.

Further information for health professionals and the public

Driver and Vehicle Licensing Authority http://www.dvla.gov.uk

Undergoing awake craniotomy

- The patient is fully awake during part or whole of the procedure.
- During surgery, once the brain has been exposed, sedation level is reduced allowing the patient to return to consciousness, able to cooperate and participate in conversation.
- With the patient awake, evoked potential electrophysiological mapping, 'functional mapping', can be performed allowing the surgeons to stimulate the brain with electrical probes to avoid damage to important structures, i.e. language, special senses, movement.
- The patient is asked to speak, count and perform other basic tasks while the mapping takes place.
- The patient remains pain free due to the lack of pain receptors in the brain and local anaesthetic to the skin edges.

Awake craniotomy

Used for:
- Resection of an epileptic focus
- Excision of tumors and AVM's
- Deep brain stimulation for PD
- Reduces the interference of anaesthetic drugs on electrocorticography (ECoG), recordings

Bupivacaine, lidocaine and adrenaline (epinephrine) are frequently used to anaesthetize the skin and provide localized nerve block to the nerves.

- A successful operation requires a thorough pre-operative assessment, taking into account the psychological and mental state of the patient.
- The patient has to remain motionless for long periods of time. Some sedation is necessary to keep the patient still and comfortable, it must be titrated so that it does not interfere with the ECoG recordings. Drugs include: propofol, fentanyl, alfentanil or remifentanil.
- Option of converting to a general anaesthetic if problems occur during surgery.

Contraindications to awake craniotomy

- Lack of resources
- Patients with learning disabilities
- Confused patient
- Young children
- Large, complex procedures
- Potentially difficult intubation if conversion required

Advantages

- Reduced morbidity and mortality
- Early discharge
- ↓ side effects from anaesthetic agents

Unstable cervical injury

The diagnosis of unstable spinal injury is frequently difficult and complex and may be as high as 33% in patients with concomitant head injuries. Failure to accurately diagnose a spinal injury can have devastating short- and long-term consequences.

❶ All spinal injuries should be considered unstable until excluded both radiologically and by the medical team.

It is important to differentiate between those patients who might be cleared through clinical examination alone and those injuries that must be investigated further using CT or MRI scanning. Assessment of ligament damage in the absence of a fracture is difficult, particularly in unconscious patients that are unable to articulate complaints of neck pain or tenderness.

A small number of spinal injuries have a second, sometimes non-adjacent, fracture within the spine.

Criteria for unstable spinal fracture
- Neurological deficit
- Posterior element injuries
- Loss of more than 50% of anterior vertebral body height
- > 25–35° of angulation
- Thoracolumbar fracture—angulation of thoracolumbar junction > 20° and spinal canal compromise > 30%

Three column instability of spinal column
- **Anterior column injury**—anterior portion of vertebral body and the connected frontal ligaments.
  - Includes compression fractures with > 25% loss of height indicating posterior ligament rupture and fractures through the vertebrae.
- **Middle column injury**—Posterior half of the vertebral body and corresponding ligaments.
  - Unstable injury may be complex with an anterior fracture or dislocation. Surgical stabilization is frequently required although upper thoracic spine injuries are generally more stable.
- **Posterior column injuries**—ligaments, laminae and spinal process.

Pre-hospital management
- Manual spinal protection should be applied immediately.
- Application of immobilization device, e.g. traction, should not take priority over resuscitation measures.

Hospital management
- The spinal board should be removed as soon as possible once the patient is on a firm trolley.
- ⚠ Prolonged use of spinal boards can rapidly lead to pressure injuries.
- Full immobilization should be maintained until the patient is stablized. Manual protection should be re-instated if restraints need to be removed for examination or procedures.

- The log-roll is the standard manoeuvre to allow examination of the back and transfer on and off back boards. Four people are required, one to hold the head and coordinate the roll, three to support the chest, pelvis and limbs. The number and degree of rolls should be kept to a minimum.
- Clinical and radiological clearance of the spine with evaluation of stability is essential.
- Spinal immobilization is a priority in multiple trauma, spinal clearance is not.
- Patients should be transferred to a specialized spinal injury unit, ideally within 24 hours of diagnosis (⊞ see Neurosurgery nursing, p 332).
- ⚠ Unconscious patients must continue with spinal precautions until fully conscious.
- Thoracolumbar spine imaging is indicated if there is pain, bruising, swelling, deformity or abnormal neurology attributable to the thoracic or lumbar spinal regions.
- The presence of a fracture anywhere in the spine demands full spinal imaging.
- Unconscious patients who cannot be clinically assessed, require radiological clearance of the whole spine.
- To facilitate early mobilization, unstable fractures may be surgically fixed with bone grafting or metal fusion.

Long-term neurological conditions

Multiple sclerosis

Incidence	7 per 100,000
Prevalence	100 to 120 per 100,000 (female:male 2:1)
Aetiology	Idiopathic autoimmune disorder possibly due to:
	• Abnormal immune response to a virus
	• Environmental toxin
	• Genetic factors

Multiple sclerosis (MS) affects up to 62,000 people in England and Wales. Average age of onset is approximately 30. Onset over the age of 60 and juvenile cases of MS are exceptionally rare.

MS is understood to be an autoimmune disorder causing progressive inflammatory damage to myelin and eventual destruction of axons.

Forms of MS

Relapsing–remitting
The most common form of MS at presentation.

A relapse or clinical attack is defined as new or recurrent neurological signs and symptoms, which last for at least 48 hours. A minimal interval of 30 days of neurological stability should exist. Relapse rate varies but the average is approximately one per year. Only 12% of people with MS will have greater than four relapses per year. Higher frequency of relapse rate and higher levels of unremitting impairment are probably associated with a poorer prognosis. Transient recurrence of previous symptoms is typical and can be associated with infection, fever, heat or exertion.

Presentation of relapse:
• Weakness: 40%
• Loss of vision (typically optic neuritis): 22%
• Paraesthesiae: 21%
• Diplopia: 12%
• Balance impairment: 5%
• Altered micturition: 5%

Secondary progressive
Progression following a period of relapsing remitting disease. Progression is defined as a sustained deterioration for at least 6 months. Relapses may still occur against a background of progression but general relapses will become less frequent. Approximately 65% of people with relapsing–remitting MS will have developed secondary progression after 15 years.

Primary progressive
10% of people with MS. Onset is usually over the age of 40. Disease activity primarily affects the spinal cord. Presentation is characterized by progression from onset without distinct attacks or remission and is typically associated with symptoms affecting lower limb function.

Life expectancy

Death as a direct result of MS is exceptionally rare to the point where MS is generally considered not to be a terminal condition. Life expectancy for the vast majority of people with MS is not affected. Premature death, when related to MS, typically occurs due to complications such as pneumonia and aspiration.

Signs and symptoms

- Cognitive impairment
- Depression
- Fatigue
- Bladder dysfunction
- Bowel dysfunction
- Balance impairment
- Sexual dysfunction
- Tremor and ataxia
- Spasticity
- Visual disturbance
- Disturbance of swallowing and speech
- Weakness
- Pain

Medical management

Disease modification

Treatment with beta interferon and glatiramer acetate is available for people with MS who experience relapses, irrespective of whether they are following the subtypes of relapsing–remitting or secondary progressive MS. Treatment criteria have been developed by the Association for British Neurologists. Natalizumab has been approved for use in the NHS by NICE.

Symptom management

The aim of management is to enhance quality of life and reduce risk of complication through the combined use of medication and a multidisciplinary team (MDT). This team would typically consist of neurologist, GP, specialist nurse, physiotherapist, occupational therapist, speech and language therapist, continence advisers. Functional and vocational goals for rehabilitation are equally important.

Relapse management

Treatment of clinical attacks should be with intravenous methylprednisolone 500mg–1g daily for between 3–5 days, or with oral methylprednisolone 500mg to 2g daily for between 3–5 days. Treatment should commence as soon as possible and be accompanied by rehabilitation from a multidisciplinary team. Treatment will positively affect speed of recovery.

Nursing care

During the diagnostic phase

- Psychological support is vital for both patient and family
- Promote concept of wellness and provide patient with information about their condition

- Advise patient about employment and refer to social services if required
- Refer to MS specialist nurse
- Provide patients with information about local support groups
- Encourage patient to avoid triggers that may exacerbate their symptoms, e.g:
  - Heat and humidity (hot bath, holidays to hot climate)
  - Infections
  - Stress
  - Anxiety
  - Sleep deprivation

During a relapse
- Assess patient's activities of living and assist in identifying trigger factors for relapse
- Administer steroids as prescribed and monitor effectiveness and side effects
- Provide psychological support to patient and their family

Spasticity and mobility problems
- Carry out moving and handling risk assessment
- Refer to physiotherapist
- Position patient to prevent spasticity
- Assess limb movement and degree of spasticity
- Avoid triggers (🕮 see Chapter 7)
- For other aspects of nursing management 🕮 see Chapter 7, pp 155–178
- Consider orthotic splinting

Fatigue
- Identify triggers for fatigue
- Promote a balance between activity and rest
- Encourage rest periods throughout the day
- Ensure adequate sleep
- Pace activities
- Avoid extremes of temperature

Bladder and bowel dysfunction
- Assess bladder and bowel function (🕮 see Chapter 3)
- Check for urinary retention and consider clean intermittent self-catheterization if the patient's residual urine volume is greater than 100ml post-void
- Prevent constipation and monitor for and appropriately manage faecal incontinence (🕮 see Chapter 7)
- Refer to continence advisory service

Speech and swallowing disturbance
- Assess speech and swallowing (🕮 see Chapter 3)
- If dysphagia or communication problems are present refer to SLT and dietitian
- Provide suitably adapted diet if required
- Assist patient with eating and drinking and monitor for signs of aspiration (🕮 see Chapter 7)

Pain

- Patients with MS may experience pain due to spasticity and painful joints or neuropathic pain
- Assess pain using an appropriate pain assessment tool (📖 see Chapter 3)
- Administer analgesia as prescribed and monitor effectiveness
- Assist patient to change to a more comfortable position and relieve spasticity which may be causing pain
- Consider other methods of pain relief (📖 see Chapter 7)

Further information for health professionals and the public

Contact the MS Society or MS Trust.

http://www.mssociety.org.uk

http://www.mstrust.org.uk

National Collaborating Centre for Chronic Conditions (2003) *Multiple sclerosis: management of multiple sclerosis in primary and secondary care.* London: NICE.

Zajicek, J., Freeman, J. and Porter, B. (2007) *Multiple sclerosis care: a practical manual.* Oxford: Oxford University Press

Parkinson's disease

Incidence	20 per 100,000
Prevalence	190 per 100,000 (male:female 3:2)
Aetiology	Idiopathic, chronic, progressive disorder. Symptoms are produced by degeneration of dopaminergic neurons in the substantia nigra (SN), part of the basal ganglia, possibly due to:
	• Genetic factors
	• Environmental facors (e.g. pesticides, heavy metals, proximity to industry, rural residence)
	• Combination of the above

120,000 PD sufferers live in UK. 10,000 are diagnosed each year, 1 in 20 of these having young-onset PD. Predominantly a disease of older age. Symptoms appear from the age of 50, but in young-onset PD can appear before 40 years. Parkinsonian features are also seen in other conditions i.e. multi-system atrophy, progressive supranuclear palsy, Lewy body dementia and Parkinsonism due to other causes.

Signs and symptoms

Slow onset. Symptoms vary and include motor and non-motor symptoms:
- Bradykinesia (slow movement)
- Resting tremor
- Rigidity
- Balance problems
- Gait disturbance—freezing, shuffling
- Micrographia (small hand writing)
- Non-motor symptoms include: low mood and other cognitive changes, constipation, anosmia (loss of sense of smell), sleep disorder, reduced facial expression, monotonous and hypophonic (low volume) speech, and occasionally on presentation dribbling and dysphagia.

Medical management

Mainstay of treatment is pharmacological.

Drug	Preparations	Action and side effects
MAO-B inhibitors	Selegiline Rasagiline	Inhibits monoamine oxidase, inhibiting breakdown of dopamine
Dopamine agonists	Bromocriptine Pergolide Apomorphine	Mimic the action of dopamine
Levodopa	Sinemet® Madopar®	Precursor of dopamine—crosses the blood–brain barrier and is converted to dopamine

(Continued)

Drug	Preparations	Action and side effects
CMOT inhibitors	Entacapone	Inhibits the breakdown of levodopa administered orally
	Tolcapone	
(anti-viral)	Amantadine	Reduces receptor activity
Anticholinergics	Older drugs and rarely used	Inhibit ACh receptors—restores the balance between dopamine and ACh

Nursing care

At diagnosis

- Accurate and sensitive 'telling' of diagnosis, supporting acceptance and understanding is essential.
- Refer to PD nurse specialist (PDNS) if this contact has not already been made.
- Provide people with Parkinson's (PWP) and carer with information regarding treatment options including conventional and complementary therapies, support agencies, driving and employment etc.
- Assess functional disability and encourage early referral to multi-disciplinary team (MDT) and (PDNS).
- Support and monitor as chosen drug treatment is initiated.

During maintenance phase of disease

- Ensure regular review of diagnosis and treatment by specialist team.
- Provide advice on self-care strategies promoting independence including exercise, diet, rest, medication concordance and individual lifestyle choices.
- Psychological support for PWP and family, symptoms are emotion-sensitive. Offer opportunity to discuss any relationship issues physical/emotional.

During complex phase of disease

This stage is characterized by advancing symptoms including dysautonomia and polypharmacy.

> ❶ Maintenance of individual's drug regime crucial. Drugs must be given on time during any hospital admission, even if this means outside of usual drug rounds.

- Mobility:
  - High risk of falls (compromised balance and postural hypotension increase risk).
  - Conduct risk assessment provide mobility and moving and handling advice for PWP and carers.
  - Seek input from physio and OT re bed mobility and gait initiation difficulties. This may include provision of handling aids/mobility devices alongside cueing strategies (e.g. counting one, two to initiate steps).

- Communication problems:
  - Loss of volume and clarity of speech, diminished facial expression—PWP can appear depressed/uninterested/even angry—discourages interaction which leads to isolation.
  - Reduce background noise, allow time to speak and listen carefully, prompting sensitively if train of thought lost.
  - Do not assume you have understood if you have not.
  - Do not finish the patient's sentences for them, this will only increase frustration.
  - Seek further advice and support from SLT.
- Nutrition:
  - PWP can become malnourished, dehydrated and lose weight; may also increase risk of infection and poor skin condition. PWP may have problems of drooling saliva and difficulty chewing/swallowing (dysphagia), dyskynesia and poor manual dexterity
  - Conduct nutritional and swallowing assessments (see Chapter 3)
  - Allow extra time for smaller more frequent drinks and meals
  - Ensure SLT/dietitian referral is made for assessment
  - Record weight monthly
  - Modify diet/thicken fluids as advised
  - PEG may be discussed.
- Elimination:
  - Due to autonomic disturbance bladder and bowel function may be affected.
  - Conduct assessment essential as problems are variable (🕮 see Chapter 3, pp 61–90)
  - Refer to community nursing team or continence specialist as required.
  - Constipation is common in PD, usually a result of the condition but may be compounded by drug side effects, reduced mobility, poor diet and fluid intake.
  - Adjust diet, give stool softeners (make sure adequate fluid intake for drugs to work) or stimulant laxatives/suppositories.
- Sleep problems:
  - Common and may be due to poorly controlled PD, nocturia, vivid dreaming and sometimes REM sleep behaviour disorder, hallucinations, restless legs syndrome, pain or cramps; can exacerbate excessive daytime sleepiness.
  - Control of PD throughout 24 hours by adherence to drug administration times.
  - Ensure a regular bedtime routine and specific advice and treatment for diagnosed sleep disorders.
- Identify and treat behavioural/psychological issues—depression, psychosis.

During palliative phase of disease
In addition to all the issues above, consider reduction of dopaminergic treatment, and involving palliative care team for further support of PWP, their family and specialist team to manage end of life care.

Managing apomorphine pumps

Apomorphine is a rescue drug for patients who are experiencing end of dose 'off' effects from levodopa. It is effective within 5–10 minutes of administration.

- Ensure patients and carers are taught how to administer subcutaneous injections or manage an apomorphine pump.
- Change the injection site daily.
- Ensure good hygiene for both injection sites and hands.

Further information for health professionals and the public

Parkinson's Disease Society http://www.parkinsons.org.uk

MacMahon, D.G., Thomas, S., Fletcher, P. and Lee. M. (2006) *Paradigm for disease management in Parkinson's disease.*

Clough, C., Chaudhuri, K.R. and Sethi, K. *Fast facts: Parkinson's disease.* http://www.fastfacts.com

Multiple system atrophy

Incidence	3 per 100,000
Prevalence	6 per 100,000
Aetiology	Unknown

Multiple system atrophy (MSA) is a sporadic, progressive neurodegenerative disorder of adult onset, characterized by any combination of autonomic dysfunction, Parkinsonism and ataxia. It is slightly more common in men than women, usually diagnosed between the ages of 40–69 years. Disease duration is 5–9 years, average survival from diagnosis is 3.5 years.

Signs and symptoms

Initially may look like or be misdiagnosed as early PD. Symptoms vary and include motor and non-motor symptoms. Patients develop other symptoms much sooner than might be expected in PD and generally have a poor long-term response to levodopa. Diagnosis of PD may be reviewed with the emergence of 'red flags':

- **Parkinsonism**: Slow and stiff, rapid deterioration in mobility.
- **Autonomic dysfunction**: Postural hypotension, bladder and bowel dysfunction, speech and swallow problems, erectile dysfunction.
- **Cerebellar disturbance**: Poor balance, coordination and postural instability.
- Other movement features may be present; spasiticty, weakness and ante-collis.

Medical management

- Limited benefit from pharmacological treatments.
- Providing symptom relief alongside supportive care, with practical strategies to manage at home and suitable options for longer term care are the most helpful plans.
- The team needs to be coordinated, honest and practical. These families do not have time to waste.
- Regular review of symptoms and treatment by specialist team.
- Advice on disease progression, self-care strategies to maintain independence and information about future service provision.
- Psychological support for the patient and family. Offer opportunity to discuss any relationship issues, physical/emotional.

Nursing care

Patients require a sensitive 'telling' of the reviewed diagnosis and considerable support in coming to terms with the prospect of rapid and unpredictable progression of their disease.

- *Mobility:* high risk of falls (compromised balance, ataxia, increasing weakness and postural hypotension increase risk):
  - conduct risk assessment
  - provide mobility and moving and handling advice for patient and carers
  - Refer to physio and OT

- *Communication:* loss of volume and clarity, diminished facial expression, speech monotone, slurred one-breath delivery, may experience complete loss of sound reproduction.
  - Reduce background noise, allow time to speak and listen carefully, prompting sensitively if train of thought is lost
  - Seek further advice and support from SLT
- *Nutrition and swallowing problems:* Due to increasing difficulty with chewing and swallowing, may become unsafe swallowing fluid, at risk of aspiration. May become malnourished, dehydrated, and lose weight; also increased risk of infection, constipation, and poor skin condition. May have problems of drooling. Problems with feeding, poor manual dexterity:
  - allow extra time for smaller more frequent drinks and meals
  - ensure SLT/dietitian assessment, Modify diet/thicken fluids as advised, PEG is very often required
  - record weight monthly
- *Elimination:* Due to autonomic disturbance bladder and bowel function are usually affected, with urgency, frequency, nocturia and retention being common in 70–80% of people.
  - Assessment essential as problems are variable (📕 see Chapter 3)
  - Refer to community nursing team or continence specialist as required
  - Often require catheterization
  - Constipation is common, usually a result of the condition but may be compounded by drug side effects, reduced mobility, poor diet and fluid intake: adjust diet, give stool softeners (make sure adequate fluid intake for drugs to work) or stimulant laxatives/ suppositories
- *Sleep problems:* Linked to autonomic dysfunction, may experience snoring, stridor, apnoea, oxygen desaturation and inspiratory sounds, many of these problems can also occur in the daytime, very distressing for the patient and family.
  - Will require specific advice and treatment for diagnosed sleep disorders
  - Identify and treat psychological issues—depression, psychosis.
- *Postural hypotension;* drop of 20mmHg systolic on standing, complaints of dizziness, fatigue, blurred vision, 'coat hanger' pain (pain across neck and shoulders). May experience altered level of consciousness, increased risk of falls. Triggers may include; eating/worse after a meal, warm environment, medications, straining on the toilet, muscular activity, changes in posture—laying–sitting–standing.
- *Temperature disturbance;* may have cold extremities. Sweating disturbance, may be unable to sweat in hot weather, core temperature not always same as skin temperature.
- *Erectile dysfunction* reported in approx 70–90% of men

Further information for health professionals and the public

Sarah Matheson Trust for Multiple System Atrophy Tel 020 788 1520 or
  http://www.msaweb.co.uk

Progressive supranuclear palsy

Incidence	Unknown
Prevalence	5 per 100,000 (but, thought to be higher, since it is one of the two most common of the Parkinson's Plus syndromes, and can be difficult to diagnose.
Aetiology	Unknown

Progressive supranuclear palsy (PSP) is a progressive neurodegenerative disease. Age of onset is usually between 55–75 years. The pathological hallmark is tau protein-positive filamentous inclusions, known as neuro-fibrillary tangles, which are found in the basal ganglia, diencephalon and brainstem. Some cases of PSP map to a polymorphism in the *Tau* gene. Life expectancy is between 5 and 10 years (median 6–7 years).

Signs and symptoms
Symptoms vary but include:
- Most common presenting symptom of PSP is several falls over a year, usually backwards with 'motor recklessness'
- Head retracted
- Low frequency blinking
- Fixed 'Mona Lisa' stare, patients are unable to look up or down to command. Vertical eye movements following a target are preserved early on. Photosensitvity
- Personality change and cognitive impairment
- Depression and apathy
- Parkinsonism usually bradykinesia (limb tremor is rare)
- Dysarthria and dysphagia (bulbar dysfunction)
- Poor response to levodopa
- Constipation, nocturia and sometimes difficulty initiating urine flow

Medical management
Pharmacological
- No specific licensed treatment
- Anti-Parkinsonian drugs may offer modest benefit, consider amantadine
- Artificial tears for dry eyes
- Botulinum toxin may be used for neck spasm and blepharospasm

Nursing care
- Symptomatic relief, maintain quality of life (QoL), speed of response important:
  - Ensure early referral to MDT and PSP Association
  - Psychological care—acceptance of diagnosis can be difficult when many have been adjusting to a diagnosis of PD
  - Refer early to physio and OT for advice and training re falls prevention and management, bed mobility and perhaps equipment.

- Dysphagia—modify diet and thicken fluids if advised after SLT/dietitian assessment. In later stages a PEG (feeding tube) may be recommended either to supplement oral intake or as method of choice for nutrition and hydration.
- Excess salivation (sialorrhoea)—can be difficult to manage—may be helped with SLT-provided reminders, low-dose amitriptyline or atropine drops to mouth. In extreme cases botulinum toxin may be considered
- Vision impairment—refer to OT and or ophthalmologist for advice and equipment to manage this problem more effectively.
- Dysarthria—early referral to SLT and dietitian, provide communication aids
- Mood changes—consider referral to mental health team (MHT) for further support and treatment as required.
- Key issues to consider:
  - Ongoing psychological support often needed in order to come to terms with condition
  - Later discuss patients wishes/advance directives/preferred place of death
  - PSP Association can help with information, advice, equipment loan and financial support. 24 hours/7 days a week phone counselling service 01327 322410
  - Respite care

MDT should have ensured

- Home physio/OT assessment for safety and aids required
- Referral to Social Services for full community assessment process
- Awareness of state benefits for disability and attendance
- Carers assessment so their support needs can be addressed
- Effective communication between all parties

Further information for health professionals and the public

The PSP-Europe Association, PSP House, 167 Watling Street West, Towcester, Northamptonshire NN12 6BX. Email: psp@pspeur.org

Burn, D.J. and Lees, A.J. (2002) Progressive upranuclear palsy: where are we now? *Lancet Neurology*, 1(6): 359–69.

Nath, U. and Ben-Schlomo, *et al.* (2003) Clinical features and natural history of progressive supranuclear palsy. *Neurology*, 60: 910–16.

Epilepsy

Incidence	80 per 100,000 per annum
Prevalence	400–1000 per 100,000 (higher numbers in developing countries)
Aetiology	30% of cases of epilepsy are idiopathic.
	Other causes include:
	• vascular disease
	• congenital malformations
	• degenerative disorders
	• sclerosis of the hippocampus
	• neoplasms
	• trauma
	• infection
	• genetic and epileptic syndromes of childhood

Epilepsy is a disorder of the brain characterized by an ongoing tendency to recurrent unprovoked seizures. Epilepsy has many forms and underlying causes, hence the use of terms such epilepsies and epilepsy syndromes. The International League Against Epilepsy has classified the epilepsies and epilepsy syndromes as follows:

1. Focal epilepsies
2. Generalized epilepsies and syndromes
3. Epilepsies and syndromes undetermined whether focal or generalized
4. Special syndromes—situation-related seizures

Mortality People with epilepsy have a 2–3 times higher death rate than the general population. Sudden unexpected death in epilepsy (SUDEP) accounts for 17% of epilepsy-related deaths

• Best prognosis is for patients with acute symptomatic seizures
• Worst prognosis seen in patients with a congenital cause
• In general, 70% of patients achieve seizure control when taking medication
• Over half of patients will achieve a 3-year remission by 10 years after diagnosis
• Some epilepsy syndromes require life-long treatment

Signs and symptoms

• Recurrent seizure activity including impairment of:
  • Motor function
  • Sensory perception
  • Autonomic function
  • Psychic phenomena with or without alteration in consciousness or awareness

Diagnosis

• Clinical diagnosis—witness/patient account of the seizure and behaviour
• Electroencephalography (EEG)

- Magnetic resonance imaging (MRI) of brain
- Electrocardiogram (ECG)—rule out cardiac causes
- Blood tests—rule out other causes

Medical management

- Pharmacotherapy
  - Anti-epileptic medication

The main antiepileptic medications used in the UK		
Carbamazepine	Levetiracetam	Rufinamide
Clobazam	Oxcarbazepine	Tiagabine
Clonazepam	Phenobarbital	Topiramate
Ethosuximide	Phenytoin	Valproate
Gabapentin	Pregabalin	Vigabatrin
Lamotrigine	Primidone	Zonisamide

- - Benzodiazepines are also used.
- Surgery—depends on localization of epileptogenic region and cause of epilepsy.
  - Curative surgery:
    - Hemispherectomy
    - Lobectomy
    - Lesionectomy
  - Radiotherapy (DXT)
  - Palliative surgery
    - Vagus nerve stimulation
    - Corpus callosectomy/callosotomy
    - Multiple subpial transection
  - Other functional surgical procedures not routinely practiced include deep brain stimulation (DBS); transcranial magnetic stimulation (TMS) and gamma-knife or proton-pencil beam surgery
- Abolish seizures
- Reduce risk of injury
- Reduce risk of social dependence
- Reduce risk of stigma associated with condition
- Key issues to consider:
  - Help come to terms with condition
  - Age and gender of patient and effect of treatment
  - Other medical problems and co-medication
  - Patients who live alone

Further information for health professionals and the public

National Society for Epilepsy (NSE) http://www.epilepsynse.org.uk
Epilepsy Action (EA) http://www.epilepsy.org.uk
International League Against Epilepsy (ILAE) http://www.ilae-epilepsy.org

Nursing care of people with epilepsy

A majority of patients with epilepsy are managed in an outpatient setting. Admission to hospital becomes necessary if there is acute exacerbation of seizures or status epilepticus. Regardless of treatment setting, it is vital for nursing staff to be aware of potential seizure-precipitating factors. These include:

- Sleep deprivation and fatigue
- Fever or ill health
- Photic stimulation in 3% of patients
- Menstrual cycle
- Metabolic disturbances
- Alcohol and alcohol withdrawal
- Emotional disturbance and stress

Other less common factors include startle, fright, dietary changes, pain, fasting, allergy, hormonal changes etc.

Aims of care

- Ensure effective seizure control
- Support the patient and family in coming to terms with the condition and its limitations
- Provide ongoing surveillance for potentially harmful side effects of AEDs
- Key issues to consider:
  - Age of the patient
  - Gender
  - Type of epilepsy/seizures
  - Epilepsy medication and other prescribed drugs
  - History of and response to previous anti-epileptic medication
  - Other medical conditions
  - Ethnicity

Nursing care

- Assess patient's seizure frequency
- Assess and ensure concordance with treatment
- Assess patient's understanding of the condition and potential seizure-precipitating factors
- Assess accessibility to pharmacy and supply of medication
- Assess general risks associated with seizure activity and take measures to control the risks

- Providing evidence-based and up to date advice and counselling on the areas contained in the table below

Treatment concordance	Insurance issues
Medication side effects	Employment and education
Seizure precipitants	Social and leisure pursuits
Driving regulations	Safety
Contraception	Associated stigma and social isolation
Menstruation	Potential for sudden unexpected death
Pregnancy	Support charities

- Administer anticonvulsants as prescribed and evaluate response to treatment
- Engage relevant agencies and other professionals to provide a holistic approach to patient care
- Ensure regular follow-up
- Ensure good communication between the responsible neurology team, patient and their GP
- ⚠ Women with epilepsy should be warned that anticonvulsants may interact with other drugs, e.g. they reduce the effect of the oral contraceptive pill. Some may also cause fetal abnormalities so pre-conceptual counseling is advised.

Useful resources

- Liverpool seizure severity scale

Further information for health professionals and the public

The National Institute for Clinical Excellence (2004) *The epilepsies—the diagnosis and management of the epilepsies in adults and children in primary and secondary care.* London: NICE.
National Society for Epilepsy (NSE) http://www.epilepsynse.org.uk
Epilepsy Action (EA) http://www.epilepsy.org.uk

Psychogenic non-epileptic seizures (pseudoseizures)

The term 'pseudoseizure' is now outdated and psychogenic non-epileptic seizures (PNES) is the preferred terminology.

Incidence	Unknown
Prevalence	Unknown
Aetiology	A number of psychological causes of PNES have been found (Moore and Baker, 1997) including: • anxiety and depression • stress • physical or sexual abuse • bereavement • family dysfunction • relationship difficulties

30% of patients with epilepsy will develop PNES, but it also occurs in others without an epilepsy diagnosis.

Females are affected more than males (4:1).

Differentiating PNES from epileptic seizures

It is very difficult to differentiate between the two but some signs may be useful:

Pseudoseizures	Genuine seizures
Pupils unchanged	Pupils dilate
P and BP unchanged	↑P and BP
Plantar downgoing	Extensor plantar
No nailbed cyanosis	Peripheral + central cyanosis
pO_2 and pH unaltered	↓pO_2 + pH
Serum prolactin normal	↑Serum prolactin
Normal EEG	Seizure activity on EEG

PNES is often said to be attention-seeking, hysterical or malingering, but it is not. Episodes of violent shaking and feigned unconsciousness occur, but this is often caused by the subconscious and the patient is not necessarily 'putting it on'.

Medical treatment

- Accurately diagnose PNES
- Convey diagnosis with sensitivity and reassure patient that they are not crazy.
- Stop/reduce unnecessary anti-epileptic drugs to reduce risk of harm from side effects
- Identify stressors
- Counselling and psychological support

Nursing care

Patients may injure themselves and have been witnessed to have a respiratory arrest during PNES so always treat as a genuine seizure and act accordingly (see previous topic).

Nurses are vital in diagnosis and the importance of good witness accounts should not be underestimated. Carefully observe and document any seizure activity.

Inform medical staff of seizure activity immediately if serum prolactin levels have been requested—blood must be taken within 15 minutes.

Treat patient with understanding—they are not malingering.

Assist with personal hygiene if the patient has been incontinent.

Provide reassurance and psychological support/counselling.

Further information for health professionals and the public

Moore, P.M. and Baker, G.A. (1997) Non-epileptic attack disorder: a psychological perspective. *Seizure*, 6(6): 429–34.

Russell, A.J.C. (2006) The diagnosis and management of pseudoseizures or psychogenic non-epileptic events. *Annals of Indian Academy of Neurology*, 9(2): 60–71.

Alzheimer's disease

Incidence	163,000 new cases throughout UK per year
Prevalence	70+ per 100,000 age 40–64 increasing to 10,000 per 100,000 age > 85 years
Aetiology	Unknown—likely to be multifactorial

Alzheimer's disease (AD) is a neurodegenerative (progressive) disease and the commonest cause of dementia in the UK, accounting for 55% of cases of dementia in older people. Amyloid plaques and neurofibrillary tangles develop in the brain causing cell death, leading to a reduced concentration of neurotransmitters, including acetylcholine. Age is the greatest risk factor. Alzheimer's disease may coexist with depression and vascular dementia: 700,000 people are living with dementia in the UK, including 15,000 affected below the age of 65. Alzheimer's lasts, on average, seven years from diagnosis to death.

Signs and symptoms
- Short-term memory loss
- Word-finding difficulties
- Confusion
- Social withdrawal
- Difficulties with reading, spelling and calculation
  Later, may include:
- Visual perception difficulties
- Behavioural and psychiatric symptoms such as wandering, aggression, delusions
- Incontinence
- Seizures

The person gradually becomes dependent on others for all activities of daily living, and may require a nursing or residential care home placement.

Medical management
Early, accurate diagnosis allows the person to access appropriate care and treatment, and plan for the future.
- Pharmacological management:
  - Alzheimer's disease cannot be cured, but treatment with cholinesterase inhibitors (donepezil, rivastigmine or galantamine) may stabilize symptoms. Treatment must be initiated by a specialist and is recommended by NICE for those scoring between 10 and 20 on Mini Mental State Examination. Side effects may include gastrointestinal disturbance, sleep disturbance, and loss of appetite.
  - Neuroleptics and benzodiazepines for behavioural and psychiatric symptoms may be used cautiously after consideration of non-pharmacological approaches. Newer antipsychotics with lower side effect profile are preferable, and even then 'start low and go slow'. The Committee on Safety of Medicines state that risperidone

and olanzapine should not be used other than short term, under specialist supervision, for severe and distressing symptoms,
- SSRIs may be useful in depression.

Medication should be reviewed at least twice annually.

Nursing care

Given the devastating impact of Alzheimer's disease on the person and their family, information must be provided in a sensitive and timely manner, and not rushed in the ward or outpatient consultation:
- Information and advice is required on:
  - (When and if the patient is ready) diagnosis and prognosis
  - Symptom management
  - Legal and financial matters: discussions on giving up driving, although essential, are not likely to be well received. The DVLA must be informed if someone has dementia or any organic brain syndrome
  - Lasting powers of attorney, and advance decisions (see Mental Capacity Act 2005), should be considered in the early stages
  - Entitlement to State benefits such as attendance allowance, or assistance with residential or nursing home fees
  - The role of statutory and voluntary support services such as the community mental health team, social services, and patient support groups such as the Alzheimer's Society and local carers' groups
- Non-pharmacological management:
  - Needs assessment to include environment and safety issues, e.g vulnerability if living alone, risk of falls
  - Ensure timely referral to OT, physio and social services
  - Behavioural and psychiatric symptoms can often be reduced following detailed assessment and a person-centred approach to interventions
  - Referral to other relevant healthcare professionals for specific advice may include an Admiral nurse and dementia nurse specialist where available, community psychiatric nurse, old age psychiatrist, neurologist, continence advisor
  - Provide supportive care for cognitive impairment (📖 see Chapter 7, pp 155–178)

Maintaining independence for as long as possible, and providing a stimulating environment, will help a person live well with Alzheimer's. Supporting family members in their caring role improves care for the person with dementia and reduces carer morbidity. Family carers of people with dementia save the UK over £6 billion a year.

Further information for health professionals and the public

Alzheimer's Society http://www.alzheimers.org.uk

National Institute for Clinical Excellence (NICE) (2007) *Donepezil, galantamine, rivastigmine (review) and memantine for the treatment of Alzheimer's disease.* http://www.nice.org.uk

Vascular dementia

Incidence	163,000 new cases throughout UK per year
Prevalence	70+ per 100,000 age 40–64 increasing to 10,000 per 100,000 age > 85 years
Aetiology	Unknown—likely to be multifactorial

Vascular dementia (VaD) is a neurodegenerative (progressive) disease and the second most common form of dementia in the UK. Risk factors are as for cardiovascular disease. Vascular dementia may coexist with Alzheimer's disease (known as mixed dementia). Mixed dementia accounts for 20% of cases of dementia in older people. Vascular dementia lasts, on average, seven years from diagnosis to death.

Signs and symptoms

Symptoms are similar to Alzheimer's disease so may include:
- Word-finding difficulties, short-term memory loss, confusion, social withdrawal, difficulties with reading, spelling and calculation, visuoperceptual difficulties, behavioural and psychiatric symptoms such as wandering, aggression, delusions, incontinence, seizures

In addition,
- If caused by stroke (single or multi-infarct), symptoms may include weakness, paralysis and slurred speech, with a 'stepwise' pattern of deterioration (symptoms constant then sudden deterioration).
- If caused by small vessel disease (subcortical) the symptoms develop more slowly and often include difficulties walking.

Depending upon the cause, the person may have a fairly stable cognitive deficit, or will become dependent on others for all activities of daily living, and may require a nursing or residential care home placement.

Medical management

Early, accurate diagnosis allows the person to access appropriate care, receive advice to prevent further transient ischaemic attack/stroke or to slow progression in small vessel disease, and plan for the future.

Medical treatment is aimed at preventing further events and slowing progression. Hypertension, hypercholesterolaemia, diabetes, heart problems and sleep apnoea need to be managed, and the patient advised that healthier lifestyle choices (e.g stop smoking) may slow progression.
- Pharmacological management:
  - Treatment with cholinesterase inhibitors (donepezil, rivastigmine or galantamine) is not recommended by NICE for vascular dementia although there is some evidence it may help, particularly if the person also has Alzheimer's disease.
  - Neuroleptics and benzodiazepines for behavioural and psychiatric symptoms may be used cautiously after consideration of non-pharmacological approaches. Newer antipsychotics with lower side effect profile are preferable, and even then 'start low and go slow'. The Committee on Safety of Medicines state that risperidone

and olanzapine should not be used other than short term, under specialist supervision, for severe and distressing symptoms,
- SSRIs may be useful in depression.

Medication should be reviewed at least twice annually.

Nursing care

Given the devastating impact of a diagnosis of vascular dementia on the person and their family, information must be provided in a sensitive and timely manner, and not rushed in the ward or outpatient consultation:

- Information and advice is required on:
  - (When and if the patient is ready) diagnosis and prognosis, including management of controllable risk factors, such as giving up smoking
  - Legal and financial matters: discussions on giving up driving, although essential, are not likely to be well received. The DVLA must be informed if someone has dementia or any organic brain syndrome. Lasting powers of attorney, and advance decisions (see Mental Capacity Act 2005), should be considered early on
  - Entitlement to State benefits such as attendance allowance, or assistance with residential or nursing home fees
  - The role of statutory and voluntary support services such as the community mental health team, social services, and patient support groups such as the Alzheimer's Society (support people with dementia of any cause, not just Alzheimer's) and local carers' groups
- Non-pharmacological management:
  - Needs assessment to include environment and safety issues, e.g vulnerability if living alone, risk of falls
  - Ensure timely referral to physio, OT and social services
  - Behavioural and psychiatric symptoms can often be reduced following detailed assessment and a person-centred approach to interventions,
  - Referral to other relevant healthcare professionals for specific advice may include an Admiral nurse and dementia nurse specialist where available, community psychiatric nurse, old age psychiatrist, neurologist, continence advisor

Further information for health professionals and the public

Alzheimer's Society http://www.alzheimers.org.uk
National Institute for Clinical Excellence (NICE) http://www.nice.org.uk

Dementia with Lewy bodies

Incidence	163,000 new cases throughout UK per year
Prevalence	70+ per 100,000 age 40–64 increasing to 10,000 per 100,000 age > 85 years
Aetiology	Unknown—likely to be multifactorial

Dementia with Lewy bodies (DLB) is a neurodegenerative (progressive) disease. Lewy bodies are protein deposits in nerve cells (also occurs in PD) that disrupt the neurotransmitters acetylcholine and dopamine. About a quarter of people with Parkinson's disease develop dementia within 10 years. DLB may coexist with depression. DLB lasts, on average, seven years from diagnosis to death.

Presentation

In addition to symptoms of both Alzheimer's disease (including memory loss) and of PD (including stiffness and tremor), dementia with Lewy bodies produces characteristic symptoms:
- Fluctuating cognition (day-to-day and even hour-to-hour)
- Extreme sensitivity to neuroleptics
- Visual hallucinations (generally very real, but non-threatening, people or animals)

Aims of care

Early, accurate diagnosis allows the person to access appropriate care and treatment, and plan for the future. Maintaining independence for as long as possible, and providing a stimulating environment, will help a person live well with DLB. Supporting family members in their caring role improves care for the person with dementia and reduces carer morbidity. Family carers of people with dementia save the UK over £6 billion a year.

Medical management
- Pharmacological management:
  - Treatment with cholinesterase inhibitors (donepezil, rivastigmine or galantamine) is not recommended by NICE for DLB, although there is some evidence it may help,
  - Anti-Parkinson's drugs may improve mobility but worsen confusion. It will be important to ascertain which symptoms are most troublesome to patient and carer.
  - Neuroleptics can be particularly dangerous for people with DLB, causing rigidity, serious difficulty with mobility and speech, and some research has linked use in DLB with sudden death. The Committee on Safety of Medicines state that risperidone and olanzapine should not be used for any form of dementia other than short term, under specialist supervision, for severe and distressing symptoms. Even more care must be taken if a person with DLB has to be prescribed a neuroleptic,
  - SSRIs may be useful in depression.

Nursing care

Given the devastating impact of DLB on the person and their family, information must be provided in a sensitive and timely manner, and not rushed in the ward or outpatient consultation:

- Information and advice is required on:
  - (When and if the patient is ready) diagnosis and prognosis
  - Symptom management. In particular, it is important that carers understand fluctuating cognition is part of the disease and not the person being intentionally difficult with some people
  - Legal and financial matters: The DVLA must be informed if someone has dementia or any organic brain syndrome, unless the person has voluntarily stopped driving. Lasting powers of attorney, and advance decisions (📖 see Mental Capacity Act 2005), should be considered in the early stages
  - Entitlement to State benefits such as attendance allowance, or assistance with residential or nursing home fees
  - The role of statutory and voluntary support services such as the Community Mental Health Team, Social Services, and patient support groups such as the Alzheimer's Society (support people with dementia of any cause, not just Alzheimer's) and local carers' groups
- Non-pharmacological management:
  - Needs assessment to include environment and safety issues, e.g. vulnerability if living alone, risk of falls (increased in people with DLB)
  - Ensure timely referral to OT, physio and social services
  - Provide pressure area care if mobility is compromised
  - Behavioural and psychiatric symptoms can often be reduced following detailed assessment and a person-centred approach to interventions. Distraction seems to work better than challenging hallucinations or misperceptions
  - Referral to other relevant healthcare professionals for specific advice may include an Admiral nurse and dementia nurse specialists where available, community psychiatric nurse, old age psychiatrist, neurologist, continence advisor

Further information for health professionals and the public

Alzheimer's Society http://www.alzheimers.org.uk

National Institute for Clinical Excellence (NICE) http://www.nice.org.uk

Woodward, S. (2005) The pathophysiology and treatment of dementia with Lewy bodies: an overview. *British Journal of Neuroscience Nursing*, 1(4): 164–9.

Creutzfeldt–Jakob disease

Incidence	1 per 1,000,000
Prevalence	Approx 10–20 per 100,000 among under 65s, increasing with age
Aetiology	Depends on the form: see below

Creutzfeldt–Jakob disease (CJD) is a rapidly progressive, neurodegenerative prion disease in which abnormally folded proteins cause spongiform encephalopathy.

Four main forms of CJD

- Sporadic—most common (85%), usually affects those aged over 50, life expectancy 4–6 months
- Familial—inherited, tends to affect younger people, life expectancy a few weeks to several years depending on the mutation
- Iatrogenic—caused by accidental transmission from infected person during medical or surgical procedure (e.g. corneal transplant, human growth hormone), life expectancy is 1–2 years
- Variant—from infected beef products, tends to affect younger people, life expectancy 14 months on average

Presentation

Depends on type. In general, however:
- Early signs are memory problems, mood and apathy
- Shortly after, clumsy, unsteady, speech affected
- Later, myoclonus, tremor, stiffness, incontinence, loss of speech.
- Behavioural and psychiatric disturbance may pre-date other symptoms

❶ The National CJD Surveillance Unit must be informed of all cases of suspected CJD via their national reporting system

Aims of care

Early, accurate diagnosis allows the person to access the appropriate care package. Care coordinators at the CJD Surveillance Unit will arrange for any shortfall in local authority care package to be made up. Supporting family members in their caring role improves care for the person with dementia and reduces carer morbidity. Family carers of people with dementia save the UK over £6 billion a year.

Medical management

- Pharmacological management:
  - Neuroleptics and benzodiazepines for behavioural and psychiatric symptoms may be used cautiously after consideration of non-pharmacological approaches.
  - Newer antipsychotics with lower side effect profile are preferable, and even then 'start low and go slow'.

- ⚠ The Committee on Safety of Medicines state that risperidone and olanzapine should not be used other than short term, under specialist supervision, for severe and distressing symptoms

Nursing care

Given the devastating impact of CJD on the person and their family, information must be provided in a sensitive and timely manner, and not rushed in the ward or outpatient consultation:

- Information and advice is required on:
  - (When and if the patient is ready) diagnosis and prognosis
  - Symptom management
  - Legal and financial matters: The DVLA must be informed if someone has dementia or any organic brain syndrome, unless the person has voluntarily stopped driving. It may be possible to discuss lasting powers of attorney, and advance decisions (📖 see Mental Capacity Act 2005), although the rapid progression of CJD may make this impossible
  - Entitlement to State benefits such as Attendance Allowance, or assistance with residential or nursing home fees
  - The role of statutory and voluntary support services such as the community mental health team, social services, and patient support groups such as the Alzheimer's Society (support people with dementia of any cause), the CJD Support Network, and local carers' groups
- Non-pharmacological management:
  - Needs assessment to include environment and safety issues
  - Behavioural and psychiatric symptoms can often be reduced following detailed assessment and a person-centred approach to interventions, involvement of the psychiatric team is likely to be needed early on in variant CJD
  - Referral to relevant healthcare professionals for specific advice may include an Admiral nurse and dementia nurse specialist where available, community mental health team, psychiatrist, neurologist, social worker, continence advisor

Further information for health professionals and the public

Alzheimer's Society http://www.alzheimers/.org.uk
National CJD Support Network http://www.cjdsupport.net
National CJD Surveillance Unit http://www.cjd.ed.ac.uk
Alzheimer's Societyhttp://www.alzheimers.org.uk
National Institute for Clinical Excellence (NICE) http://www.nice.org.uk

Other dementias

There are over 200 causes of dementia, although more than half of the dementias in older people are caused by Alzheimer's disease. Cognitive impairment is associated with other disorders such as HIV, paraneoplastic syndromes, leukodystrophies, Wilson's disease, motor neuron disease, multiple sclerosis, Parkinson's disease, prolonged alcohol abuse, Down's syndrome.

The prevalence of all cases of dementia is 1:1400 age 40–64 years, rising to 1:6 at 80 years. 700,000 people are living with dementia in the UK, including 15,000 affected below the age of 65.

Mild cognitive impairment

Mild cognitive impairment (MCI) is a form of memory loss which can be demonstrated on neuropsychological testing, but does not cause significant difficulties in planning, attention or everyday living.

MCI is not dementia and poor neuropsychological test results could be explained by stress, anxiety, depression or physical illness. However, people with MCI seem to be at greater risk of developing Alzheimer's disease, or other dementia.

Frontotemporal degeneration

Frontotemporal degeneration (FTD) accounts for 5% of all cases of dementia in older people. Variants of FTD include Pick's disease, primary progressive aphasia and primary non-fluent aphasia.

Unusual presentations of Alzheimer's disease

Include posterior cortical atrophy and biparietal Alzheimer's disease.

Genetic

There are familial forms of Alzheimer's disease (less than 1% of all Alzheimer's is inherited), vascular dementia (known as CADASIL) and Huntington's disease.

Nursing Care

Nursing care would be similar to that for other dementias
  📖 See also Assessment of cognition, p 78, and Caring for a confused patient, p 157.

Further information for health professionals and the public

Alzheimer's Society http://www.alzheimers.org.uk
Genetic Interest Group http://www.gig.org.uk
Pick's disease support group http://www.pdsg.org.uk
Woodward, S. and Mestecky, A.-M. (2009) *Evidence-based neuroscience nursing.* Oxford: Wiley-Blackwell.

Stroke

Incidence	150,000 people per annum in the UK
Prevalence	250,000 people live with disability following stroke in the UK
Aetiology	Ischaemia: thrombus or embolus Haemorrhage

Stroke is sometimes referred to as a brain attack. It occurs as a result of the loss of blood supply to a part of the brain (ischaemia), resulting in neuronal cell damage and death.

Stroke is the commonest cause of long-term disability in the UK, occurring once approximately every 5 minutes, and considerable government attention is now being paid to effective stroke care as it costs the NHS budget around £2.8 billion every year.

The new National Stroke Strategy was published by the DH in December 2007 and aims to modernize stroke service provision. The DH have previously set a target to reduce the death rate from stroke in people under 75 by 40% by 2010 (DH, 2004) and this remains a high priority for healthcare. The strategy focuses on the need to educate the public to recognize a stroke and to act quickly as 'time is brain'.

Service provision has changed and stroke is now treated as a medical emergency, with an emphasis on early recognition, 24-hour access to hyperacute care, thrombolysis and care within a stroke unit, as evidence that patients have higher morbidity and mortality if they are not cared for in a stroke unit has emerged.

The following topics reflect the emphasis in the National Stroke Strategy on:
- Early recognition of stroke
- Emergency management of transient ischaemic attack (TIA) and secondary prevention
- Hyperacute care and thrombolysis
- Quality rehabilitation

Further information for health professionals and the public

DH (2004) *National standards, local action: health and social care standards and planning framework 2005/06–2007/08*. London: Department of Health.

DH (2007) *National stroke strategy*. London: Department of Health.

The Stroke Association: http://www.stroke.org.uk

Stroke: FAST and stroke recognition

The FAST tool—face, arm, speech time—was developed to aid early recognition of the signs and symptoms of stroke and has a high sensitivity and specificity in the pre-hospital setting (up to 93%). It was designed to be quick and easy to use for pre-hospital care including by members of the public. The FAST test is promoted by The Stroke Association and further information is available via their website. The Joint Royal Colleges' Ambulance Liaison Committee (JRCALC) clinical practice guidelines recommend the use of FAST and this is monitored by the Healthcare Commission.

Is there sudden onset of:
- **Facial weakness**—can the person smile? Has their mouth or eye drooped?
- **Arm weakness**—can the person raise both arms?
- **Speech problems**—can the person speak clearly and understand what you say?
- **Time to call 999**—stroke is a medical emergency.
- By calling 999 early treatment can be given which can prevent further brain damage.
- A FAST test will assess three different functions, but any one of these symptoms can be a sign of a stroke.

Actions on suspecting a stroke

▶▶If a stroke is suspected on a FAST test, a 999 call should be made. Many ambulance services now respond to stroke as a medical emergency and have pre-hospital guidelines on managing stroke patients.

Assessment in A&E

On arrival at hospital a more detailed assessment of stroke signs and symptoms needs to be undertaken. The ROSIER (recognition of stroke in the Emergency Room) tool (Nor et al, 2005) can be used as a part of this. The tool provides points for signs and symptoms to identify the likelihood of stroke as a diagnosis.

Usual emergency assessment of airway, breathing, circulation and observations should also be undertaken.

Stroke mimics

There can be a number of conditions which present with a similar onset to stroke, called stroke mimics, but in general stroke:
- is sudden in onset (not progressive)
- is not spreading e.g. from one limb to another
- is presents with 'negative' symptoms e.g. loss of function, loss of speech

Some stroke mimics
- Seizure—can be partial complex or tonic clonic producing limb weakness and reduced conscious level
- Migraine—e.g. causing spreading sensory disturbance of the face and arm
- Space-occupying lesions—producing focal neurological deficits

- Hypoglycaemia—producing focal neurology and reduced conscious level
- Peripheral nerve lesions—peripheral nerve distribution of deficits, e.g. Bell's palsy

Further information for health professionals and the public

The Stroke Association: http://www.stroke.org.uk

Nor, A.M. *et al.* (2005) The Recognition of Stroke in the Emergency Room (ROSIER) scale: development and validation of a stroke recognition instrument. *Lancet Neurology*, 4(1): 727–34.

Management of TIA and secondary prevention of stroke

Some patients with an initially positive FAST test may have resolved or be rapidly resolving at assessment in A&E—these are likely to be TIA. There is a high risk of stroke within the first month after a TIA and around 1 in 4 patients will have a completed stroke by one month, many in the first week.

Focal neurology which lasts longer than around 40 minutes to 1 hour is likely to cause cerebral ischaemia which would be visible on MRI scan.

Assessment

Risk of a stroke event, e.g. using ABCD2 tool and rapid access to imaging, echocardiogram carotid dopplers and urgent carotid endarterectomy if indicated

Management

Carotid endarterectomy if needed, secondary prevention including lifestyle advice/support and medication management

Secondary prevention of stroke

Secondary prevention should be focused on the likely cause of the stroke. This will incorporate aspects of lifestyle and medication management. Secondary prevention is often a nurse-led area of care and nurses should support patients with:

Lifestyle management
• Smoking cessation
• Dietary changes including increased fibre, reduced fat and salt intake
• Increased physical activity and weight loss
• Alcohol reduction to within recommended limits

Medication management
• Anti-platelets—usually aspirin with dipyridamole or clopidogrel where indicated
• Anti-coagulation—for atrial fibrillation or other indication
• Anti-hypertensive agents—to maintain BP within recommended limits
• Cholesterol-reducing agents—often statins
• Maintain good diabetic control

Further information for health professionals and the public

National Collaborating Centre for Chronic Conditions (2008) *Stroke: National clinical guideline for diagnosis and initial management of acute stroke and transient ischaemic attack (TIA)*. London: Royal College of Physicians.

Stroke: hyperacute care and thrombolysis

There is now clear evidence that providing thrombolysis with alteplase for acute ischaemic stroke is beneficial for selected patients (Cochrane Collaboration 2007).

Alteplase is a fibrinolytic agent which, whilst relatively inactive systemically, acts upon any thrombus causing local breakdown of the fibrin holding the thrombus together. It has a fairly short half life of around 5 minutes.

Criteria for use

- Treatment should commence within 3 hours of the start of stroke symptoms and should not be given to those following recent surgery or GI bleed.
- The patient must have a CT brain scan and a full neurological examination prior to treatment to exclude intracerebral haemorrhage.

Administration

- Give 10% of the total dose by bolus over 1–2mins then the remaining 90% of the dose administered via infusion pump over 1 hour.
- It is important to flush the infusion tubing at the end of the infusion to avoid discarding some of the active drug.

Complications

Complications include: anaphylactoid reactions, intra- and extracranial haemorrhages

⚠ The signs and symptoms to observe for include:

- Oropharyngeal oedema, hypotension, facial oedema, respiratory wheeze, agitation, restlessness
- Gradual or sudden drop in GCS or limb function
- Increasing difficulty obtaining same GCS
- New incontinence
- Headache , nausea and vomiting
- Abdominal pain, haematemesis or malaena

Post-thrombolysis nursing care

Patients must be cared for in a high-dependency area where appropriate neurological and cardiovascular monitoring can be undertaken ideally on an acute stroke unit.

- Carry out neurological observations every 15 minutes for the first 2 hours, ½ hourly for a further 6 hours then hourly until 24 hours post-thrombolysis
- Ensure active management of hypertension post-thrombolysis (180/110mmHg) e.g. using labetalol
- Avoid invasive procedures such as suction or catheterization
- ⚠ Caution with mobilization due to risk of falls and potential damaging effects post-thrombolysis

- Observe for and manage any post-thrombolysis complications including immediate access to repeat CT if intracranial haemorrhage is suspected

The patient should have a repeat CT or MRI at around 24 hours post-thrombolysis to identify any local or remote haemorrhage.

Nursing care in the hyperacute/acute stage of stroke

Maintenance of normal physiological parameters

Protocol based care including:

- Blood pressure management—avoid actively lowering BP in the acute ischaemic stroke, avoid and treat hypotension and consider active lowering of BP in intracerebral haemorrhage using labetalol or glyceryl trinitrate (GTN)
- Respiratory management—maintain O_2 sats above 95%, maintain upper airway and observe the rate, depth and pattern of respiration
- Neurological monitoring—frequent observations to identify any deterioration in GCS or functional deficits
- Cardiovascular monitoring—continuous cardiac monitoring, observation for atrial fibrillation (AF) or other dysrhthymias
- Temperature management—active pyrexia management including anti-pyretics and septic screen. Haemorrhage can also cause pyrexia.
- Blood sugar management—maintain safe level using sliding scale if needed—ideally 7–10mmol/L.

Prevention, detection and management of complications

- Assess swallowing using a validated tool and keep the patient NBM if swallowing is unsafe (☐ see Swallowing assessment, p 72). If there are signs of aspiration from admission consider antibiotic treatment, supplementary oxygen, positional changes and indications of retained secretions and the need for suctioning and/or chest physio (☐ see Swallowing problems (dysphagia), p 164).
- Deep vein thrombosis (DVT)—generally avoid prophylactic heparin due to the potential risk of haemorrhagic changes in the acute stroke phase. The use of anti-embolic stockings in stroke patients may offer some prophylaxis. Observe for signs of DVT.
- Monitor fluid intake and hydration. Provide additional fluids where necessary either by encouraging oral intake or using intravenous fluids.
- Urinary tract infections—avoid catheterization unless confirmed retention or need for critical fluid monitoring. If inserted remove as soon as no longer required.
- Pressure area management including risk assessment and use of equipment and position changes.
- Positioning including those positions which prevent spasticity.
- Maintenance of appropriate nutritional intake either by oral route or using nasogastric feeding where needed to prevent malnutrition.
- Assess mobility and ensure early mobilization.
- Ensure early referral to appropriate therapy staff.

Further information for health professionals and the public

NICE (2007) *Alteplase for the treatment of acute ischaemic stroke.* London: National Institute for Health and Clinical Excellence.

Quality stroke rehabilitation

Following a period on the stroke unit, many patients will continue to require ongoing management either for rehabilitation, adapting to disability, or secondary prevention.

Rehabilitation

This may happen at home, in an outpatient setting or as an inpatient in a specialist neuro-rehabilitation facility. Rehabilitation after stroke unit care can include:

- Adapting to disability in the home environment
- Accessing social, transport and leisure facilities
- Returning to work or household activities
- Adapting to cognitive or emotional effects of stroke

There may be some benefit for patients being able to re-access a further period of rehabilitation months or years after the stroke to improve their functional abilities.

Adapting to disability

Long-term effects of stroke can include spasticity, post-stroke pain and post-stroke epilepsy. Patients often require ongoing management to help them maintain function, prevent deterioration and aid their adjustment to their disability.

It is vital to involve patients and carers/family in planning for discharge home.

Headaches

Headaches are the commonest neurological condition. The only pain receptors inside the cranium exist within the meninges and cerebral arteries and pain is transmitted via the trigeminal nerves. The brain tissue itself does not feel pain.

Headaches from raised ICP

Patients often fear that they have serious neurological problems with repeated headaches (e.g. brain tumours), but this is rarely the case. Headaches associated with raised ICP are caused by tension on the meninges and cerebral blood vessels.

These serious headaches have the following characteristics:

- Generalized
- Worse when waking in the morning (due to collection of CSF in the cranium overnight while lying down)
- May improve on sitting/standing
- Exacerbated by bending or coughing (which increases ICP)
- Progressively worsen over time
- May be associated with projectile vomiting later

Classification of headaches

There are many types and causes of headaches, some occurring much more frequently than others.

The following topics outline the care and management of patients with specific headache types.

Classification and frequency of common headache types (not a complete classification)

Headache type	Frequency
Primary headaches	
• Tension-type headache	Most common—affects 69% of males and 88% of females and accounts for approx 90% of all headaches
• Migraine	Affects 16% of females and 5% of males
• Cluster headache and other primary trigeminal autonomic cephalalgias	Cluster headache affects 50–100 per 100,000. Male:female ratio 4:3
• Other primary headaches e.g. thunderclap headache	
Secondary headaches	
• Headaches attributable to cranial or cervical vascular disorder (e.g. giant cell arteritis)	

Further information for health professionals and the public

International Headache Society (2007) *The international classification of headache disorders*, 2nd edn. Available from http://ihs-classification.org/en/02_klassifikation/ accessed 27 July 2008.

Kernick, S. and Goadsby, D. (2008) *Headache: a practical manual*. Oxford: Oxford University Press.

Tension-type headaches

This is the most common type of headache. They are caused by prolonged muscular tension and contraction, e.g. frowning, clenching teeth. There are pain receptors within these muscles, which become stimulated and cause the pain.

Characteristics of tension-type headaches
- Dull aching
- Generalized
- May feel tight 'band' round scalp
- Worsened by touching scalp
- Exacerbated by noise
- Last hours to days
- Associated with stress and maybe depression

Medical treatment
- Psychological support
- Reduce analgesic overuse
- Antidepressants

Nursing care
- Assess pain (📖 see Pain assessment, p 74)
- Encourage the patient to keep a headache diary to aid diagnosis
- Reassure the patient about the nature of the headache
- Offer counselling and provide psychological support
- Suggest methods for relaxation and managing stress
- Administer simple analgesia as prescribed if required and monitor effectiveness
- Administer antidepressants as prescribed
- Encourage patient not to overuse analgesia and only take it when absolutely necessary

Migraine

Migraine is a common and debilitating type of headache. There is often a family history, suggesting a genetic susceptibility. It is thought to be due to vasoconstriction or vasodilation of the cerebral arteries. Lack of serotonin is also implicated in the onset of migraine due to cerebral vasodilation. The pain receptors within these vessels then become stimulated and the migraine is felt.

Characteristics of migraine

- May occur with or without aura (e.g. flashing lights)
- Usually unilateral
- Throbbing
- Worsened by light
- May induce nausea and vomiting (due to reduced stomach emptying and gut transit)
- Relieved by sleep
- Lasts between 2–48 hours
- Affects more women than men (2:1)
- May be associated with other symptoms depending on the vessel affected e.g visual field defects, vertigo, hemiparesis

Precipitating factors

- Diet (e.g. chocolate, cheese, alcohol)
- Hormonal influence (e.g. oestrogen fluctuation)
- Sleep deprivation
- Stress
- Fatigue

Medical treatment

- Simple analgesia
- Anti-emetics
- Serotonin agonists (e.g. sumatriptan) to reduce vasodilation
- Prophylaxis in severe cases

Nursing care

During an acute attack

- Assess pain (📖 see Pain assessment, p 74) and encourage the use of a headache diary
- Administer analgesia as prescribed if required
- Administer anti-emetics with analgesia (usually metoclopramide to increase gut motility and stomach emptying)
- Ensure oral analgesia is administered as soon as symptoms are perceived—due to reduced gut motility and stomach emptying drug absorption may be affected later. IM/IV administration may be required
- Provide a dark environment in which the patient can lie down and sleep

Patient education

- Assist the patient to identify and avoid possible triggers
- If patient experiences recurrent, debilitating attacks they may be prescribed migraine prophylaxis—ensure the patient is aware of the correct dosage and administration of medication, including possible side effects of treatment

- Encourage patient to achieve regular sleep pattern
- If stress is implicated suggest methods to reduce stress (e.g. relaxation therapies)
- Some patients find acupuncture helpful (may stimulate release of endorphins)
- Some patients are deficient in magnesium—advise regarding dietary intake of leafy greens, peas and beans, seafood, nuts and wholegrains

Further information for health professionals and the public

Lindsey, K.W. and Bone, I. (2004) *Neurology and neurosurgery illustrated*, 4th edn. Edinburgh: Churchill Livingstone.

The Migraine Trust http://www.migrainetrust.org

Migraine Action Association http://www.migraine.org.uk

Cluster headaches

Cluster headaches can be excruciating and patients will often describe wanting to bang their head against the wall. They are often experienced by allergy sufferers and are more common during summer months when the pollen count is high. Histamine levels rise during attacks and they are often therefore referred to as histamine cephalgia.

Characteristics
- Unilateral
- Often focused around the eye
- Watery eye
- Associated with rhinorrhoea (runny nose)
- Often wake the patient in the early hours
- Last 2–10 hours
- Occur in clusters
- May be precipitated by alcohol

Medical treatment
- Antihistamines are ineffective
- Ergotamine
- Prednisolone in acute attack for severe cases (30–40mg daily reducing over 2 weeks)

Nursing care
- Assess pain (📖 see Chapter 3) and encourage the use of a headache diary
- Administer analgesia as prescribed if required
- Ensure 100% oxygen is prescribed and administer this during an acute attack
- Stay with the patient if possible and reassure them during an acute episode
- Assess effectiveness of analgesia
- Encourage the patient to refrain from alcohol if this is a known precipitant.
- Administer steroids as prescribed and ensure the patient is aware of any potential side effects.

Further information for health professionals and the public

Lindsey, K.W. and Bone, I. (2004) *Neurology and neurosurgery illustrated*, 4th edn. Edinburgh: Churchill Livingstone.

Trigeminal neuralgia

Trigeminal neuralgia is a type of facial pain (also known as tic douloureux). It is usually caused by nerve root compression of the trigeminal nerve or possibly due to demyelination. Women over 50 are most commonly affected. The pain is severe, can be intractable and reduce patients to tears. Social withdrawal and depression may result.

Characteristics

- Severe stabbing pain
- Sharp and shooting
- Short duration
- Spasmodic attacks (may last for days–weeks)
- Affects distribution of one or more branches of trigeminal nerve (ophthalmic, maxillary or mandibular)
- Usually unilateral
- Triggered and exacerbated by chewing, washing face, brushing teeth, cold wind, speaking

Medical treatment

Drug treatment

- Anticonvulsants e.g. carbamazepine, phenytoin, lamotrigine, gabapentin
- Others, e.g. baclofen

Surgical and other invasive treatment

- Nerve blocks (with phenol or alcohol)
- Microvascular decompression (via posterior fossa craniectomy)—sponge inserted between artery and nerve to relieve compression
- Surgical division of the nerve root
- Radiofrequency thermocoagulation (under GA)—causes permanent lesion of nerve

Nursing care

- Assess pain (📖 see Chapter 3) and encourage the use of a pain diary
- Administer analgesia as prescribed if required
- Monitor effectiveness of analgesia and report to medical staff
- Assist patient to identify triggers
- Assist patient in identifying ways to avoid triggers that have been identified
- Ensure patient receives adequate nutrition (some patients will avoid eating for fear of triggering the pain)
- Provide emotional support

Specific post-operative nursing care

- Regular neurological assessment until stable
- Observe for facial asymmetry
- Provide eye care if facial weakness develops and protect the cornea
- Prevent the patient from rubbing their eye and observe for redness and inflammation of cornea (pain sensation from cornea may be lost)
- Administer artificial tears as prescribed if required
- Provide a soft diet and prevent chewing on the affected side

Giant cell (temporal) arteritis

This is an autoimmune disease that affects older people. The artery becomes infiltrated with 'giant cells' and may become occluded.

Characteristics
- Unilateral
- Throbbing over temporal artery on affected side
- Artery becomes thickened and tender to touch
- May be associated with stroke
- Pain when chewing (due to ischaemia of muscles of mastication)
- Causes temporary blindness (may become permanent if not treated early—due to occlusion of ophthalmic artery)
- Double vision (diplopia)
- Headache is continuous and intractable until treated

Medical treatment
- Confirm diagnosis—temporal artery biopsy is often performed
- Steroids—prednisolone 60mg daily or high dose IV—reducing over several weeks
- 25% of patients require long-term steroids

Nursing care
- Assess pain (📖 see Pain assessment, p 74)
- Prepare and care for patient undergoing temporal artery biopsy (usually performed under local anaesthetic):
  - Check consent has been obtained
  - Document allergies
  - Assist patient to wash and dress in a gown ready for theatre
  - Explain procedure to patient
  - Post-op observe wound for bleeding and ensure dressing remains intact
  - Record vital signs
- Administer steroids as prescribed and ensure the patient is aware of any potential side-effects, especially if long-term use is prescribed.

Further information for health professionals and the public

Lindsey, K.W. and Bone, I. (2004) *Neurology and neurosurgery illustrated,* 4th edn. Edinburgh: Churchill Livingstone.

Antiphospholipid syndrome

Antiphospholipid (Hughes) syndrome (APS) was identified in 1983. APS patients may have been misdiagnosed with MS. It is an autoimmune disorder in which the patient produces antibodies to their own body proteins and phospholipids. The antibodies cause platelet activation and aggregation, leading to clot formation. They may also cause neurological damage directly as well as the cerebrovascular effects.

Clinical history

- Recurrent venous and/or arterial thrombosis (e.g. DVT—implicated in approx 1 in 5)
- Recurrent miscarriages
- Neurological diagnosis (e.g. stroke—may account for 1 in 5 under age of 45)
- Presence of AP antibodies in blood
- Skin abnormalities
- Renal problems
- Thrombocytopaenia

Epidemiology

- Predominantly females
- Approx 1 in 500 affected
- Family history has been suggested—many patients have a family history of migraine

Common neurological consequences

- Intractable migraine
- Cognitive impairment (e.g. memory impairment)
- TIA and stroke
- Seizures
- MS-like symptoms

Medical treatment

- Screening for APS in young stroke patients
- Differential diagnosis from MS
- Anticoagulation with either aspirin or warfarin

Nursing care

Prepare patient for investigations while the diagnosis is being investigated, e.g:

- MRI scan
- Blood tests

Ensure anticoagulation medication is administered as prescribed.

Ensure that the patient is aware of side effects of medication and the actions to take in the event of bleeding. If patient is taking warfarin ensure they have a follow-up appointment in the anticoagulation clinic.

Reassure the patient that memory and cognitive problems may improve once anticoagulation is commenced.

Assist the patient to recover from migraine by:
- Administering analgesia as prescribed
- Allowing them to lie quietly in a dark environment

Further information for health professionals and the public

Woodward, S. (2007) Antiphospholipid (Hughes) syndrome. *BJNN*, 3(1): 16–18.

Spinal infarcts

The main blood supply to the spinal cord is from the anterior and posterior spinal arteries or branches from these vessels. The posterior spinal artery supplies the posterior $^1/_3$ of the cord and the anterior artery supplies the anterior $^2/_3$.

The areas of the cord supplied by the anterior spinal artery receive less collateral supply from other vessels, so these are the areas that are usually damaged by vascular conditions.

In effect the same pathological processes that cause stroke (e.g. arteriosclerosis leading to thrombosis or embolus) can affect the spinal arteries and result in an infarct of the spinal cord. The signs and symptoms depend on the level affected.

Signs and symptoms of anterior spinal artery infarct
- Radicular pain at time of infarct (pain radiating along the dermatome supplied by the affected nerve root)
- Sudden paralysis below level of lesion
- Initially muscle flaccidity progressing to spasticity over a period of a few days in affected limbs
- Loss of sensation to pain and temperature below level of lesion (proprioception and vibration sensation are intact as these tracts are supplied by the posterior artery)
- Urinary retention (initially due to an areflexic bladder, but then detrusor–sphincter dyssynergia may occur)
- Constipation/faecal incontinence

Medical management
- Investigate to exclude other causes of paralysis (MRI)
- Identify cause of ischaemia and infarct
- Symptomatic treatment

Nursing care
- Essentially the care is similar to that for patients who have suffered a spinal cord injury (🔲 see p 332) although there is not the same need to prevent further trauma due to movement—the damage has already been done!
- Reassure patient and provide emotional support—they have experienced a sudden and catastrophic paralysis and are likely to be extremely distressed and anxious
- Assess pain (🔲 see Pain assessment, p 74)
- Administer analgesia as prescribed if required and assess effectiveness
- Catheterize to drain retained urine—may use an indwelling uretheral catheter initially, but clean intermittent self-catheterization is preferable asap if the patient is able
- Conduct moving and handling assessment and assist patient to position themselves in a comfortable position
- Pay attention to pressure area care—turn at least 2 hourly and observe pressure areas regularly

- Apply TED stockings especially during flaccidity (patients are at risk of developing DVT)
- Assess bowels and develop an individual bowel management programme (remember that manual removal of faeces may be necessary)
- Assist with personal hygiene
- Ensure patient receives adequate oral intake of diet and fluids
- Refer to OT and physio and liaise re treatment—continue to support therapy interventions while the patient is on the ward, e.g. moving and handling techniques/patient positioning
- May need to refer to social services for financial and other advice, e.g. funding for care packages long-term, grant applications for home adaptations

Motor neurone disease

Incidence	1–2 per 100,000
Prevalence	4–6 per 100,000
Aetiology	Unknown

Motor neurone disease (MND) is a progressive neurodegenerative disease affecting up to 5000 adults in the UK and favours males slightly more than females: 1.7:1. Age at onset is usually 55–70 but can occur in any adult. 95% of cases are sporadic, 5–10% are familial with an autosomal dominant inheritance.

There are four main phenotypes of MND:
- Amyotrophic lateral sclerosis (ALS)—most common (75%)
- Progressive bulbar palsy (PBP)
- Progressive muscular atrophy (PMA)
- Primary lateral sclerosis (PLS)—least common (<5%)

Life expectancy is generally 2–5 years from onset of symptoms but can vary, PLS has a much longer prognosis of >10 years.

Presentation

Symptoms vary according to phenotype but include:
- Muscle weakness, wasting and fasiculations
- Increased muscle tone, brisk reflexes, cramps
- Emotional lability
- Dysarthria and/or dysphagia
- Weight loss
- Cognitive changes, mild to moderate in up to 50% of people (usually executive dysfunction and memory problems)
- Dementia—rare, occurs in less than 5% of all cases

The disease affects limb, bulbar and respiratory muscles and is progressive in nature. Heart muscle, eyesight, hearing, bowels, bladder, sexual function and senses remain intact.

Medical treatment

Only disease-modifying therapy currently is riluzole 50mg b.d. which has a moderate effect of prolonging survival or time to ventilation by a matter of months.

Aims of care

A coordinated multidisciplinary approach is required to meet the rapidly changing physical and psychosocial needs of both the patient and carer, optimal symptom management may even extend survival time. Early referral to a specialist centre or MDT is essential. Quality of life and patient autonomy should be central to decisions regarding interventions and future plans.

Nursing management

Dysphagia

- Assess swallowing (📖 see Chapter 3)
- Early referral to SLT/dietitian for assessment of swallowing and dietary needs
- Start discussions early about possibility of gastrostomy, use radiologically sited gastrostomy in people who may not tolerate lying flat for the procedure

Dysarthria

- Ensure referral to SLT
- Consider use of communication tools early so the patient is familiar with their use

Sialorrhoea

Excessive drooling is a very socially isolating and distressing symptom, but does respond to anticholinergic drugs such as hyoscine (sublingual or transdermal) atropine or tricylcic antidepressants (amitriptyline) and beta-blockers. Another alternative is glycopyrronium bromide which has slightly less side effects and can be administered via a gastrostomy tube.

Pain

Pain is often related to immobility and spasms.
- Ensure accurate pain assessment (📖 see Chapter 3)
- Use baclofen/tizanidine for spasms, quinine for cramp
- Early referral to physiotherapist for passive exercises, walking aids provision and assessment for collars
- Fasiculations can be distressing and respond to small dose clonazepam

Dyspnoea

- Position upright to assist weak diaphragm
- Early morning headaches are indicative of nocturnal hypoventilation. If FVC < 50% consider non-invasive ventilation, which can aid symptom management and should be discussed early on
- Refer to palliative care services if not already known at onset of respiratory difficulties
- Access to medication to relieve anxiety such as The Breathing Space kit may be necessary at home. Be aware carer burden increases with provision of specialist equipment. Consider referral to social services for carer support.

Emotional lability

Related to upper motor neurone damage. Exhibited in excessive inappropriate crying or laughing, responds well to SSRI group of antidepressants.

Psychological distress

Grief-like reaction to diagnosis is a normal psychological process and supportive counselling may be helpful. Maintaining hope and living with changing expectations puts huge demands on both patients and carers. Access to specialist palliative care services to help with psychological distress is recommended.

Equipment
- Ensure early referral to OT for home assessment
- Provide pressure relieving cushions, riser/recliner chairs, hoists, splints and small aids
- Ensure prompt referral to wheelchair service as appropriate

Advance care planning

Referral to palliative care is encouraged early on to discuss
- End of life discussions/advance care planning/preferred place of care
- Patient's wishes concerning life-prolonging treatments/interventions
- Respite care/continuing care funding application

Social issues

- Ensure referral to social services for provision of benefits/access to community transport/re-housing/domiciliary alarm systems and carers assessment and provision of carers
- MND Association can help with provision of some equipment and small financial grants
- Good communication remains central to facilitating coordinated care in the community.

Further information for health professionals and the public

MND Associaiton http://www.mndassociation.org

Genetic and inherited neurological conditions

With recent advances in our understanding of human genetics, knowledge of neurological inherited disorders is growing and many disorders are being identified as having a genetic aetiology.

The following section presents the care of patients with several of the more common neurological disorders that may be seen in practice. This is far from a comprehensive list and where relevant the genetic predisposition to develop a particular condition is identified within the relevant topic elsewhere in the book.

Huntington's disease

Incidence	< 0.1 per 100,000
Prevalence	0.1 per 100,000
Aetiology	Genetic mutation: autosomal dominant inherited condition

Huntington's disease (HD) is an inherited, incurable neurodegenerative disorder. Age of onset is usually during the fourth or fifth decade of life but first symptoms can more rarely be seen in children and the elderly. Being autosomal dominant, it affects both male and female alike with each child of an affected parent having a 1:2 risk of inheriting HD.

There is a genetic test which can accurately determine whether a person carries the gene. However, it can't predict the age of onset and in the absence of a cure; many at risk choose not to take this test. Everyone who carries the gene will develop HD.

It is caused by a change in the gene that produces the huntingtin protein. Certain brain cells are vulnerable to this change, leading to severe movement disorder, psychiatric symptoms, and cognitive impairment.

Life expectancy: 15–20+ yrs from onset of symptoms. Children who develop the juvenile form rarely live to adulthood. Complications such as infection or choking are frequently the cause of death.

Presentation
Symptoms usually progress slowly and are often described as a triad of motor, cognitive and psychiatric. They can vary between individuals—some of the most common are as follows:

Motor
- Involuntary movements (e.g. chorea, dystonia, tics)
- Impairment of voluntary movement: walking, speech, swallowing
- Poor coordination and balance

Cognitive
- Slowing of thought processes
- Diminished ability to plan activities and decreased concentration
- Perseveration (being fixed on one thought or action)
- Impulsiveness (unable to wait) and lack of insight
- Impairment of short-term memory

Psychiatric or behavioural
- Depression
- Bipolar disorder
- Obsessive compulsive disorders
- Schizophrenia-like disorders
- Anxiety, apathy and irritability

Nursing care

- Administer medication to assist with severe involuntary movements. This needs to be monitored carefully as side effects are common.
- Assess risk of and prevent falls.
  - ⚠ Take care not to interrupt the person with HD whilst they are focusing on walking. A safe environment and introduction of aids/specialist equipment can help.
- Speech generally deteriorates—ensure referral to SLT for measures to allow the individual to maintain control are vital.
- Assess swallow and nutritional status: choking is a real risk so an experienced caregiver is essential when an affected person is to be fed. Insertion of a feeding tube may be considered.
- Refer to physio. Physiotherapy can help with coordination and balance.
- Cognitive changes often present the most difficulties for the caregiver to consider. Understanding the changes in the brain and the subsequent possible changes in behaviour helps.
- Allow the affected individual more time to respond to instruction or complete actions.
- Routine, schedules, and consistency may reduce confusion and increase independence.
- Creativity and individual problem solving is often required.
- Depression in HD can frequently be treated and the role of the caregiver is to help in its detection.
- Changes in mood can be common, including aggressive outbursts. Low arousal techniques can be successful as attempts to reason, intervene or persuade can make matters worse.
- Key issues to consider:
  - Genetic and ongoing counselling, advocacy and support for individuals and families.
  - Employment, implications for finances including insurance.
  - Future wishes, advance directives and potential loss of capacity.
  - Discussion about maintaining independence, personal care, respite care and long-term care needs.
  - Training and education for professional staff as level of knowledge and experience with client group may be low.

MDT should have ensured

- Specialist nurse input for full assessment
- Neuropsychological and psychiatric input
- OT assessment for adaptations/mobility aids and housing
- Physiotherapy, exercise and fitness
- Speech/language therapy and dietitian input
- Awareness of State benefits for disability and attendance
- Carers assessment and support needs addressed
- Often safety issues with driving and smoking

Further information for health professionals and the public

Huntington's Disease Association http://www.hda.org.uk
Scottish Huntington's Association http://www.hdscotland.org

Freidreich's ataxia

Freidreich's ataxia is the commonest inherited neurological ataxic condition. It affects approximately 1 in 50,000 people although 1 in 20 could be carriers of the affected gene. The genetic mutation causing this condition is autosomal recessive.

The mutation results in a spinal cord that has a shrunken appearance, with degeneration and demyelination of some tracts (e.g. corticospinal and spinocerebellar tracts). Changes are also seen in the peripheral nerves and cerebellum.

Signs and symptoms

- Balance disturbance
- Musculoskeletal problems and scoliosis/kyphosis
- Progressively ataxic/spastic gait
- Lack of coordination in the limbs
- Limb weakness
- Cardiomyopathy—leading to dysrhythmias and heart failure
- Visual problems and deafness
- Diabetes is common
- Onset before age 25 (usually at puberty)

Medical management

Management is symptomatic and should be multidisciplinary.

Nursing care

Nursing care will vary depending on the stage of progression of the ataxia and the dependency of the patient

- Urinalysis and blood sugar monitoring may be required if diabetes is suspected or present
- Administer cardiac drugs and insulin as prescribed if required
- Observe patient if they are walking—falls are a risk—ensure a safe environment and remove any obstacles
- Ensure the patient has access to their mobility aids
- Refer to OT and physio for provision of wheelchair and seating assessment
- Liaise with OT and physio re patient positioning, moving and handling, application of splints etc.
- Observe for pain and assess if it occurs (📖 see Pain assessment, p 74)
- Pressure area care and observation is important, especially of spine where scoliosis may cause pressure points
- Provide emotional and psychological support for patient and their family
- Genetic counseling may be required—refer if necessary

Fabry disease

This is an inherited lifelong metabolic disease, which can lead to serious organ problems and ultimately death. This is one of a group of lysosomal storage disorders in which enzymes that are normally present within lysosomes are lacking. This leads to increasing levels of the lipids normally broken down by the enzymes accumulating in the body and becoming toxic to the eyes, kidneys, autonomic nervous system and heart.

The gene is X-linked.

Incidence in the general population is 1 in 117,000 and 1 in 40,000 males.

Signs and symptoms

Early (childhood)
- Pain in extremities, e.g. burning sensation in the hands
- Reduced sweating
- Gastrointestinal hyperactivity (causing stomach pain, nausea and diarrhoea), especially after eating
- Skin rashes

Later
- Kidney failure
- Heart failure and myocardial infarction
- Stroke

Medical management

- Mainstay of treatment is enzyme replacement therapy. This is given as an intravenous infusion every 1–2 weeks for life
- Anticonvulsants (e.g. carbamazepine) are administered for the neuropathic pain in hands and feet
- Dialysis and renal transplantation may be required
- Metoclopramide may help gastrointestinal dysfunction
- Skin rashes may be treated with laser surgery to remove them

Nursing care

- Administer anticonvulsants as prescribed.
- Administer analgesia as prescribed for pain, following detailed pain assessment (see Chapter 3).
- Some patients find a low-fat diet helps gastrointestinal symptoms.
- Some patients experience fatigue—advise on energy conservation and balance of activity and rest throughout the day.
- Peripherally inserted central catheter (PICC) line may be inserted for long-term administration of IV infusions
- Patients should be monitored for infusion reactions during infusions administered in a hospital setting.
- If the patient is stable on the infusions and concordant with therapy home infusion should be considered, but only after a number of infusions have been administered within the hospital setting.
- The catheter insertion site should be monitored for signs of inflammation and infection.

- Monitor for pyrexia, which could be indicative of a line infection—check blood cultures and seek advice about whether the line should be removed or not, before removing it if necessary.
- If a line is removed—send the tip to the laboratory for microscopy, culture and sensitivities (MCS).

Further information for health professionals and the public

Cousins, A., Lee, P., Rorman, D. *et al.* (2008) Home-based infusion therapy for patients with Fabry disease. *BJN*, 17(10): 653–7.

Neurofibromatosis

Neurofibromatosis is an autosomal dominant inherited disorder of multiple organs, but significantly produces tumours. There are two main types: type 1 and 2, but other rare variants exist. Family history of the disease is common, but it may also occur due to a new mutation.

Type 1 (NF1)

- Incidence 1:2500
- Characterized by *café au lait* spots and neurofibromata, commonly seen as pea-sized skin lesions lying along the distribution of peripheral nerves
- The lesions are caused by overgrowth of embryological tissue and produce non-cancerous tumours of meninges, vascular system, skin, viscera, PNS and CNS
- Occasionally plexiform neurofibromas may become malignant
- Rarely astrocytomas may develop
- Scoliosis (spinal curvature) and other orthopaedic problems may occur
- May cause hypertension
- Stroke may occur

Type 2 (NF2)

- Incidence 1:50,000
- Characterized by bilateral acoustic neuromas (schwannomas)
- Other intracranial tumours may occur

Medical management

- Superficial skin lesions may be removed for cosmetic reasons—usually by specialist plastic surgeons and scarring and regrowth may occur
- Acoustic neuroma and other intracranial lesions are surgically removed/treated as they occur (see Chapter 9)
- Optic gliomas may cause visual problems and are monitored by an ophthalmologist

Nursing care

- Embarrassment due to altered body image is a particular problem and most people will continue to develop new lesions as they age. Psychological support is required to help the patient come to terms with the disfigurement.
- Patients may require referral to a service that teaches them how to apply camouflage make-up if the skin lesions are obvious and cannot be removed
- Advise patients to use high-factor sun-block to prevent exacerbation of the lesions with age and sun exposure.
- Advise the patient to monitor the growth of lesions obvious under the skin (plexiform neurofibroma) which may rarely become malignant. Watch for rapid growth, where this has previously been slow, development of pain which cannot be explained or change in texture.
- Advise patient to have their blood pressure monitored annually for hypertension.

- Pain and headaches may occur—administer analgesia as prescribed and refer to specialist pain services for assessment and management of chronic pain.
- Female patients who are considering pregnancy may require referral to genetic counselling services for advice

Further information for health professionals and the public

The Neurofibromatosis Association http://www.nfauk.org/

Meningitis

Meningitis is an inflammation of the meninges (dura, arachnoid, and pia mater) that cover the brain and spinal cord. This inflammation may be due to:
- Bacteria
- Chemical toxins
- Viruses
- Fungi
- Other infective organisms e.g. tubercle bacillus (TB)
- Carcinoma

Chemical or viral meningitis is often also referred to as aseptic meningitis as no causative organism is identified.

Bacterial meningitis

Bacteria may enter the cranium from the nasopharynx (following an upper respiratory tract infection), from bacterial infection elsewhere that causes bacteraemia, via sinuses or open skull fractures.

Once beyond the blood–brain barrier the body's natural defences are unable to mount sufficient defence and the organisms multiply. Purulent exudate is produced and cerebral oedema with raised intracranial pressure can develop.

Signs and symptoms
- Headache
- Fever
- Neck stiffness
- Photophobia
- Characteristic rash with meningococcal infection that does not disappear under pressure from a glass
- Impaired level of consciousness
- Seizures may occur

If the onset of meningococcal meningitis is sudden and causes septicaemia, there is a 10% risk of mortality.

Diagnosis
- CT scan to exclude mass lesion
- LP—CSF examination to identify causative organism
- Chest and skull X-rays to identify origin of infection may be performed

Medical management
- Treatment begins immediately, without waiting for culture and sensitivities, with either penicillin G or a cephalosporin antibiotic.
- Four days of dexamethasone 10mg every 6 hours will be prescribed.
- Once the causative organism and sensitivities are known the antibiotic prescription may be revised.
- CT scanning/MRI may be required if the patient deteriorates to detect mass effects and hydrocephalus.
- Close contacts of patients with meningococcal meningitis will need to be traced and offered prophylactic antibiotics.
- Other symptomatic management may be required.

Nursing care
Patients with bacterial meningitis are often acutely unwell and are treated as a medical emergency.
- Nurse in a single room for the first 24 hours of antibiotic therapy to minimize the risk of cross-infection, but do not compromise patient safety—they may require 1-to-1 supervision if very unwell in a high-dependency setting.
- Ensure antibiotics are administered as prescribed and on time—these will usually need to be given IV.
- Carry out frequent, serial neurological and systemic observations—at least half hourly for first 24 hours of antibiotic therapy, then reduce as

the patient's condition allows. Monitor for signs of raised intracranial pressure (📖 see Rising intracranial pressure and coning, p 132).
- Report any deterioration to medical staff immediately.
- Ensure an accurate fluid balance is maintained and encourage fluid intake, particularly if the patient is febrile.
- Patients will often be prescribed intravenous fluids if they are unable to maintain sufficient oral intake.
- Administer anti-pyretics and paracetamol as prescribed if required and monitor effectiveness.
- Assess headaches (📖 see Pain assessment, p 74) and administer analgesia as prescribed if required.
- Ensure a patent airway is maintained and monitor for signs of respiratory distress. Monitor O_2 saturations, chest auscultation and respiratory rate and depth.
- Administer humidified oxygen as prescribed and provide mouth care at least 2 hourly
- If the patient has a chest infection suctioning may be required—position the patient to facilitate postural drainage from lungs and maximal respiratory function, suction as required and refer to the physio for chest physiotherapy.
- Observe for and manage seizure activity (see earlier in this chapter).
- Patients may become confused and aggressive. Ensure patient safety as well as that of others. Restraint may be required following discussion with medical staff and the patient's family (📖 see p 152).
- Provide for the patient's hygiene needs.
- Assess pressure areas and provide pressure area care every 2 hours if the patient is unable to turn themselves in bed.
- Observe for signs of adrenal insufficiency (e.g. hypotension and respiratory failure) if the patient becomes septic and report to medical staff immediately.
- Provide psychological support for the patient and their family, who may be particularly anxious during the acute stages of the illness and fearful for the survival of the patient.

Further information for health professionals and the public

The Meningitis Trust http://www.meningitis-trust.org/
Meningitis UK http://www.meningitisUK.org

Other meningitis

Viral meningitis

This is the commonest viral infection of the CNS although it is not as problematic and serious as viral encephalitis. Recovery is usually spontaneous within 1–2 weeks of the onset of symptoms without treatment.

Signs and symptoms
- Sore throat and general malaise may precede other signs
- Meningism (headache, photophobia, neck stiffness)
- Occasionally diarrhoea

Medical management
- Provide symptomatic relief

Nursing care
- Provide symptomatic relief
- Patients are more comfortable on bed rest
- Encourage fluid intake
- Administer analgesia as prescribed for headache and monitor effectiveness
- Darken the environment if photophobia is a problem
- Monitor systemic observations and administer anti-pyretic medication as prescribed if required

TB meningitis

This is seen in adults following respiratory TB and also in people who are immunocompromised, e.g patients with HIV disease.

Signs and symptoms
- Fever
- Lethargy
- Confusion
- Seizures
- Cranial nerve palsies
- Meningism: headache, photophobia and neck stiffness
- Vasculitis—results in stroke
- Deteriorating level of consciousness and eventually coma

Medical management
- Diagnosis is based on clinical history and presentation, + identification of TB in the cerebral spinal fluid (CSF)
- Treatment is with antituberculous therapy +/– steroid therapy
- Provide symptomatic relief
- Perform ventriculoperitoneal (VP) shunting if hydrocephalus develops

Nursing care
- Ensure antituberculous medication is administered as prescribed
- Educate the patient about their drug regime and the importance of concordance with this—they will be on long-term therapy (between 6–24 months)
- Warn patient about and monitor for side effects of medication
- Provide symptomatic relief (see previous topic)

Subacute/chronic meningitis

The onset of meningeal symptoms is often insidious and protracted.
It may be caused by:
- Fungi (e.g. *Cryptococcus, aspergillus*)
- Carcinoma (e.g. metastatic spread, leukaemia, lymphoma, CNS primary
  tumours)
- Chemical toxins (e.g. intrathecal drug administration or contrast media)
- Parasites (e.g. toxoplasma)
- SLE

Signs and symptoms
- Similar to TB meningitis

Medical management
- Fungal infections are treated pharmacologically with drugs that will
  destroy the causative organism, e.g. amphotericin or fluconazole
- Carcinomatous meningitis may be treated with radiotherapy
- Provide symptomatic relief

Nursing care
- Depends on cause
- Administer medication as prescribed
- Monitor neurological and systemic observations
- Provide symptomatic relief and assist with activities of living as
  previously discussed in this and the previous topic
- Provide psychological support—especially if the patient is given a new
  cancer diagnosis.

Encephalitis

Encephalitis is an inflammation of the brain tissue, usually caused by a viral infection. The most common causative organism is herpes simplex (incidence 1:250,000), but it can also occur following an infection with mumps, measles or rubella, *varicella zoster* (chicken pox) and with Epstein–Barr virus.

Patients are usually acutely ill, with frequent seizures, acute confusion and may require high-dependency care.

Signs and symptoms
- Patients commonly present with seizures
- Headache and myalgia
- Pyrexia
- Confusion and altered level of consciousness
- Ataxia
- Autonomic disturbance
- Behavioural changes, e.g. aggression
- Cerebral oedema
- Coma (poor prognosis)

Medical management
- Mainstay of treatment is with antiviral agents, e.g. acyclovir
- Symptomatic relief

Nursing care
Nursing care is very similar to that for patients with acute bacterial meningitis, but isolation in a single room is not required.

Nurse the patient where they can be easily observed—usually near to the nurses' station.
- Ensure antivirals are administered as prescribed and on time—these will usually need to be given IV for quite some time, before switching to oral administration
- Carry out frequent, serial neurological and systemic observations—at least half hourly for first 24 hours of antiviral therapy, then reduce as the patient's condition allows. Monitor for signs of raised intracranial pressure (□ see p 132)
- Report any deterioration to medical staff immediately
- Ensure an accurate fluid balance is maintained and encourage fluid intake, particularly if the patient is febrile
- The patient may require an intravenous infusion to maintain fluid intake
- Administer anti-pyretics and paracetamol as prescribed if required and monitor effectiveness
- Assess headaches (□ see p 74) and administer analgesia as prescribed if required.

- Ensure a patent airway is maintained and monitor for signs of respiratory distress. Monitor O_2 saturations, chest auscultation and respiratory rate and depth
- Administer humidified oxygen as prescribed and provide mouth care at least 2 hourly
- Observe for and manage seizure activity
- Patients may become confused and aggressive. Ensure patient safety as well as that of others. Restraint may be required following discussion with medical staff and the patient's family
- Provide for the patient's hygiene needs
- Assess pressure areas and provide pressure area care every 2 hours if the patient is unable to turn themselves in bed
- Psychological support needs to be provided to both the patient and their family. Patients may have some insight into their condition and the confusion they experience may be distressing

Neurological manifestations of HIV disease

Neurological manifestations of HIV disease usually present once the patient has reached a certain level of immunocompromise later in the stages of the disease. This is measured by assessing CD4 cell counts.

These include:

- Cryptococcal meningitis
- Toxoplasmosis
- Primary CNS lymphoma
- Cytomegalovirus (CMV) encephalitis
- TB meningitis
- Tuberculoma
- Spinal TB
- HIV dementia

Medical management

- Investigation to confirm diagnosis (LP, brain biopsy)
- Treatment with antiretroviral therapy (based on CD4 levels). This usually consists of Highly Active AntiRetroviral Therapy (HAART), using a combination of drugs
- In addition antibiotics, antiviral agents and anti-TB drugs for example may be used to treat the specific infection/problem
- Symptomatic relief

Nursing care

Nursing management for patients who develop CNS infections, tumours or other neurological complications as a result of HIV is no different to the care for patients with those conditions who have not got HIV disease. Please refer to relevant topics.

In addition patients with HIV need the following specific care:

- Pay particular attention to patient confidentiality, due to the stigma associated with an HIV diagnosis.
- Counselling is required before any HIV test is conducted.
- Post-test counselling should also be arranged if the test is positive.
- Psychological care and management of anxiety are paramount
- Do not avoid physical contact with the patient or avoid talking to them, this will only make them feel more stigmatized and alienated.
- Educate patients regarding their antiretroviral therapy—concordance is essential even if the patient feels well as non-compliance with HAART will enable the virus to develop increased resistance.
- Ensure that medication is administered as prescribed and on time— ensure that the drug regime the patient is prescribed is continued if they are admitted to hospital from the community.

- Ensure that universal precautions are followed during any contact with blood or body fluids—as should be the case for all such contact. No other specific precautions are required.
- Reverse barrier nurse patients who are severely immunocompromised to minimize the risk of them developing an opportunistic infection
- Ensure that aseptic technique is maintained when dealing with invasive lines etc.

Further information for health professionals and the public

Woodward, S. and Mestecky, A.-M. (2009) *Evidence-based neuroscience nursing*. Oxford: Wiley-Blackwell.

Idiopathic intracranial hypertension

Formerly known as benign intracranial hypertension (BIH) or pseudotumour cerebri, idiopathic intracranial hypertension (IIH) produces raised intracranial pressure, without the presence of a mass lesion, hydrocephalus or other known cause of raised ICP, hence the term idiopathic, i.e. no known cause.

Incidence is 1–2 per 100,000 and more women are affected than men. It is commonly associated with obesity and pregnancy.

Signs and symptoms

- Headaches
- Double vision (diplopia) and other visual disturbances (obscurations—blurred vision—and impaired acuity) due to papilloedema (swelling of the optic disc due to raised ICP).
- Visual field defects
- Nausea and vomiting
- Disorientation and loss of visuospatial awareness
- Ataxia

Medical management

- Serial lumbar punctures to drain CSF and reduce ICP
- Weight loss
- Acetazolamide (diuretic used to reduce CSF production)
- Optic nerve decompression in extreme cases to protect vision, although this remains controversial
- Lumbar peritoneal shunt if conservative measures are insufficient and to protect vision as a last resort

Nursing care

- Ensure acetazolamide is administered as prescribed and monitor for side effects (tingling of fingers and toes, may cause hypotension)
- Explain the importance of concordance with the medication to the patient
- Assess headache pain (📖 see p 74) and administer analgesia as prescribed
- Monitor effectiveness of analgesia and liaise with medical staff to review if this is ineffective
- Discuss weight loss and healthy eating and refer patient to dietitian for further advice
- Monitor weight weekly while in hospital and on each admission
- Prepare patient for and assist with repeated lumbar punctures if these are performed (📖 see p 108)
- Ensure environment is kept free of obstructions to prevent trips and falls due to visual deficits or ataxia
- If the patient is pregnant ensure that midwifery services are informed of the admission so that routine ante-natal care can continue in the hospital if required.

Further information for health professionals and the public

Idiopathic Intracranial Hypertension UK http://www.iih.org.uk

Myasthenia gravis

Myasthenia gravis is an autoimmune neurodegenerative disorder. Patients experience muscular fatigue and weakness due to damage to the neuro-muscular junction.

The body recognizes acetylcholine receptors on the post-synaptic (muscle) cell as foreign and they are attacked by antibodies and destroyed. This reduces neuromuscular transmission of impulses, resulting in the fatigue and weakness.

The thymus gland is implicated in many cases (this produces T lymphocytes and normally curls inwards and reduces in size during puberty). Many patients with myasthenia have an intact thymus gland into adult life.

Signs and symptoms

- Muscular weakness worsens with repeated muscular activity
- Drooping upper eyelid (ptosis)
- Dysphagia
- Positive response to edrophonium (Tensilon®) test —an acetylcholinesterase inhibitor—weakness improves when this short-acting drug is administered
- Respiratory failure in severe cases and myasthenic crisis

Medical management

- Confirm diagnosis from history, clinical examination (fatiguability on testing of muscle groups), positive tensilon test and EMG
- Anticholinesterase inhibitors (allow ACh to 'sit' in the synapse in a greater quantity and for a longer time as the enzyme that breaks it down is inhibited), e.g. pyridostigmine
- Steroids—need to be started at low doses and gradually increase to prevent worsening of myasthenia.
- Immunosuppressants
- Thymectomy
- Plasmaphoresis (plasma exchange) or IV immunoglobulin (IVIg) for emergency treatment, but the effects only last about 6 weeks
- Manage myasthenic and cholinergic crisis as medical emergency.
- Manage respiratory failure through intubation and ventilation if required

Myasthenic crisis	Cholinergic crisis
Sudden worsening of myasthenic symptoms and respiratory failure	Acute and profound generalize weakness and respiratory failure
Often precipitated by infection	Due to toxic effects of anticholinesterase medication
Intubate and ventilate until condition stabilizes	May be preceded by abdominal cramps and diarrhoea
	Intubate and ventilate—monitor respiratory function

Nursing care

- During edrophonium test:
  - Accompany medical staff when edrophonium is administered
  - Ensure that crash trolley is outside patient's bed area/room, but out of sight of the patient so as not to cause alarm
  - Prior to administration of edrophonium ensure that a syringe of atropine and one of normal saline is drawn up ready in case this is needed to counteract the effects of the edrophonium.
  - Reassure patient and prepare them for the test—explain what is going to happen.
- Administer prescribed medication on time—pyridostigmine is needed at regular intervals and often outside of regular drug rounds.
- Ensure that pyridostigmine is administered prior to meals etc, so that the patient is not fatigued and experiencing muscle weakness when trying to chew or swallow for example.
- Explain to patient the importance of timing of activity and rest throughout the day to coincide with administration of medication doses.
- Monitor respiratory function for signs of neuromuscular respiratory failure using regular FVC measurement (🕮 see p 136).
- If respiratory function deteriorates treat as a medical emergency and inform medical staff and anaesthetist immediately (🕮 see p 136).
- Assess swallowing and refer to speech and language therapist and dietitian if required.
- Monitor for signs of aspiration (🕮 see p 138).
- Administer steroids as prescribed and monitor for side effects. Explain the importance of the medication to the patient and that they should not be suddenly withdrawn.
- Provide psychological support and manage the patient's anxiety and fears by providing information and education about the condition and its management.
- Ensure that patients know how to recognize both myasthenic and cholinergic crisis and to treat these as a medical emergency, calling an ambulance.
- Advise patient to wear a medical identification tag bracelet.

Further information for health professionals and the public

Myasthenia Gravis Association http://www.mgauk.org/

Guillain–Barré syndrome

Guillain–Barré Syndrome is an autoimmune acute demyelinating disease affecting peripheral and some cranial nerves. It is thought to be a post-infective problem caused by an abnormal response to a virus. It usually occurs 1–3 weeks following upper respiratory tract or gastrointestinal infections.

The incidence is 1:200,000. The disease is usually self-limiting and patients make a full neurological recovery without recurrence. Generally speaking, the quicker the onset, the quicker the recovery. Only 3–5% of patients will experience recurrence.

Patients with severe symptoms (those with respiratory failure) are more likely to be left with residual disability (20%) due to axonal damage and neuronal destruction.

Signs and symptoms
- Ascending weakness and sensory loss from fingers and toes towards the trunk in a 'stocking and glove' distribution
- Eventually complete paralysis of limbs and other skeletal muscles may occur and disease progression usually halts after 3 weeks
- Muscle wasting may occur as the muscles lose innervation and become flaccid
- Neuromuscular respiratory failure
- Autonomic dysfunction due to vagus nerve involvement (postural hypotension, labile BP, tachycardia and dysrhythmias, urinary retention)
- Dysphagia if cranial nerves are involved, also poor lip seal and facial muscle weakness/paralysis may occur

Medical management
- Diagnosis from CSF (LP performed) and clinical history + nerve conduction studies (see Chapter 4)
- IVIg administration
- Plasma exchange
- Supportive management:
  - Intubate and ventilate if FVC falls below approx 1–1.5L
  - May require tracheostomy for long-term ventilation
  - DVT prophylaxis

Nursing care
- Monitor respiratory function using forced vital capacity (FVC) at least 4-hourly and increase frequency if condition deteriorates (🕮 see p 136).
- Use face mask rather than mouthpiece with spirometer if poor lip seal is an issue due to facial weakness.
- Inform medical staff immediately if deterioration in respiratory function is detected so that elective intubation can be planned, rather than as an emergency when the patient has respiratory arrest.
- Patients may require to be nursed in a high dependency or ITU for long-term invasive ventilation (up to six months).
- Consider cardiac monitoring to detect dysrhythmias due to autonomic involvement.

- IVIg is a blood-derived product: Record half-hourly systemic obs during IVIg infusions, increasing the rate slowly due to risk of anaphylaxis, and observe for side effects (flu-like symptoms, unstable vasodilation and vasoconstriction, congestive heart failure, stroke, myocardial infarction (MI), renal failure)
- Assess swallowing (📖 see p 72) and refer to SLT and dietitian to ensure nutritional requirements are met if dysphagia is an issue.
- If patient is assessed to be at risk of aspiration, keep NBM and consider NG feeding.
- Monitor progression of sensory loss and weakness—conduct moving and handling assessment.
- Monitor urine output—if the patient goes into retention an indwelling urethral catheter is required.
- Nurse in a profiling bed and ensure that knees are supported at all times.
- Foot drop may occur—do not tuck bedclothes in tightly—consider using a bed cradle to lift the weight off the legs. This may also be helpful if the patient experiences parasthesia and hypersensitivity during recovery.
- Prevent DVT—administer subcutaneous heparin as prescribed. Patients will not normally be taken off heparin until they are mobile for 50% of their norm.
- Ensure TED stockings are worn at all times.
- Refer to physiotherapist and OT for help with mobilizing during rehabilitation and also for orthotic splints to support limbs in a functional position.
- Carry out passive limb exercises to prevent stiffness and ensure patient is always supported in a functional position.
- Assess pain (painful joints are a problem due to lack of support of the joint from flaccid muscles leading to hyperextension injuries as well as parasthesia and neurogenic pain during recovery) and administer analgesia as prescribed.
- Provide psychological support to patient and family—anxiety and fear of death may be a problem, especially if respiratory involvement occurs.

Further information for health professionals and the public

Guillain–Barré Syndrome Support Group http://www.gbs.org.uk

Chronic inflammatory demyelinating polyneuropathy

Chronic inflammatory demyelinating polyneuropathy (CIDP) is a chronic remitting relapsing disorder related to Guillain–Barré syndrome (GBS). The two are similar and only distinguished by the rate of onset of symptoms and recovery. While GBS has an acute onset and is at its worst within 4 weeks, patients with CIDP often deteriorate more slowly and over a longer period of time.

This rarely involves respiratory muscles or cranial nerves.

It is very rare with the incidence 1:5,000,000.

Signs and symptoms

- Fatigue
- Sensory loss (tingling or numbness in extremities)
- Progressive weakness in limbs
- Chronic deterioration over a long period of time

Medical management

- High-dose steroids initially for moderate disease (60mg prednisolone orally then tapering doses)
- IVIg or plasma exchange
- Immunosuppressants, e.g. azathioprine +/– cyclophosphamide in severe cases

Nursing care

- Administer steroids as prescribed and monitor for side effects. Explain the importance of the medication to the patient and that they should not be suddenly withdrawn.
- IVIg is a blood-derived product: Record half-hourly systemic obs during IVIg infusions, increasing the rate slowly due to risk of anaphylaxis, and observe for side effects (flu-like symptoms, unstable vasodilation and vasoconstriction, congestive heart failure, stroke, MI, renal failure).
- Monitor progression of sensory loss and weakness—conduct moving and handling assessment.
- Advise patient to avoid infections wherever possible—these have been known to trigger relapse.
- Some exercise is important, but this needs to be balanced with periods of rest to avoid fatigue.
- Refer to physiotherapist and occupational therapist for assessment and exercises etc to maximize functional ability, including home assessment if required.
- Psychological support for patient and family is essential—patients will initially be anxious and may go on to develop depression.
- Provide psychological support and manage the patient's anxiety and fears by providing information and education about the condition and its management.

- Encourage the patient to talk to their partner about relationship issues and sexual functioning. Patients may experience erectile dysfunction or vaginismus and should be encouraged to seek advice if this occurs. Muscle weakness and fatigue can also affect libido and sexual relationships.

Further information for health professionals and the public

Guillain–Barré Syndrome Support Group http://www.gbs.org.uk

Neuropathies

Peripheral nerve damage (neuropathy) may be caused by a number of factors including:
- Drugs (e.g. some anti-TB or cytotoxic medication)
- Environmental toxins (e.g. lead and organophosphates)
- Nutrition deficiency (e.g. vitamin B)
- Alcohol and other substance misues (e.g. heroin, solvents)
- Cancer
- Rheumatoid arthritis
- Systemic lupus erythematosis (SLE)
- HIV
- Metabolic disorders (e.g. diabetes, uraemia)
- Hereditary disorders

Signs and symptoms
- Loss of sensation
- Parasthesia (pins and needles)
- Neuropathic painful sensations (e.g. hypersensitivity to pain or even allodynia—perception of pain from a non-painful stimulus)
- Muscle weakness and loss of tone
- Loss of reflexes in affected limb
- Autonomic symptoms in autonomic neuropathies (e.g. postural hypotension, bladder and bowel dysfunction)

Medical management
- Identify degree of neuropathy (EMG, nerve biopsy and nerve conduction studies)
- Investigate and identify cause
- Treatment is dependent on cause (e.g. diabetic neuropathy requires better diabetic control)
- Symptomatic relief

Nursing care
- Assess pain, motor and sensory loss (📖 see Chapter 3, pp 61–90).
- Administer analgesia for pain as prescribed and monitor effectiveness.
- If patient has sensory loss, advise and educate about monitoring for injury that may not be felt, e.g. scalds from bath water that is too hot, wounds from ill-fitting shoes and other foot injuries. This is especially important if the neuropathy is due to poorly controlled diabetes, due to the incidence of ulceration and poor wound healing should such injuries occur. Diabetic patients should receive regular foot assessment from a chiropodist—refer if required and never cut the patient's toenails for them, even if you are asked.
- Conduct a moving and handling risk assessment if lower limb weakness is causing reduced mobility.
- Foot drop may occur due to muscle weakness—do not tuck bedclothes in tightly.
- If the neuropathy results in reduced mobility prevent DVT—administer subcutaneous heparin/dalteparin as prescribed. Ensure TED stockings are worn at all times or consider the use of sequential compression devices.

- Refer to physiotherapist and OT for help with mobilizing during rehabilitation and also for orthotic splints to support limbs in a functional position.
- Carry out passive limb exercises to prevent stiffness and ensure patient is always supported in a functional position.
- If the neuropathy is due to poor diabetic control nurses must advise and educate the patient about improving their self-management of the condition—advise re diet and correct glycaemic control, monitoring blood sugar and refer to diabetic nurse specialist for review and support if required.

Further information for health professionals and the public

Lindsey, K. and Bone, I. (2004) *Neurology and neurosurgery illustrated*, 4th edn. Edinburgh: Churchill Livingstone

Bell's palsy

Bell's palsy is an idiopathic neuropathy affecting the facial nerve due to inflammation leading to possible ischaemia and demyelination in response to an infection with herpes virus. Incidence is approx 15–30 per 100,000 and males and females (especially during pregnancy) are equally affected. Peak onset is in the 40s. Patients may have a one-off episode, but it may recur, and recovery is often spontaneous.

Signs and symptoms
- Weakness/paralysis down one side of the face
- Lower eyelid droops and eyelids do not close
- Reduced tear production
- Difficulty chewing
- Pooling of food and saliva on affected side of mouth
- Dribbling

Medical management
- Investigate possible differential diagnoses
- Corticosteroids (prednisolone 60mg per day reducing over 10 days)

Nursing care
Psychological support
Psychological support is essential while the condition is being investigated—similar symptoms may be produced by MS, tumours, stroke and Guillain–Barré syndrome, so patients may be anxious about diagnosis.

Altered body image affects these patients—facial disfigurement (albeit temporary) is very distressing and patients may avoid social contact or eating in front of others.

Nutrition
Patients often withdraw from eating and find chewing difficult.
- Provide an appetizing menu and offer smaller portions
- Check that food is not pooling in the affected cheek
- Assess swallowing
- Monitor nutritional and fluid intake

Eye care
The eye is at risk of corneal irritation and ulceration—artificial tears may need to be administered as prescribed and regular eye care is required. If the palsy is not resolved, tarsorrhaphy may be required in which the eyelids are sutured closed at the outer edge to protect the eye.

Further information for health professionals and the public

Tiemstra, J.D. and Khatkhate, N. (2007) Bell's palsy: diagnosis and management. *American Family Physician*, 76: 997–1002.

Salinas, R.A., Alvarez, G. and Ferreira, J. (2004) Corticosteroids for Bell's palsy (idiopathic facial paralysis). *Cochrane Database of Systematic Reviews*, Issue 4.

Myositis

Myositis is an inflammatory myopathy and is thought to be autoimmune. Two common forms of such inflammatory myopathies are polymyositis and dermatomyositis.

Incidence is 8:100,000 and they can affect any age group.

They may occur in conjunction with cancer or SLE.

Signs and symptoms

- Painful muscles
- Muscle weakness
- Dysphagia and dysphonia with involvement of bulbar muscles
- Cardiac and respiratory muscles may be affected—cardiac and respiratory failure
- In addition dermatomyositis produces a skin rash

Medical management

- Steroids
- IVIg for polymyositis
- Immunosuppression with azathioprine for dermatomyositis

Nursing care

- Administer steroids as prescribed (long term) and monitor for side effects. Explain the importance of the medication to the patient and that they should not be suddenly withdrawn.
- Administer IVIg as prescribed.
- IVIg is a blood-derived product: Record half-hourly systemic obs during IVIg infusions, increasing the rate slowly due to risk of anaphylaxis, and observe for side effects (flu-like symptoms, unstable vasodilation and vasoconstriction, congestive heart failure, stroke, MI, renal failure).
- Assess swallowing (📖 see p 72) and refer to SLT and dietitian to ensure nutritional requirements are met if dysphagia is an issue.
- If patient is assessed to be at risk of aspiration, keep NBM and consider NG feeding.
- Monitor for signs of respiratory and cardiac failure.
- Psychological support for the patient and the family is essential. Patients are likely to experience anxiety, especially as they may also be being investigated for cancer.

Ataxia

Ataxia or unsteadiness of gait is associated with a number of neurological conditions. It is often due to damage to the cerebellum, which normally helps to coordinate smooth voluntary movement through a number of feedback mechanisms.

If the cerebellum is damaged, movement can become uncoordinated and unsteady.

Ataxia can be seen in:
- MS
- Cerebellar degeneration
- Spino-cerebellar ataxia (degenerative and often inherited disorders e.g. Friedreich's ataxia)
- Multi-system atrophy
- Intracranial tumours
- CNS infections (e.g. abscess)
- Metabolic disorders (e.g. vitamin B deficiency, alcohol misuse, hypoxia)
- Vascular disorders of the cerebellum (e.g. infarct or haemorrhage)
- Drug toxicity (e.g. anticonvulsants, barbiturates, diazepam)

Signs and symptoms
- Ataxic gait (broad-based with jerky steps)
- May be accompanied by nystagmus

Medical management
- Depends on cause—see other topics throughout this text
- Review of medication
- Vitamin B injections if this is the cause

Nursing care
- Observe patient if they are walking—falls are a risk—ensure a safe environment and remove any obstacles
- Conduct a falls and moving and handling risk assessment
- Ensure the patient has access to their mobility aids
- Liaise with OT and physio re patient positioning, exercise regimes, moving and handling, etc.
- Refer to OT and physio for provision of wheelchair and seating assessment
- If ataxia is causing reduced mobility, pressure area care and observation is important.
- Provide emotional and psychological support for patient and their family

Narcolepsy

Narcolepsy is a disorder of wakefulness and rapid-eye-movement (REM) sleep. It is thought to have a genetic origin, which leads to autoimmune changes in the hypothalamus.

Prevalence is 1:2000 and it affects both men and women.

Signs and symptoms

Narcolepsy is characterized by the four main symptoms below, although not all patients experience cataplexy.

- Excessive daytime sleepiness and sleep attacks
- Disturbed and abnormal REM sleep
- Cataplexy (sudden temporary muscle weakness and loss of tone)
- Parasomnias (e.g hallucinations, sleep walking, nightmares and other vivid dreams)
  In addition patients may experience:
- Change in energy levels
- Altered metabolism and appetite (sugar craving)
- Obesity

Medical management

- Treatments for excessive daytime somnolence (e.g. modafinil, sodium oxybate)
- Tricyclic antidepressants for cataplexy
- Low-carbohydrate diet

Nursing care

- Patient education is required—patients are at risk of injury at work if they suddenly experience sleepiness while working with machinery and should be advised to discuss this with their employer if necessary.
- Social withdrawal is seen due to fears of falling asleep in public.
- Psychological and emotional support is required as patients may become depressed due to the impact of narcolepsy on their quality of life. Help the patient explain the condition and its effects to their family.
- Advise patients that they must inform the DVLA of the condition, but they may not necessarily lose their driving licence. Document this discussion in the notes.
- Administer medication as prescribed.
- Inform the patient about their medication including possible side effects (e.g. headaches, nausea).
- Refer patient to dietitian for advice about low-carbohydrate ketogenic diet (similar to Atkins diet).
- Promote good night-time sleep, by avoiding afternoon sleeps, avoid dietary and fluid stimulants prior to bedtime (e.g. alcohol and caffeine), stick to a regular night-time routine.
- Advise the patient to create a relaxing bedroom atmosphere, e.g. do not have TV or computers/workstations in a bedroom.
- Patients may be advised to sleep alone to avoid disturbing their partner's sleep and putting further strain on a relationship.

Further information for health professionals and the public

Cook, N.F. (2008) Understanding narcolepsy, part 1: epidemiology and neurophysiology. *BJNN*, 4(3): 108–14.

Cook, N.F. (2008) Understanding narcolepsy, part 2: accurate diagnosis and effective management. *BJNN*, 4(4):170–6.

Chronic fatigue syndrome

Chronic fatigue syndrome (CFS) is characterized by excessive fatigue, that is not relieved by sleep, or rest, is long-lasting and impacts on daily living and quality of life.

CFS was formerly known as myalgic encephalomyelitis (ME).

Prevalence is estimated at 1:200 and it is more common in females. Peak age of onset is during the early 20s to mid-40s, but children as young as 13 may be affected.

It was originally thought to be a post-infective disorder, usually following a viral infection, but it is now known that genetic and other factors (exhaustion, mental stress, depression and traumatic life events) play a part in onset of CFS.

Signs and symptoms

Symptoms last months to years and include:
- Extreme mental and physical fatigue
- Muscle pain (myalgia)
- Joint pain (arthralgia)
- Headaches
- Poor concentration and memory
- Lymph node inflammation
- Irritable bowel symptoms
- Sleep disturbance
- Panic attacks and depression

Medical management

- Symptomatic relief e.g. analgesia
- Cognitive behavioural therapy (CBT)
- Antidepressants
- Complementary therapies, e.g. homeopathy, osteopathy, nutritional therapy

Nursing care

- Explain to patient the importance of balancing activity and rest throughout the day, with planned sleep/rest periods vital and activity and rest tailored to how their energy levels feel.
- Advise the patient to avoid stressful situations.
- Refer to physiotherapist for advice about moderate exercise regimes.
- Encourage the patient to avoid alcohol, caffeine, sugar and sweeteners as well as other foods that may trigger and exacerbate symptoms.
- Provide small and regular meals—eating a large meal may exacerbate fatigue during digestion.
- Teach relaxation techniques, e.g. deep breathing and progressive muscle relaxation. Patients may like to try guided imagery tapes to assist with relaxation.
- Encourage the patient to contact a local support group.
- Provide psychological care for the patient and their family—explain symptoms and the impact of the condition. There is often a misconception that patients are being lazy.

Further information for health professionals and the public

SupportME http://www.supportme.co.uk provides an online resource for sufferers of CFS, including details of support groups.

Stiff man syndrome

Stiff man syndrome (SMS) (sometimes referred to as stiff person syndrome) is a rare, autoimmune disorder that results in destruction of an enzyme glutamic acid decarboxylase (GAD). The loss of this enzyme results in difficulty with neurotransmission leading to painful muscle spasm and rigidity.

It affects approx 1 in 200,000 individuals and affects both males and females, although women are more frequently affected.

It is commonly associated with insulin-dependent diabetes mellitus or thyroid disease.

Signs and symptoms

The main symptoms of the disease are:
- Rigidity
- Startle response (to ordinary stimuli—sights, sounds, flash photography)
- Painful muscle spasm (especially in the back, stomach, neck and thighs)
- Falls (especially on windy days)
- Anxiety
  These symptoms occur during everyday activities e.g.:
- Walking downstairs
- Crossing over a pedestrian crossing
- Walking down a slope or on a slippery surface
- Unexpected events (e.g. sights or sounds—door slamming, balloon bursting)

Medical management

- Confirm diagnosis –antibody testing for anti-GAD and EMG
- High doses of muscle relaxants (diazepam) and anti-spasmodics (baclofen) in combination
- Some anticonvulsants may be prescribed
- Steroids
- IVIg
- Plasma exchange

Nursing care

- Provide a walk-in shower with hand rails rather than a bath.
- If a patient falls, do not help them up, allow them to instruct you when they are ready to get up and they will usually be able to manage this themself by using something to hold onto.
- Ensure the environment is clear of obstructions to minimize risk of falls during mobilizing and conduct falls assessment.
- Do not make any sudden unexpected noises around the patient.
- Administer enemas as prescribed if required to prevent bowel movements triggering spasms
- Administer medication as prescribed and monitor for side effects
- IVIg is a blood-derived product: Record half-hourly systemic obs during IVIg infusions, increasing the rate slowly due to risk of anaphylaxis, and observe for side effects (flu-like symptoms, unstable vasodilation and vasoconstriction, congestive heart failure, stroke, MI, renal failure)

- Administer steroids as prescribed and monitor for side effects. Explain the importance of the medication to the patient and that they should not be suddenly withdrawn.
- Provide psychological support and manage the patient's anxiety and fears by providing information and education about the condition and its management.
- Refer the patient to the SMS support group. With rare conditions they may feel extremely isolated and contact with other sufferers can help.

Further information for health professionals and the public

Stiff Man Syndrome Support Group http://www.smssupportgroup.co.uk/

Restless legs syndrome

Restless legs syndrome (RLS) is characterized by an irresistible urge to move the legs (and rarely the arms) due to parasthesia (pins and needles) or other unpleasant sensations.

It can occur during the day, but is a particular problem when settling for the night and can cause severe sleep disturbance.

Prevalence is estimated between 3–10:100 population, although it is not sufficiently severe in all cases to result in healthcare-seeking behaviour.

Primary (idiopathic) RLS is thought to have a genetic component, but it can also occur secondary to other conditions:
- Iron deficiency
- Pregnancy
- End-stage renal failure
- Parkinson's disease
- Diabetes
- Drug effects (e.g. anti-emetics, anti-psychotics, anticonvulsants)

Signs and symptoms
- Irresistible urge to move legs due to unpleasant sensations
- Painful legs/discomfort
- Sleep disturbance
- Daytime sleepiness and fatigue
- Anxiety and depression
- Poor quality of life

Medical management
- Review causative factors
- Treatment of underlying cause e.g. iron supplements, medication review
- TENS
- Short-term use of sedatives (e.g. temazepam)
- Dopamine agonists (pramipexole or ropinirole)

Nursing care
- Assess sleep duration and quality (could use Epworth sleepiness scale for more objective assessment).
- Provide psychological care for the patient and their family—explain symptoms and the impact of the condition as well as self-management techniques.
- Massaging affected limbs with mint or herbal cream may help.
- Promote good night-time sleep, by avoiding afternoon sleeps, avoid dietary and fluid stimulants prior to bedtime (e.g. alcohol and caffeine), stick to a regular night-time routine.
- Advise the patient to create a relaxing bedroom atmosphere, e.g. do not have TV or computers/workstations in a bedroom.
- Ensure a comfortable ambient temperature in bedrooms.
- Patients may be advised to sleep alone to avoid disturbing their partner's sleep and putting further strain on a relationship.
- Encourage the patient to try yoga or long walks, which may relieve symptoms.
- Administer medication as prescribed and monitor effectiveness.

- Assist patient to apply and use TENS machine if they are using this to provide a counter-stimulation and reduce the perception of the unpleasant sensations from the legs.

Further information for health professionals and the public

Thomas, S. and MacMahon, D. (2006) Restless legs syndrome: a condition in search of recognition. *BJNN*, 2(5): 222–6.

Wilson's disease

Wilson's disease is an autosomal recessive inherited neurological disorder. It is characterized by a build up of copper within the body resulting in liver and neurological damage.

The liver develops cirrhosis and the basal ganglia are affected.

Prevalence is 1–4:100,000

Signs and symptoms

- Liver symptoms:
  - Fatigue
  - Hepatic encephalopathy (results in confusion, coma and cerebral oedema)
  - Ascites
  - Acute liver failure—deranged liver function and jaundice
  - Clotting disorders
- Neurological symptoms:
  - Cognitive impairment and behavioural changes, eventually dementia
  - Parkinsonism (bradykinesia, rigidity, tremor)
  - Psychosis
  - Dystonia
  - Ataxia
  - Seizures
  - Migraine

Medical management

- Lifelong medication to reduce copper absorption (e.g. penicillamine initially followed by a zinc preparation when levels have returned to normal)
- Dietary manipulation
- Liver transplant may be required

Nursing care

- Educate patient about reducing copper intake in diet—eliminate foods high in copper (e.g. mushrooms, chocolate, nuts, dried fruit, shellfish and liver)
- Refer to dietitian for dietary advice
- Administer medication as prescribed and observe for side effects (e.g. anaphylaxis, rashes, joint pain, drug-induced myasthenia)
- Observe for seizure activity or migraine (refer to other topics within this chapter for management)
- Assess cognitive function and refer to occupational therapist or neuropsychologist as required.
- Provide psychological care for the patient and their family—explain symptoms and the impact of the condition.
- Refer patient to the Wilson's disease support group (see Further information). With rare conditions patients may feel extremely isolated and contact with other sufferers can help.

Further information for health professionals and the public

The Wilson's Disease Support Group http://www.wilsonsdisease.org.uk provides advice and support for patients and their families in the UK.

Torticollis

Torticollis (wry neck) is a form of dystonia, affecting the sternomastoid muscle. It usually affects one side of the neck and the abnormal tone and muscular contraction causes the head to be turned towards the unaffected side. It is sometimes referred to as cervical dystonia.

20% of patients will go into remission, but the dystonia may spread to other muscles.

Torticollis may be congenital or acquired following neck trauma, with tumours at the skull base, or antipsychotic medication for example, or simply from sleeping in an awkward position.

Prevalence is approx 3:10,000 and both males and females are affected equally. Peak age of onset is during middle age.

Signs and symptoms
- Turning of the head to one side
- Increased tone in sternomastoid on affected side
- Hypertrophy of sternomastoid
- Pain

Medical management
- Anti-inflammatory analgesia and muscle relaxants
- Anticholinergics
- Botulinum toxin injections for spasmodic torticollis

Nursing care
- Assess pain (📖 see p 74)
- Administer analgesia as prescribed and monitor effectiveness
- Refer to physiotherapist for advice about low-impact neck exercises to strengthen muscles
- Patients sometimes find shiatsu massage and application of heat helpful.
- Teach patients to use 'geste antagoniste'—press with one finger against the chin on the unaffected side. This may cause the head to return to a neutral position
- Provide psychological care for the patient and their family—explain symptoms and the impact of the condition
- Refer patient to the Dystonia Society for support (see Further information)

Further information for health professionals and the public

The Dystonia Society provides information and support for patients and their families with torticollis and other forms of dystonia: http://www.dystonia.org.uk

Neurosurgery nursing

Cerebral oedema formation

Cerebral oedema is an abnormal increase in the volume of fluid in the intracellular and extracellular spaces in the brain and is a major cause of death in patients following any insult to the brain. The additional cerebral volume increases the intracranial pressure, reducing cerebral perfusion and adversely affecting the level of consciousness.

Oedema may be:
- Localized—surrounding a tumour or haematoma.
- Generalized—spread throughout the cerebral hemispheres.

Clinical signs

Early signs
- Raised intracranial pressure
- Headache
- Behavioural changes and confusion
- Cranial nerve compression—loss of upward gaze

Late signs
- ↓ level of consciousness
- Sluggish or absent pupil reflexes
- Cushings response—↑ BP, ↓ Pulse, ↓ respirations
- Abnormal posturing, i.e. extension

Types of cerebral oedema
- Vasogenic oedema
- Cytotoxic oedema
- Interstitial oedema

Vasogenic oedema
- Occurs as a result of a breakdown in the blood–brain barrier, allowing fluid to leak into the extracellular space.
- Vasogenic oedema is present around tumours, cerebral infarcts or cerebral abscesses.
- Corticosteroids are effective for treating oedema surrounding tumours.
- Osmotic diuretics (mannitol), are useful in the acute stage.

Cytotoxic oedema
- An increase in fluid within the neurons and glial cells
- Occurs as a result of damage to the ATP-dependent sodium–potassium pump
- Associated with hypoxic injuries—post-cardiac arrest, drowning
- Corticosteroids are largely ineffective
- Osmotic diuretics may be useful

Interstitial oedema
- Caused by acute hydrocephalus.
- Excess CSF within the ventricles is forced into the surrounding cerebral tissue.
- Corticosteroids and osmotic diuretics are ineffective.
- Management includes insertion of a temporary external ventricular drain or a permanent ventricular–peritoneal shunt.

Medical management of raised intracranial pressure

Surgical treatment

Skull fractures

- Deep depressed skull fractures will require elevation and removal of penetrating boney fragments.
- Cranioplasty—repair of bone defect with original bone or titanium mesh plate.

Haematomas

- Extradural haematoma—craniotomy and removal of haematoma.
- Acute subdural haematoma (SDH)—craniotomy, evacuation of haematoma ± partial lobectomy to control pressure effects.
- Chronic SDH can be aspirated through a burr hole once the haematoma has reverted back to fluid.
- Intracerebral haematoma—routine surgical evacuation remains controversial and depends on the location and degree of pressure effects on the remaining brain tissue.

Contusions and lacerations

- Conservative management involving intensive care support and control of ↑ ICP.
- Treat complications resulting from ↑ ICP e.g. hydrocephalus.

Diffuse axonal injury and oedema

- Radical decompressive craniectomy to prevent further ischaemia and infarction.

Medical treatment

Neurological support

- Intracranial pressure monitoring.
- Aim for an ICP <25mmHg and CPP >60–70mmHg.
- External ventricular drain to relieve hydrocephalus.
- Anticonvulsant therapy may be prescribed.
- Therapeutic cooling <33–36°C reduces the number of raised ICP episodes but increases risk of developing coagulopathy and pneumonia—the intervention remains controversial.
- Repeat CT scan to monitor progress.
- Administer diuretics: mannitol, furosemide or hypertonic saline (similar action to mannitol).

Mannitol (osmotic diuretic)	Furosemide (loop diuretic)
Dose: 0.25–1.0g/kg, (approx 100ml)	Dose: 20–40mg 4–6-hourly
Requires intact blood–brain barrier	Inhibits CSF production and enhances absorption
Decreases cerebral oedema	
Discontinue when plasma osmolarity level 310–320mOsmol/kg	

Respiratory support
- Elective intubation and ventilation (neuromuscular block, sedation).
- Serial arterial blood gas analysis.
- SaO_2 > 97%
- PaO_2 > 12kPa
- $PaCO_2$ at 4.3—4.5 kPa—↑ CO_2 dilates cerebral blood vessels, increasing blood volume and subsequently raises ICP.
- Jugular bulb venous saturation monitoring ($SjvO_2$ >55%).
- Monitor levels of serum haemoglobin (Hb) and haemocrit (HCT) to optimize O_2 delivery at capillary level.
- Consider thiopental if all other measures have been ineffective.
- Excessive hyperventilation can induce vasoconstriction increasing vascular resistance and reducing cerebral blood flow.

Cardiovascular support
- Central line inserted for monitoring of fluid/drug therapy.
- Optimise cerebral perfusion pressure (CPP) >60mmHg (in adults), with fluids, colloids or inotropic support.
- Maintain MAP > 90–100mmHg.
- Maintain systolic blood pressure 140–160mmHg.
- CVP > 8–10mmHg.
- Correct any coagulopathy.
- Aim for serum osmolarity <320mOsm.
- Fluid replacement using isotonic saline. Avoid dextrose solutions that metabolize to lactic acid, lowering pH, decreasing plasma osmolality and exacerbating ischaemic brain injury.

Renal function
- Urine osmolarity <320mOsm.
- Control hyperglycaemia with sliding scale insulin and avoid hypoglycaemia.
- Monitor electrolyte levels—specifically sodium and potassium.
- Treat diabetes insipidus (DDAVP) 1–4ug I.M/I.V

Further information for health professionals and the public

Harris, O.A., Calford, J.M., Good, M.C. *et al.* (2002) The role of hypothermia in the management of severe brain injury; a meta-analysis. *Archives of Neurology*, 59(7): 1077–83.

Nursing management of raised intracranial pressure

Oxygenation
- Record ventilator parameters—avoid hypoxia and hypercapnia.
- Titrate IV sedation and opiates with level of consciousness and ICP observations.
- Control hyperpyrexia—antipyretic medication, cooling therapy.
- Observe for signs of seizure activity—cerebral function monitors (CFM).
- Monitor O_2 saturations >12kpa, CO_2 >4.3–4.5 kPa.
- Ensure endotracheal tube or tracheostomy tapes do not compress or occlude venous drainage.

Endotracheal suctioning
- Consider ICP, mean arterial BP, CPP, SaO_2, end tidal CO_2, prior to suctioning procedure.
- Suctioning must be based on clinical need, e.g. increased inflation pressures, deteriorating blood gases and auscultation.
- Limit amount of time and numbers of passes with suction catheter.
- Pre-oxygenate with 100% O_2 prior to suctioning.
- Allow at least ten minutes between each suction procedure.

Neuro management
- Assume an unstable spinal/neck fracture.
- Monitor ICP, aim to maintain ICP <20mmhg and optimise cerebral perfusion pressure (MAP–ICP = CP).
- Perform effective, repeated neurological observations.
- Document limb movements, sensation, power and tone.
- Monitor cranial nerve function and integrity.
- Record vital signs—respiratory rate and pattern, pulse and BP.
- Record pupil reactions at least hourly.
- Continuous monitoring of ICP—consult with medical staff if ICP remains high, despite all active interventions.
- Monitor levels of sedation—CFM or BIZ, sedation scoring.

Fluid management
- Maintain normovolaemia—potassium and sodium levels.
- Give colloids to maintain CVP and CPP.
- Administer vasoactive drugs to maintain CPP.
- Maintain an accurate fluid balance.
- Initiate enteral feeding as soon as practicably possible.
- Record urine output hourly and report signs of diabetes insipidus (give desmopressin if necessary).
- Record bowel action, avoid constipation or initiating valsalva manoeuvre.
- Administer anti-emetics for nausea if required.

Temperature control

- Pyrexia increases cerebral metabolism.
- Exclude alternative causes of pyrexia—blood cultures, swabs (IV lines, urine, wounds) for culture and sensitivity.
- Paracetamol 1g 6hrly.
- Implement adjuncts to cooling therapy; cooling blankets, fanning.
- Monitor skin integrity whilst using hypothermia guidelines.

Positioning

- Elevate head of bed to 15–30°.
- Optimise head positioning—neutral position, avoiding extreme flexion or rotation of head or neck.
- Alter position using 'log rolling' technique.
- Avoid extreme hip flexion.
- Coordinate patient movement (bathing, linen changes) with therapists.
- Consider bolus sedation prior to any changes in position.
- Postpone care if ICP not controlled or within acceptable limits.
- Refer to therapists for splinting to reduce foot drop.
- Provide continuous explanation and psychological support to ensure compliance with therapy.

Noxious stimuli

- Limit painful procedures whenever possible.
- Avoid unnecessary touch and disturbance.
- Avoid unnecessary noise.
- Educate family to benefits and hazards of over-stimulation.
- Ensure the family are kept informed of treatment plan, progress, and potential prognosis and outlook.
- Involve family and carers in assisting with basic care whenever possible.
- Liaise with multidisciplinary team in preparation for eventual transfer or discharge.
- Avoid over-sedation that may cloud neurological assessment or induce hypotension.
- Remember to explain all procedures to the patient – they may still be able to hear.

External ventricular drains

An external ventricular drain (EVD) allows excess cerebrospinal fluid (CSF) to drain from the ventricles to reduce the intracranial pressure of the brain. Following acute trauma or some neurosurgical procedures, the intracranial pressure (ICP) can rise to dangerous levels above normal levels.

Indications for use

- Acute hydrocephalus (due to either excess production, blockage to the flow of CSF in the ventricles or malabsorption).
- Meningitis or encephalitis (preventing the re-absorbtion of CSF through the arachnoid granulations).
- Tumours of the 3rd or 4th ventricle (which cause compression and blockage of the flow of CSF).
- Closed head injury where the ICP is difficult to control.
- Subarachnoid haemorrhage (reducing the flow of CSF through the ventricular system and preventing re-absorption).
- Reyes' syndrome (more common in children).

Insertion technique

A soft catheter is inserted into the lateral ventricles via a burr hole and connected to an external drainage system. The wound is sutured and covered with a sterile occlusive dressing.

Complications

- Infection—risk of developing meningitis or ventriculitis.
- Over-drainage of CSF, may collapse the ventricles resulting in headaches (often called a low-pressure headache), and possible subdural haematoma.
- Haemorrhage due to coagulopathy.
- Pain and discomfort at the drain site.
- Accidental removal in the confused and agitated patient.

Management of an EVD

Levelling of drain

- The drain is calibrated to read zero at the intraventricular foramen of Munroe (IFM) corresponding with the external auditory meatus.
- A laser system or leveling ruler must be readily accessible.
- The drainage chamber of the manometer system is set at the height prescribed by the medical staff e.g. +10cm (10cm above the zero point on the scale).
- If the drain is raised it will decrease the amount of CSF drained and if it is lowered, it will increase the amount of CSF drained.
- The amount of drainage should be recorded hourly. Drainage of 5–15ml per hour is within normal limits.
- Empty the collection chamber hourly and document amount.
- Increases of 10ml above the patients normal drainage amount should be reported—might be due to inaccurate zeroing of the drain, change of position of the patient or a sudden rise in intracranial pressure.
- CSF description—colour and clarity should be documented.

- Patency of the drain should be checked and documented hourly—look for pulsation and oscillation of CSF within the drainage tube.
- The CSF collection bag should be handled as infrequently as possible and changed when ¾ full, using universal precautions.

Management
- Glasgow Coma Scale observations are recorded at a minimum of 2hrly to detect neurological changes.
- Temperature, pulse and respirations are performed and recorded 4hrly to detect early signs of infection.
- Intrathecal medication is usually administered by an experienced doctor.
- Flushing of the ventricular catheter should only be performed by the medical staff.
- During therapy, the drain is normally elevated rather than clamped to prevent over-drainage.
- The confused and agitated patient will require increased supervision or 1:1 nursing care to avoid inadvertent removal (sedation may be indicated in some cases).
- The patient and carers should have an opportunity to discuss the rationale and progress of the CSF drainage system.

CSF sampling
- CSF sampling is collected under strict aseptic technique.
- 2ml of CSF should be sent for culture, gram stain, cell count, glucose and protein as per local protocols.
- Ensure that the drainage system has not been left clamped off accidentally following sampling.

Transfer of patients
The drain should be clamped for the minimal amount of time required and then re-zeroed and unclamped as soon as possible.

The drip chamber must be emptied prior to laying the system horizontally on the bed to prevent blocking of the hydrophobic filter with fluid.

Removal
The incidence of catheter-related infection increases significantly after five days *in situ*.

Drains are removed as soon as clinically indicated—wound site may requiring minor suturing.

Further information for health professionals and the public
Woodward S., Addison C., Shah S., Brennan F., MacLead A., and Clements M. (2002) Benchmarking best practice for external ventricular drainage. *British Journal of Nursing* 11(1): 47–53.

Traumatic brain injury

Traumatic brain injury (TBI), occurs when a sudden or violent trauma causes damage to the brain.

The damage may be localized (confined to one area of the brain), or more diffuse, spreading throughout the brain. TBI may present as a *closed head injury,* when the head violently hits an object but the skull remains intact, or as a *penetrating/open head injury* when the skull is fractured and brain tissue is exposed (📖 see p 132).

Classification

Symptoms of a TBI can be mild, moderate, or severe, depending on the extent of the damage to the brain

Severity
- Mild GCS 13–15
- Moderate GCS 9–12
- Severe GCS 3–8

Some symptoms will be immediately obvious, while other symptoms may take several days or even weeks to become apparent.

Clinical features

Mild TBI symptoms include
- Headache
- Confusion and disorientation
- Fatigue and lethargy
- Insomnia
- Behavioural and mood swings
- ↓ Concentration
- Short-term memory difficulties
- Dizziness, and tinnitus
- Blurred vision

Moderate TBI symptoms include
- Persistent headache (post-concussion syndrome)
- Vomiting or nausea
- Seizures
- Lack of coordination
- Varying level of confusion
- Young children may be difficult to console or to be reassured

Severe TBI symptoms include
- Fluctuating levels of consciousness
- Focal neurological deficits
- Pupil changes—decreased light reaction, impaired eye movement
- Physiological signs and symptoms of ↑ICP. (Cushings triad—↑blood pressure, bradycardia, changing respiratory pattern—**very late signs**)

Indications for urgent CT scan
- Deteriorating GCS.
- Loss of motor function—abnormal posturing.
- Epileptic seizures.
- CSF rhinorrhoea or otorrhoea.

- Basal skull fracture—'battle' signs (bruising behind the ears) or 'panda eyes' (orbital swelling).
- Possible penetrating injury.
- Difficulties performing an accurate assessment due to alcohol or substance abuse.

Causes and risk factors for TBI

- Road traffic accidents.
- Trips and falls, particularly in the elderly.
- Assaults.
- Sports injuries.
- At least half of TBI incidents involve alcohol or substance abuse.

Types of TBI

- 'Concussion'—a short period of unconsciousness.
- Depressed skull fracture.
- Contusions—necrosis and oedema.
- Diffuse axonal injury—caused by shearing forces and damage to neurons and axons.
- Haematomas—extradural, subdural and intracerebral haematomas.
- Hypoxic injuries—post cardiac arrest, head and neck injuries, asphyxia.

Causes and types of head injury

Head injury refers to any trauma to the head, and most specifically to the brain itself. Injuries range from very minor to potentially fatal. Outcome following head injury depends upon the initial severity of the injury and the subsequent developing complications.

Causes

- Trauma is the leading cause of death for people under the age of 45
- In the UK approximately 1,500 per 100,000 attend A&E with a head injury (2007).
- The incidence of disability in adults following head injury is very high:
  - Road traffic accidents 40–50%
  - Domestic/individual accidents 20–30%
  - Sports and recreational injury 10%
  - Assaults 10%

Primary injury

Irreversible, structural, and functional damage sustained at the moment of injury. Contusions, lacerations and diffuse axonal injuries adversely damage the neurons that are particularly susceptible to the effects of hypoxia and hypoperfusion.

Secondary injury

Results from delayed complicating factors that may occur minutes or hours after the initial injury, e.g.

- Haematomas
- ↑ ICP
- Cerebral oedema
- Hydrocephalus
- Infection
- Epilepsy and seizure activity
- ↓ Cerebral perfusion
- Systemic hypotension
- Pyrexia
- Electrolyte derangement
- Hypoxia and hypercarbia

Types of injury

1. Blunt Injuries

- Coup—directly under the area of impact, e.g. from a club.
  - Disrupts the blood–brain barrier with loss of autoregulation and development of vasogenic oedema.
- Acceleration/deceleration—damage inflicted at the opposite side of the brain to the direct impact (contra-coup). Produced by the movement of the brain occurring at different rates within the skull following a sudden impact.
  - Brain damage tends to be diffuse.
  - Contusions and lacerations.
  - Rotation of the axons.
  - Lateral flexion and hyperextension causes shearing of axons.

- The initial appearance of the CT scan frequently underestimates the extent of the brain injury and repeat CT scanning is required.

2. Skull fractures
- Tend to be linear.
- May cross vascular lines.
- May be compound.

3. Crush or compression injuries
- Diffuse damage across the hemispheres.
- Severe cerebral oedema.

4. Sharp/penetrating
- E.g. from knives, screwdrivers, scissors.
- High risks of infection—clinical meningitis, abscess.

5. High-velocity injury
- Gunshot wounds—damage depends on the size, shape and velocity of the bullet and the structures involved.
- High risk of necrosis, contusions, oedema, infection, abscesses.

6. Scalp
- Abrasions.
- Contusions.
- Haematoma.

Skull fractures and haematomas

Skull fractures

Involve the bone surrounding the brain or other structures within the skull. They frequently cross vascular lines resulting in extensive bleeding and trauma. Skull X-rays will quickly highlight any boney fractures, particularly if CT scanning is unavailable.

Linear skull fracture
- A simple break in the skull that usually follows a straight line.
- May occur following a relatively minor head injury, frequently involving the frontal/temporal bone where the bone is much thinner.
- May not be a serious injury, providing the underlying brain is not compromised.
- A common injury, especially in children.

Depressed skull fracture
- Occurs following direct force with a blunt object.
- Fractures that extend below the skull line are usually surgically elevated for cosmetic reasons and to reduce the possibility of developing epilepsy.
- May be comminuted with tearing of the scalp and dura.

Basal skull fracture
- A serious fracture frequently occurring as a result of a severe blunt head injury.
- May arise from extension of a linear fracture into the anterior and middle fossa.
- Surgery is not always indicated unless CSF continues to leak out or air enters the brain causing compression and ↑ICP (dural repair) or other injuries are suspected.
- Avoid inserting a nasogastric tube (pass an orogastric tube if tolerated).
- CSF leaks may spontaneously heal within 7–10 days.

Signs and symptoms of a skull fracture
- Inadequate history from the patient or witnesses.
- Loss of consciousness or amnesia.
- Fluctuating level of consciousness.
- Nausea and vomiting.
- Extensive scalp laceration.
- Palpable 'boggy' swelling under the scalp.
- CSF or blood leakage from the nose or ear.
- Periorbital bruising (panda eyes), bruising behind the ear (Battle, signs).
- Facial palsy and hearing loss from local nerve compression or damage.

Complications
- Rhinorrhoea—CSF leakage from the nose.
- Otorrhoea—CSF leakage from the ear.
- Infection—abscess, meningitis, osteomyelitis.
- Carotid-cavernous sinus compression or fistula formation.

Haematomas

Extradural haematoma (EDH)

- Arterial bleeding between the dura mater and the inner aspect of the skull, frequently occurring when the posterior branch of the middle meningeal artery is severed.
- Most commonly affects the temporal–parietal region of the brain.
- Strips the dura away from the skull, appears on CT as a biconvex lesion. Around 75% are associated with skull fractures.
- Typically occurs following a relatively minor injury, followed by a lucid interval of up to 36 hours delay before the onset of symptoms.

Acute subdural haematoma (ASDH)

- An acute arterial or venous bleed from cortical vessels lying between the brain and the dura mater.
- Occurs after a significant high impact injury such as road traffic accident (RTA) or fall.
- Frequently there is an immediate loss of consciousness with developing neurological deficits.
- Rarely, may take up to 48 hours to develop.

Sub-acute subdural haematoma (SASDH)

- May develop from an underlying contusion.
- May take 48 hours to 2–3 weeks to develop.

Chronic subdural haematoma (CSDH)

- Stretching and tearing of 'bridging veins' between the brain and dura mater.
- Chronic subdural haematomas develop more slowly after a moderate or minor head injury.
- Presents more frequently in the elderly where the bridging veins are more fragile and stretched.
- There is a progressive decline in Glasgow Coma Score over weeks or months following the initial injury (e.g. forgetfulness, confusion and incontinence).

Intracerebral haematoma (ICH)

- Describes bleeding into the actual brain tissue itself.
- Develops from major contusions or vascular injuries.
- May also occur spontaneously, secondary to hypertension, tumours, coagulopathy or ruptured aneurysms.
- Small haematomas are managed conservatively; however larger haematomas usually require surgical removal.

Traumatic subarachnoid haemorrhage

- Following a severe head injury, blood breaches the ventricular system.
- Severe subarachnoid haemorrhage or ICH.

Emergency and acute management

Initial management—primary survey

Airway

Always identify the potential for cervical spine injury and maintain the spine in a safe neutral position until clinical examination and radiological findings exclude injury.

- Assess and protect the airway:
  - Examine airway with suction.
  - Chin lift or jaw thrust.
  - Naso/oropharyngeal airway.
  - Intubation.
- Intubate and ventilate if:
  - Airway or breathing compromised.
  - High risk of aspiration.
  - GCS <9.
  - Severe maxillofacial injuries.
- Maintain normothermia

Breathing

- Assess the chest—look, listen and feel.
- Oxygenate—100% oxygen at 15l/min.
- Caution—tension pneumothorax, haemothorax, flail chest, tamponade.

Circulation

- Control excessive external bleeding.
- Assess skin colour, temperature and capillary refill.
- Observe for enlarged neck veins, pulse rate and character.
- Monitor blood pressure.
- Insert at least two large bore (>16g) IV cannulae.
- Fluid management—isotonic saline.
- Cardiac monitoring, O_2 saturation.

Disability

- Baseline neurological assessment using GCS scoring (📖 see p 64).
- Pupil response—equal and reacting briskly.
- Changes in level of consciousness or further neurological deterioration.

Exposure

- Thorough examination.
- Medical history—mechanism of injury.

Proceed to secondary survey after:

- Primary survey completed.
- Reassess ABCDE.

Acute care

Airway

- Maintain a patent airway and adequate oxygenation.
- Agitated, uncooperative patients may require elective ventilation for CT scanning.

Breathing
- Maintain PaO_2 > 12kPa.
- Maintain $PaCO_2$—4.3—4.7 kPa.
- Jugular bulb venous saturation monitoring (SjO_2) if available.

Circulation
- Fluids replacement.
- Routine bloods (FBC, glucose, biochemistry, cross match, toxicology).
- Maintain a mean arterial blood pressure at more than 90mmHg to reduce adverse effect of hypotension and maintain an adequate CPP.

Disability
- Cervical fractures—apply inline immobilization and rigid collar.
- Monitor ICP—aim to maintain ICP <20mmHg and opitimise cerebral perfusion pressure >60mmHg. (CPP = MAP–ICP) (📖 see p 358).
- Support blood pressure with vasoactive drugs if necessary.
- Administer mannitol 0.5g/kg over 15 minutes depending on CPP measurements (monitor plasma osmolarity levels).
- GCS observations.
- Observe pupillary reflexes.
- Assess limb function.
- Observe for signs of cerebral herniation and ↑ICP.
- Refer to neurosurgical unit.

Adjuncts to assessment
- Chest and pelvic X-rays.
- Ultrasound.
- Arterial blood gas analysis.
- Urinary catheters—monitor urine output.
- Nasogastric tube—unless contraindicated, e.g. basal skull fracture.

Further information for health professionals and the public

NICE (2007). *Triage, assessment, investigation and early management of head injury in infants, children and adults.* NICE, London.

Nutrition in head injury

The commencement of early nutritional support together with ongoing monitoring of nutritional status is seen as a high priority for management of head injured patients. Failure to instigate an adequate feeding regime within 48 to 72 hours following the injury will increase the risk of developing a range of complications, resulting in longer hospital admissions and poorer outcomes:

- Degeneration of the mucosal lining in the intestines.
- Skeletal muscle mass atrophy.
- Hypercatabolism causing protein depletion.
- Bacterial translocation (movement of bacteria or endotoxins across the intestinal epithelium precipitating sepsis and nosocomial pneumonia).
- Immunosuppression and poor wound healing.
- increased risk of multi-organ failure.

Physiology

- Nitrogen is the major component of amino acids (essential for the production of protein in the body).
- One gram of nitrogen provides 6.25 grams of protein creating 30 grams of lean body mass.
- A patient requires an average of 25–35kcal/kg/day of ideal body weight and 1.5–2.5g/kg/day for protein, calculated as: 1.0g–2.5g protein/kg/day depending upon the type and stage of patients condition.
- Most serum nitrogen is carried as ammonia (NH^3) and converted in the liver to urea i.e. blood urea nitrogen (BUN).
- Metabolic rate represents the energy produced by all normal activity and chemical reactions (measured in calories—Kcal).
- Basal metabolic rate (BMR), can be 60–90% of the total metabolic rate and is the energy consumed by the body at rest to maintain essential activities, calculated by number of calories used each hour per kilogram of body weight.
- Surface area, muscle mass and pyrexia increases BMR.
- A combination of all these measurements are used to assess the possible risk of developing subsequent complications.
- Serious trauma triggers a stress response resulting in hypercatabolism, hypermetabolism and increased nutritional demands, (severe protein and calorie malnutrition).
- It has been estimated that 5–10% weight loss over a month or 10–20% over 6 months is associated with increased complications.

Delays in feeding may be attributed to:

- Intubation and ventilation.
- Confusion.
- Cranial nerve involvement ↓ swallow and cough reflex → dysphagia.
- Difficulties placing a nasogastric tube.
- Poor patient tolerance of NG or orogastric tube.
- Diarrhoea, nausea and vomiting.
- Impaired renal function.
- Restricted fluid intake.
- Fasting prior to procedures or investigations.
- Refeeding syndrome.

Management strategies

- The dietitian will recommend the most appropriate feeding regime and nutritional goals, taking into consideration dietary history, food allergies or preferences, premorbid physical condition and weight history e.g. recent intentional weight loss and current physical condition.
- Patient weight and BMI should be recorded weekly unless there is severe fluid retention.
- All biochemical markers should be monitored including serum calcium, potassium, phosphorus, blood urea, nitrogen, and creatinine.
- Maintain an accurate recording of fluid intake and output.
- Ryles tube should be replaced by a fine bore tube to aid comfort as soon as critical condition improves.
- Nutritional requirements vary considerably depending upon the patient's physical build, current and past physical condition and age.
- Feed should be commenced at 30ml/hr full strength feed for 4hrs gradually increased as tolerated until target rate is achieved.
- It is important not to reduce or discontinue feeding unless aspirate volume >200ml.
- If large aspirates continue, commence metoclopromide and/or erythromycin. Jejunal tube feeding may also help improve absorption.
- Parenteral nutrition should be considered if there are delays in enteral feeding or where there are problems with the gastrointestinal tract, e.g. bowel obstruction, ileus or malabsorption.
- Consider inserting a percutaneous endoscopic gastrostomy tube for maintaining prolonged enteral feeding.
- Over-feeding may precipitate hyperglycaema, hypokalaemia or fatty liver degeneration.
- Phenytoin binds to protein resulting in decreased absorption of the drug—carefully monitor levels. Requires a 2-hour feed break before and after administration, unless given intravenously.

Complications associated with enteral feeding

- Misplacement of feeding tube.
- Tube migration for patients with basal skull fractures.
- Regurgitation and aspiration of gastric contents into the lungs.
- Nausea and vomiting.
- Diarrhoea—may be due to large volume feed, bolus feeding, high osmolality, antibiotic therapy, fibre content of feed or bacterial infection.
- Constipation.
- Electrolyte imbalance.
- Hyperglycaemia, hypoglycaemia—affected by feed rate and length of feed breaks.

Further information for health professionals and the public

Mestecky A. (2006) Metabolic responses after severe head injury and how to optimise nutrition: a literature review. *British Journal of Neuroscience Nursing* 2(2): 73–79.

Prognosis and rehabilitation

Clinical features and outcome

Disabilities resulting from head injury depend upon a number of factors:
- Age of the patient.
- Pre-existing illness or disease.
- Severity and location of the injury.
- GCS following primary injury.
- Period of hypoxia or hypotension (<90 systolic), immediately post-injury.
- Length of time of post-traumatic amnesia (PTA)—impaired memory of events that occurred following the injury, is a useful indicator of potential recovery.
- Early intervention linked to rehabilitation by the multidisciplinary team or care in a specialist rehabilitation team.

Post-traumatic amnesia
- Very mild, <5min.
- Mild, 5–60min.
- Moderate, 1–24 hours.
- Severe, 1–7 days.
- Very severe, 1–4 weeks.
- Extremely severe > 4 weeks.

Glasgow Coma outcome chart	
Good outcome	Minimal disabling sequelae but returns to independent functioning and to full time job comparable to pre-injury level.
Moderate disability	Capable of independent functioning but not returned to independent functioning.
Severe disability	Dependent on others for some aspects of daily living
Persistent	No obvious cortical function.
Vegetative state Dead	

Jennett (1975)

Rehabilitation

- Disabilities present as physical, behavioural, cognitive or psychological problems.
- Rehabilitation is a major part of the recovery process, although access to specialized units is extremely limited.
- The primary aim is to improve the patient's functional abilities and optimise their quality of life.
- Rehabilitation therapy begins from the moment the patient is taken off the ventilator in the critical care unit.

- Rehabilitation programmes must be tailored to meet the individual needs of the patient and may include a package of care for support in the home, inpatient or outpatient treatment or supportive living programmes.
- Programmes must use the knowledge and skills of the multidisciplinary team—nurses, physiotherapy, occupational therapy, speech and language therapy, psychiatry, psychologists, and social workers.
- Recovery from cognitive deficits is greatest within the first 6 months after the injury.
- Involve the family/carers in all decision-making processes.
- Referral to third sector voluntary organizations.

Complications

Table 9.1 Immediate or short-term complications

Intracranial haemorrhage	Miscellaneous:
Cerebral oedema	dural tears
	fat emboli
Infection:	carotid cavernous fistula
meningitis	skull defects
abscess	aerocoele
osteomyelitis	carotid dissection
subdural empyema	traumatic aneurysm
Epilepsy	Post-concussion headache
Hydrocephalus	
Cranial nerve deficits:	
olfactory	
trigeminal	
facial	

Reference

Jennet, B., Bond, MR. (1975) Assessment of outcome in severe brain damage: a practical scale. *Lancet* 1, 480–484.

Table 9.2 Long-term complications

Diffuse brain damage	Aggression
Focal brain damage	Cognitive disabilities
Personality changes	Inability to cope with pressures
Poor short-term memory and inability to form new ones	Lack of inhibitions
Problems performing executive functions, e.g. planning, organizing, abstract reasoning, problem-solving, and making judgements	Social inappropriateness
Lack of concentration and reasoning	Epilepsy
Tiredness	Difficulties with coordination
Depression and anxiety	Language and communication difficulties
Moodiness	Lack or excessive sexual drive
	Unrealistic about capabilities
	Sensory problems—vision, hearing, smell, taste, or touch
	Headaches

Other long-term problems associated with a TBI

Development of long-term chronic illness later in life—Alzheimer's disease (AD), Parkinson's disease and other movement disorders, dementia (chronic traumatic encephalopathy), more common in sportsmen.

Further information for health professionals and the public

Jennet, B. and Bond, M. (1973) Assessment of outcome after severe brain damage. *Lancet*, 1: 480–4.

Wade, D. and Halligan, P.W. (2007) Social roles and long-term illness: is it time to rehabilitate convalescence? *Clinical Rehabilitation*, 21: 291–8.

Subarachnoid haemorrhage

A subarachnoid haemorrhage (SAH) involves bleeding into the space between the arachnoid mater and the surface of the brain. It is one of the few lesions capable of causing sudden death in otherwise healthy people.

Most prevalent in ages 40–60 years. Occurs in approximately 1:10,000 population/year. Not a true diagnosis but a symptom of an underlying pathology.

Aetiology

- Berry or saccular aneurysms—due to maldevelopment of the media in the cerebral arterial bifurcation where the muscular coat is incomplete
- Traumatic aneurysms—associated with penetrating head injuries, skull fractures.
- Infectious cerebral aneurysms (endocarditis with septic embolisms, vasculitis or cardiac valve disease).
- Blood disorders—anticoagulant therapy, anti-platelet drugs.
- Arteriovenous malformations (AVM)—congenital knot of blood vessels within the capillary network.

Location of aneurysms

- 40–60%—anterior circulation of the Circle of Willis (internal carotid artery, anterior cerebral and communicating arteries).
- 20–30%—middle cerebral aneurysms.
- 10–15%—posterior circulation (vertebral and basilar arteries).
- 15% of aneurysms are multiple.

Contributory factors

- Cigarette smoking.
- Alcohol.
- Substance abuse.
- Hypertension.

Clinical presentation

- Headache—violent, sudden and severe.
- Nausea and vomiting.
- Altered level of consciousness—varies from mild confusion to completely unresponsive.
- Meningeal irritation—neck stiffness and photophobia.
- Nuchal rigidity and a positive Kernig's sign.
- Seizure activity.
- Focal neurological signs—hemiplegia, dysphasia.
- Signs of ↑ ICP.
- 3rd nerve palsy in association with posterior communicating artery or superior cerebellar artery aneurysm.
- Hypothalamic disturbance—pyrexia.

Size
Microscopic, <1 cm; large, 1–2.5 cm; giant, >3 cm

Table 9.3 WFNS scale for grading SAH

Grade/class	GCS score	Deficit
0	15	Unruptured aneurysm.
1	15	Asymptomatic or patient has a mild headache and neck stiffness.
2	14–13	Moderate to severe headache, nuchal rigidity, may have oculomotor palsy—patient is awake and alert.
3	14–13	Drowsy and confused, frequently mild focal signs.
4	12–7	Stupor, moderate to severe neurological deficits.
5	6–3	Deep coma, moribund and/or extensor posturing.

Diagnosis
- Clinical presentation and history (strong index of suspicion).
- CT scans—blood in the Sylvian fissure, interhemispheric fissure, basal cisterns.
- Lumbar puncture (only performed if CT negative), shows uniform blood staining of CSF or evidence of xanthochromia.
- CSF spectrophotometry for bilirubin and oxyhaemoglobin levels (chemical gold standard).
- Cerebral angiography.

Treatment options
- Direct approach—surgical clipping involves a craniotomy and the placement of a titanium clip across the neck of the aneurysm.
- Indirect approach—aneuryms embolized endovascularly with platinum coils.
- Conservative, supportive management.

Complications (☐ See Chapter 6, p 146)
- Intracerebral or subdural haematomas
- Vasospasm
- Loss of autoregulation
- Communicating hydrocephalus
- Electrolyte imbalance
- Cerebral oedema
- Neurological disability due to infarction and ischemia
- Seizures
- Rebleeding—associated high mortality

Prognosis
- The lower the GCS on presentation, the worse the prognosis.
- Risk of re-bleeding is highest during the first 30 days post initial bleed.
- One-third of survivors will remain dependent on carers.

Subarachnoid haemorrhage: surgical management

Initial management

Emergency evacuation of a subdural or intracerebral haematoma is sometimes indicated to reduce immediate pressure effects, depending on the location of the bleed, age and premorbid condition of the patient.

Blood pressure control—systemic hypertension should not be actively treated unless severe (systolic pressure >220–230mmHg).

Subsequent management

- Treatment options depend on the location, size and shape of the aneurysm, and the presence of any thrombus.
- Endovascular treatment has developed as an important first line treatment for cerebral aneurysm.
- Surgical clipping involves a craniotomy, the dissection of the blood vessel to visualize the sac and the placement of a titanium clip across the neck of the aneurysm.
- Surgery may be indicated following:
  - Failed endovascular therapy.
  - May be partially clipped to reduce the size or shape of the aneurysm so that is more suitable for endovascular treatment.
  - Removal of a local haematoma may help to reduce subsequent vasospasm.

Timing of surgery

The timing of surgery is controversial and is dictated by:
- Clinical grade of the patient.
- Underlying medical pathology.
- Available resources—specialist neurosurgeons.
- Technical factors—bypass techniques
- Surgical risk is higher in the intra and post-operative period due to risk of premature rupture and development of vasospasm.
- Delays in treatment reduces the risk factors, but increases the risk of rebleed which is highest during the first 14 days.

Surgical adjuncts

- Wide variation in the angles, sizes and shapes of clips available.
- Skull-based surgery may optimise visualization of the aneurysm.
- Extracranial–intracranial bypass technique (EC–IC), end to end anastamosis of the artery.
- Deep hypothermic circulatory arrest refers to two techniques reserved for technically difficult aneurysm. Hypothermia attempts to reduce the metabolic rate of oxygen ($CMRO_2$) to the brain to provide cerebral protection. Cardiac standstill is used to reduce the tension within the aneurysm intraoperatively by placing the patient on cardio-pulmonary bypass or very rarely pharmacologically through administration of short-acting adenosine that induces a profound hypotension, (both carry significant risks).

- Angiography and microvascular dopplers may be used during the procedure to confirm cerebral perfusion and security of the clip.
- The application of temporary clips placed either side of the aneurysm can reduce catastrophic bleeding during placement of the clip.
- Aneurysm may be wrapped in gauze, providing additional support to the arterial wall—rarely used.
- Multiple aneurysms—priority given to the aneurysm that has bled, two aneurysms on same side may be clipped simultaneously but usually a further craniotomy is arranged for a later date.
- Surgery may be indicated as an adjunct following failed or incomplete coiling (📖 see p 306).

Complications
- Raised intracranial pressure and cerebral oedema (📖 see Rising intracranial pressure and coning, p 132).
- Intracerebral and subdural haematomas.
- Re-bleeding with significant risk of mortality.
- Acute obstructive hydrocephalus due to blood in CSF.
- Loss of autoregulation and maintenance of cerebral perfusion pressure.
- Vasospasm in >40% of patients, 4–12 days following initial bleed.
- Hyponatraemia and inappropriate anti-diuretic hormone (ADH) secretion.
- Hypovolaemia.
- Seizure activity.
- Neurological disability due to infarction and ischaemia.

Subarachnoid haemorrhage: nursing management

Priorities of care
- Provide psychological support to the patient, relatives, and carers.
- Give information and explanations in a timely manner.
- Provide adequate pain control.
- Maintain adequate cerebral perfusion to prevent secondary brain injury.
- Glasgow Coma Scale observations to detect signs of deterioration.
- Maintain normal electrolyte values.
- Manage neurological complications promptly and effectively.

General management

Airway and cardiovascular management
- Oxygen saturation 95–100%. PaO_2—>14.0kPa
- Carbon dioxide levels maintained within acceptable limits 4.3–5.0kPa
- $PaCO_2$ <3.5 will trigger vasoconstriction leading to ischaemia.
- Cardiac monitoring—common arrhythmias may include ST changes, prolonged Q-T interval and elevated T waves.

Neurological assessment
- Consistent, repeated Glasgow Coma Scale observations.
- Full neurological assessment including: level of consciousness, pupil reaction, cranial nerve involvement, limb assessment.
- Vital signs—hypotension and bradycardia. Trends and fluctuations in blood pressure and pulse might indicate development of vasospasm.
- Observe for signs and symptoms of hydrocephalus—↓ level of consciousness, ↑ headache, pronator drift.
- Manage effects of neurological deficits—both physiological and psychological and refer to therapists, neuropsychologists.

Positioning
- Maintain bed rest, ideally in a quiet or darkened area of the ward.
- Raise head of bed to 15–30° angle to maximize cerebral venous drainage.
- Routine nursing care including frequent repositioning to reduce complications of prolonged bed rest.
- Avoid extreme neck flexion, extension or rotation that may restrict venous drainage.
- Prophylactic DVT therapy (anti-embolic stockings, sequential compression boots).

Medication
- Anti-thrombotic agents once the aneurysm has been secured.
- Analgesia—codeine phosphate oral, IM or subcutaneously, ± paracetamol.
- Opiates may affect pupil size, ↓LOC, ↓respiratory rate.
- Nimodipine 60 mg, 4-hourly or intravenously 0.02% in 50ml at 5–10ml/hr via a central line.

- Anticonvulsant therapy—may be prescribed prophylactically—
  e.g. phenytoin loading dose of 15mg/kg to control seizure activity.

Core temperature
- Exclude all contributory causes of pyrexia, i.e. chest infection, indwelling urinary catheter, invasive lines.
- Control pyrexia—paracetamol, active cooling measures (there is a 10% increase in O_2 consumption for every $1°$ celsius rise in temperature).

Fluid management
- Maintain an accurate fluid record.
- Maintain adequate perfusion and hydration (approx 2.5–3.5 litres), allowing for insensible loss from pyrexia, vomiting.
- Isotonic saline is recommended to maintain sodium levels (if less than 125 mmol/L 1.8 or 3% saline may occasionally be prescribed.
- The use of glucose is contraindicated (precipitates acidosis that may trigger infarction and ischaemia).
- Monitor blood electrolyte levels (observe for hyponatremia, cerebral salt wasting or hyperglycaemia).
- Record hourly urine output—large volumes of dilute urine may be a symptom of diabetes insipidus (low urine osmolarity in the presence of low serum osmolarity).

Nutrition
- Commence oral or enteral nutritional support as soon as practicable.
- Monitor blood glucose values—consider commencing sliding scale insulin.

Psychological support
- Provide opportunity for patients and relatives to discuss results of investigations and proposed management plan.
- Try to offer reassurance and allay patient's anxieties.
- Early commencement of discharge planning.
- Involve family and carers in future arrangements, preparing them for the management of potential complex health care needs.
- Refer to specialist rehabilitation services.

Interventional radiology coil embolization

Involves insertion of a catheter into the femoral artery. Tiny electrical detachable platinum coils are threaded through the catheter and positioned into the aneurysm, preventing blood flow into the sac.

The numbers of patients referred for interventional radiology increased following the ISAT trial (2001) that compared survival rates and quality of life for two treatments following subarachnoid haemorrhage—neurosurgical clipping and endovascular coiling.

The study found that in patients equally suited for both treatment options, endovascular coiling produced significantly better patient outcomes in terms of survival and reduced levels of disability at one year.

The relative risk of death or significant disability at one year for patients treated with coils was significantly lower than in surgically treated patients.

- Average hospital stay is often twice as long following surgery compared with coiling.
- Recovery time for non-invasive techniques is considerably less (12 months compared with average of 27 days).
- Less invasive and avoids the need for head shaving.
- Surgery still required for complex aneurysms not suited to endovascular therapy.

Choice of treatment depends upon:
- Age of the patient.
- Size and shape of the aneurysm.
- Location of the aneurysm.
- Neurological condition of the patient.
- Previous medical history.

Investigations
- CTA and magnetic resonance angiography (MRA) now provide rapid accurate images of the aneurysm.
- Catheter angiography confirms diagnosis and enables therapeutic procedures.

Priorities of post-procedure care
- Careful monitoring of vital signs
- Glasgow Coma Scale observations
- Observe for signs and symptoms of ischaemia and vasospasm (headache, photophobia, vomiting, ↓ level of consciousness and confusion).
- Instigate triple H therapy (hypervolaemia, haemodilution and hypertension) for vasospasm.
- Monitor puncture site in the groin for haematomas or bleeding.
- Check pedal pulse to ensure adequate perfusion.
- Monitor for signs of abdominal pain, ↓ BP, ↓ haemocrit, that may be an indication of internal bleeding.

Future considerations
- Different types and techniques of coiling are evolving but long-term complications are not yet evident.
- Insufficient data yet to support surgery versus coiling in poor grade patients.

Further information for health professionals and the public

Mitchell *et al.* (2008) Could late rebleeding overturn the superiority of cranial aneurysm embolization over clip ligation seen in the International Subarachnoid Aneurysm Trial? *J Neurosurgery*, 108; 437–22.

Cerebral vasospasm and complications

Vasospasm refers to a sudden decrease in the internal diameter of a blood vessel due to contraction of smooth muscle within the vessel, decreasing the blood flow in the parent vessel and its branches.

Signs and symptoms

- Pyrexia.
- Headache.
- Neck stiffness.
- Fluctuating level of consciousness throughout the day identified in changes in GCS observations.
- Varying levels of confusion.
- Focal neurological signs.
- 50% of patients will be asymptomatic.
- Reduced vessel diameter on angiography.
- ↑ White cell count.
- Labile BP

Incidence

Occurs in 40–70% of patients, 4–12 days after the initial haemorrhage.

Diagnosis

- Clinically obvious neurological signs and symptoms.
- Radiology—identified on angiography, transcranial doppler (TCD).
- CTA/MRA scan.
- Scans will exclude hydrocephalus, oedema or a further bleed.

Treatment options

Surgical

Removal of the blood clot surrounding the aneurysm may help to reduce the incidence of vasospasm.

Pharmacological

Nimodipine—a calcium channel blocking agent—60mg 4-hrly. Decreases the rate of development of vasospasm by 25%, preventing the entry of calcium ions into the vascular muscle cells in the cerebral arteries.

Medical

Triple H therapy—hypertension, hypervolaemia, haemodilution.

- **Hypertension**—increases blood pressure, blood flow and cerebral perfusion pressure.
  - Fluid volume—maintain normovolaemia with isotonic saline.
  - Administer colloids such as dextran and modified gelatin to improve blood flow and viscosity.
  - Vasoactive drugs to induce hypertension (only when fluid volume has been replaced) and used with caution in unsecured aneurysms.
- **Hypervolaemia**—Increases central venous and arterial pressure, increasing cerebral perfusion pressure and collateral blood flow.
  - Increase systemic volume—minimum of 3L/24hrs.

- Maintain systolic blood pressure—160–180 mmHg, or at least 30mmHg greater than patients baseline, (MAP between 105–120mmHg.)
- Maintain central venous pressure at 8–10mmHg.
- **Haemodilution**—Increased fluid volume improves cerebral perfusion and reduces adverse effects of erythrocyte aggregation in smaller vessels (least important component of triple H therapy).
  - Administer isotonic saline if Na > 125mmols/L.
  - Hypertonic saline 1.8% or 3% may be useful in mild hyponatremia.
  - Avoid glucose solutions—↑ metabolic acidosis.
  - Aim for haemocrit level of 30–33%.

Respiratory
- Maintain good oxygenation and normal arterial blood gas values.
- Elective ventilation if respiratory function inadequate.
- Avoid over-sedation.

Cardiovascular
- Administration of IV fluids to maintain normal electrolyte level.
- Routine blood monitoring—at least daily.
- Cardiac monitoring—observe for ECG changes (ST depression, inverted T waves, prolonged QT intervals).

Neurological
- Control of seizures.
- Record Glasgow Coma Scale observations.
- Observe for signs of vasospasm.
- Record vital signs—signs of ↑ ICP, bradycardia and widened pulse pressure.
- Administer nimodipine (60mg 4-hrly or 0.02% in 50mL).

Complications
- Associated with high levels of mortality and morbidity.
- Cerebral ischaemia and infarction.
- Exacerbation of existing neurological deficits.

Further information for health professionals and the public

Mestecky A. (2005) Modes of treatment for cerebral vasospasm following aneurysmal subarachnoid haemorrhage. *British Journal of Neuroscience Nursing* 1(1): 20–28.

Intracranial tumours

A large number of brain tumours arise from the brain paranchyma, largely from the glial supporting cells, i.e. astrocytes, oligodendrocytes, ependymal or microglial cells. Primary tumours affecting neuronal tissue are rare. Other tumours grow from the meningeal layers, embryonic tissue or metastatic lesions primarily from the lungs, breast, kidneys, prostate and melanoma.

The diagnosis of brain tumours has improved significantly over recent years, largely due to improved neuroimaging techniques and greater access to specialist neuroscience units.

Common signs and symptoms of a brain tumour

- Patients with brain tumours typically develop neurological signs and symptoms over a period of weeks or months.
- Patients may complain of symptoms such as chronic seizure activity for years prior to diagnosis or onset may be very sudden.
- Symptoms result from increased intracranial pressure, tumour invasion and infiltration, hydrocephalus, visual field loss, sensory or motor disturbance or increase in endocrine activity.
- Symptoms may be generalized, localized or referred from other areas.

Headache (📖 see also p 216)

- Although headache is a common symptom of a brain tumour, many patients are asymptomatic.
- New, persistent headache in patients >40 years old should be investigated.
- Headache can be non-specific, occurring in patients with or without raised ICP. Typically the headache may be:
  - Worse on waking, improving over the course of the day.
  - Exacerbated by coughing, sneezing or bending.
  - Accompanied by nausea and vomiting.

Generalized signs and symptoms

- Dizziness and tinnitus.
- Papilloedema may be identified as an incidental finding.
- Confusion and short-term memory disturbance.
- Behavioral or personality changes

Localizing signs

- Seizures—occur in up to one-third of patients.
- Focal neurological signs—depend upon the site of the lesion, hemiparesis, aphasia, visual field loss and sensory changes.
- Localized neurological symptoms, i.e. leg weakness, dysphasia.
- Cranial nerves dysfunction, particularly involving I, III, IV, VI VIII
- Cerebellar signs—ataxia, nyastagmus.

Diagnosis

- MRI.
- Specific characteristics identified on scanning may give a good indication of histological diagnosis.

- Functional MRI—allows mapping of the brain to facilitate maximal resection of the lesion.
- CT—Identifies calcified lesions such as meningiomas or oligodendrogliomas.
- PET—a research technique that uses radioactive isotopes (📖 see p 98).

Pathology

Although neuroimaging may be suggestive of a specific diagnosis, ideally biopsy will provide a definite histology.

Results will be reviewed by a multidisciplinary team who consider other factors such as age, previous medical history and quality of life before deciding on a course of treatment.

Treatment

- Stereotactic biopsy—useful for biopsy of deep brain lesions, e.g. pineal tumours.
- Surgery using advanced image-guided navigation systems.
- Decompression of the tumour.
- Complete resection.
- Developments and improvements in technology and equipment over recent years have enabled neurosurgeons to resect lesions that were previously graded as inoperable. In many cases such radical surgical procedures can give patients months and sometimes years of good quality family life. (📖 see Treatments for brain tumours, p 322)
- Radiotherapy.
- Chemotherapy.
- New treatment options.

Supportive care

This element is perhaps the most important aspect when patients have been diagnosed with a brain tumour. Most neuro-oncology units have a clinical nurse specialist who acts as a liaison between the different specialities involved with the patient throughout their treatment pathway. The nurse is an invaluable source of practical information and psychological support to both the patient and their family. Patients are given information, verbal and written, along with contact numbers which the patient or their family can access. Symptom control and psychological support is perhaps the main focus of patient care.

Meningiomas

Meningiomas are brain tumours that develop from the meningeal layers of the brain and account for approximately 15–30% of all brain tumours.

90% of the tumours grow around the cerebral hemispheres, at the base of the skull or around the brainstem. The remaining meningiomas arise in the optic nerve sheath and around the spinal cord.

They most frequently occur in middle-aged or elderly adults and are more common in women than men.

Classification

Classification is based upon their histological appearance, position in the brain and the likelihood of recurrence. Three grades of tumour include:

Grade I or benign meningiomas

Slow-growing tumors that have well-defined borders and do not appear to invade the adjacent normal brain. Due to their low mitotic index, the tumours can grow to a large size over a number of years before they become detected.

Grade II or atypical meningiomas

Contain cells with a higher mitotic index that tend to grow more rapidly. Recurrence relates to degree of surgical resection combined with histological grade.

Grade III or malignant meningiomas

Known as anaplastic meningiomas, these are most likely to recur following initial treatment. Consist of 1 to 3% of all meningiomas.

Prognosis

Low-grade tumours respond well to surgery.

Malignant meningiomas may suffer with recurrence within 2–5 years of initial diagnosis.

Contributory factors

Neurofibromatosis type 2—a rare inherited disease that affects the skin and the nervous system. Patients may develop multiple meningiomas (see p 240).

Previous radiation therapy to the head or spine, particularly childhood cancers.

Associated with changes in female hormones e.g. breast cancer, menopause (hormone replacement therapy [HRT]), pregnancy.

Symptoms

- Depend on the size and location of the meningioma—visual changes, ↓ hearing, subtle changes in personality, motor impairment.
- Seizures—occur in 30–40% of patients.
- Obstructive hydrocephalus

Diagnosis

- MRI or CT.
- Tissue biopsy.

Treatment

- Surgery—resection depends on the size, location and involvement of other structures.
- Local embolization of blood vessels may reduce intra-operative haemorrhage.
- Radiotherapy—may be used in conjunction with partial surgical removal.
- Stereotactic radiosurgery—delivered as a single, high-dose, constricted beam of radiation to the tumour. Used increasingly for smaller lesions.
- Conservative management—older patients may not benefit from surgery, particularly if the lesion is small, the patient has few symptoms or the tumour is slow-growing.

Gliomas

Classification of primary CNS tumours

The pathophysiological classification of CNS tumours is complex and is based on the type of cell from which the tumour originates. Brain tumours are the most common primary CNS malignancy, with spinal cord tumours accounting for only 10–15% of primary tumours.

Gliomas

An umbrella term used to describe primary brain tumours including astrocytomas, oligodendrogliomas and ependymomas, microgliomas/lymphomas. They all arise from the glial or supporting cells within the brain tissue.

Gliomas are classified according to the WHO grading system, according to the malignancy of the cells, and their ability to cause necrotic and haemorrhagic lesions. (Grade 1 is the least malignant, and grade 4 is the worst.)

Astrocytomas

- Astrocytomas account for around 70% of all primary brain tumours. They generally arise within the cerebral hemispheres, but can occur in the spinal cord.
- The incidence of these tumours is approx 2–3 per 100,000 of the population per year.
- Grade 1 and 2 tumours are typically well differentiated, whilst grade 3 and 4 tumours show higher levels of necrosis and vascular changes.
- The most malignant form of glioma is known as a glioblastoma multiforma and is particularly difficult to treat.
- Glioblastomas can present as the primary, or they may be secondary to a low-grade tumour that has transformed to a higher malignancy, in which case the prognosis is generally poor.

Oligodendrogliomas

- Account for approximately 5% of primary brain tumours.
- Produced by the oligodendrocytes in the CNS, responsible for the formation of myelin surrounding the axons.
- They are usually slow-growing tumours, commonly occurring in the frontal/temporal lobes.
- Treatment is with surgical incision. Some oligodendrogliomas have a particular genetic make-up that makes them more sensitive to chemotherapy and therefore they have significantly better prognosis.

Ependymomas

- Arise from the ependymal glial cells, and account for around 6% of all brain tumours.
- They can occur in adults, but are more common in children. They are unusual in that they can spread (via the CSF) to the spinal cord.
- Spinal cord ependymomas account for more than 50% of all primary spinal tumours.

Primary CNS lymphoma

- Account for less than 1% of primary brain tumours and are much more common in immunosuppressed patients, e.g. following organ transplantation or HIV infection.
- Primary treatment is usually with chemotherapy. Radiotherapy may be used as a second line treatment.

Tumour group	Treatment	5-year survival (%)
Low-grade astrocytoma (grade 1 and 2)	Surgery radiotherapy	50–60
High-grade astrocytoma (grade 3 and 4)	All treatments	<5
Oligodendroglioma	Surgery + radiotherapy	56–80
Ependymoma	Surgery + radiotherapy	45–80
Meningioma	Surgery	45–80
CNS lymphoma	All treatments	3

Further information for health professionals and the public

Cancer BACUP (2005) *Understanding brain tumours*. Cancer BACUP.
Abrey, E.L. and Mason, W.P. (2003). *Brain tumors*. FF Fast Facts. Health Press Limited.

Pituitary tumours

The pituitary gland is a small oval-shaped gland at the base of the brain lying underneath the optic chiasm. It is divided into two parts: the anterior and posterior lobes. Tumours are classified by the type of hormones they secrete.

The anterior pituitary produces:
- Growth hormone.
- Prolactin, stimulates the production of milk following childbirth.
- ACTH (adrenocorticotrophic hormone) stimulates production of hormones from the adrenal glands.
- TSH (thyroid-stimulating hormone).
- FSH (follicle-stimulating hormone).
- LH (leuteinizing hormone), stimulate the ovaries and testes.

The posterior pituitary produces:
- ADH (anti-diuretic hormone), reduces the amount of urine excreted by the kidneys.
- Oxytocin, stimulates the contraction of the uterus during childbirth and the production of milk for breastfeeding.

Tumours
- Pituitary adenomas make up nearly 10% of all brain tumours. They are most commonly found in young or middle-aged patients.
- Tumours may be benign or malignant.
- Malignant tumours invade surrounding brain tissue in comparison to benign lesions that have a more local effect.
- Pituitary tumours are either secreting or non-secreting tumours.
- Secreting tumours release excess amounts of hormones, e.g. growth hormone, prolactinoma.

Signs and symptoms
- Caused by direct pressure from the tumour on surrounding tissue or changes in the normal endocrine function.
  - Visual disturbance or bitemporal hemianopia.
  - Endocrine disturbance—amenorhoea, impotence.
  - Growth hormone—gigantism (pre-puberty or closure of epiphyses), acromegaly , hypertension and diabetes.
  - TSH—secreting tumours—disrupts normal metabolism.
  - ACTH-secreting tumours—Cushing's syndrome, weight gain, facial hair, depression.
  - FSH or LH—infertility.
  - Posterior pituitary tumours—diabetes insipidus.

Diagnosis
- CT scan—shows abnormal sella turcica region.
- MRI scan.
- Visual fields.
- Routine bloods and endocrine levels.

Treatment options

Surgery
- Transnasal hypophysectomy—access through the sphenoid sinus into the base of the pituitary gland.
- Craniotomy for larger lesions.

Drug management
- Bromocriptine or cabergoline suppresses the production of prolactin.
- Steroid replacement (hydrocortisone)—essential therapy for hypopituitary patients. Must be commenced pre-operatively and gradually reduced post-operatively following consultation with endocrinologists.

Radiotherapy or stereotactic radiosurgery

Complications
- Pituitary apoplexy—acute onset of ophthalmoplegia, blindness, coma, high mortality rate.
- Electrolyte imbalance.
- Intra-operative complications.
- Haemorrhage.
- Most patients need HRT post-operatively.

Acoustic neuromas

A slow-growing, benign tumour that develops from the lining of the VIII cranial (vestibular cochlear/acoustic) nerve, responsible for balance and hearing.

The acoustic neuroma or Schwannoma arises from the Schwann cells that form the myelin sheath surrounding the nerve.

More common in women than men, aged between 30–60 years old.

Causes
- Unknown.
- Approximately 5% are inherited, called 'Type II neurofibromatosis'
- Affects young people, who may also demonstrate other types of neuromas, particularly on the skin.

Early symptoms
- Tinnitus.
- Gradual loss of hearing.
- Ataxia, vertigo, dizziness.

Late symptoms
- Paraesthesia and facial muscle weakness.
- Hoarseness and dysphagia.
- Hydrocephalus.
- Headaches.
- Signs and symptoms of ↑ICP.

Investigations
- CT scan
- MRI scan
- Audiometry

Treatment
Depends on the size and position of the tumour.
- Conservative management—small, slow-growing tumours may not progress to cause symptoms and therefore require close monitoring.
- Stereotactic radiotherapy—gamma knife, directs high-dose radiation to the tumour, preserving surrounding tissues.
- Surgery—craniotomy, translabyrinth, retrosigmoid and middle fossa approaches can be used.
- Bilateral lesions will require more than one procedure.
- Radiotherapy—very effective if diagnosed and treated early.
- Auditory brainstem implants—now recommended as an aid to improve auditory function where hearing preservation surgery has not been possible.

Complications
- Cranial nerve damage.
- Damage to the facial nerve is often inevitable—may be temporary or permanent. Facial reanimation surgery (facial–hypoglossal anastamosis) may be considered where facial nerve injury occurs. Functional aids such as eye drops, tarsorraphy and gold weights inserted into the eye lids help to prevent corneal ulceration.
- Decreased or absent corneal reflex (causes corneal ulceration).

Metastatic brain tumours

- About one-third of patients with cerebral metastases have not been previously diagnosed with cancer. Their neurological symptoms may be the first indication that they are ill, although the primary site may never be isolated.
- Multiple cerebral tumours are more likely to be metastatic lesions.
- Men—80% of metastatic tumours spread from the lungs, gut or kidney.
- Women—80% of lesions arise from the breast, lung, colon or skin.
- Management is focused on aggressive local treatment with surgery or radiosurgery where there are no more than two lesions, with follow-up radiotherapy.
- Long-term survival is influenced by age and pre-existing morbidity of the patient.
- Prior to radical surgery, investigations to locate the primary lesion must be undertaken.

Treatment options

- Steroids—dexamethasone helps to reduce vasogenic oedema
- Radiotherapy.
- Surgery.
- Combination of treatments.
- The main aim when treating secondary brain tumours is to improve the symptoms and improve the quality of the patient's life for as long as possible.

Spinal tumours

Spinal column tumours account for approximately 10–15% of primary CNS tumours.

Pathology
- Extradural, intradural–extramedullary, and intramedullary lesions.
- Extrinsic tumours invading from vertebral body.
- Tumours are classified histologically, e.g. ependymomas, astroctyomas, meningiomas.
- A large percentage are metastatic, most commonly from breast, lung, prostate gland, lymphoma and myeloma.

Presenting symptoms
- Back pain—may be intense, progressive, often neuropathic.
- Neurological deficits—ataxia, unsteady gait, numbness and tingling.
- Autonomic dysfunction—urinary retention, incontinence, constipation.

Diagnosis
- Medical history combined with presenting signs and symptoms.
- Neurological examination.
- CT and MRI scan.

Complications
- Neurological deficits—particularly motor signs.
- Diagnostic delay—need to have a high index of suspicion.
- Spinal cord compression.

Management
Surgery
Image-guided biopsy to optimise future management.
- Total excision via a laminectomy and spinal fusion to maintain spinal stability.
- Partial debulking followed up with radiotherapy.
- Vertebrectomy—removal of vertebral body and replacement with a titanium spinal cage to preserve neurological function.

Steroids
- High dose dexamethasone regime.

Radiotherapy
- Palliative radiotherapy may help to relieve severe pain symptoms.

Prognosis
- Depends on the patients pre-existing medical condition.
- Histology of tumour.
- Extent of surgical excision.

Further information for health professionals and the public
Tadman M., Roberts D. (2007) *Oxford Handbook of Cancer Nursing*, Oxford University Press: Oxford.

Treatments for brain tumours

Steroids

Dexamethasone is primarily used to reduce vasogenic oedema caused by either the tumour or the side effects of radiotherapy.

Side effects include, obesity, myopathy, diabetes, skin bruising and oral candida. Mood changes may also occur, such as feeling 'high', overactive, depressed and insomnia.

When taking steroids for a long period of time it is advisable to take stomach-protecting medication such as ranitidine or lansopresole as steroids can damage the lining of the stomach.

Radiotherapy

This is perhaps the most effective treatment for brain tumours. Radiotherapy treats cancer cells by using high-energy, ionizing radiation beams from a linear accelerator, to target and destroy malignant cells. The aim of radiation is to damage the genetic structure of the cells, the DNA (deoxyribonucleic acid).

These machines operate at different voltages, the location of some brain tumours may be deep and complicated, planning is required to treat them.

Treatment planning is carried out on a simulator machine, current and previous scans are fused together to maximize the accuracy of the treatment. Accuracy is very important because the beams are aimed in a manner that administers a high dose of radiation to the tumour, whilst trying to reduce the exposure of healthy tissue to the damaging rays.

Headshells

With all external beam radiation treatment it is essential that the patient lies still during treatment. A perspex headshell is the best way of achieving immobilization, so treatment can be given more accurately.

Each headshell is made individually from a plaster impression to allow the patient to breathe and see normally, but some patients may still feel claustrophobic. For patients with secondary brain tumours or patients having a short course of radiotherapy, a mould may not be necessary.

Radiotherapy can be given following surgery, alone or in combination with chemotherapy. Most patients tolerate this treatment very well and the side effects are minimal.

Side effects of radiotherapy to the head:
- Headaches
- Hair loss
- Tiredness
- Skin changes
- Somnolence
- Lethargy

The length of treatment will depend on the person's age and performance status. Treatment is normally given over a 2–6-week period.

Patients are monitored daily by the radiographers and weekly by the oncologist. Blood counts are checked weekly.

Chemotherapy

Chemotherapy is more commonly used for recurrent disease, to limit disease progression and minimize symptoms. In some patients it is given as an adjuvant treatment following radiotherapy, or given concomitantly with the radiotherapy. Concomitant chemotherapy is given in the form of tablets and is taken about one hour before the radiotherapy treatment.

The use of chemotherapy for the treatment of brain tumours is often difficult, because of intrinsic chemoresistance, and problems of drug delivery across the blood–brain barrier. All chemotherapy for brain tumour patients is palliative.

Informed consent needs to be established prior to commencing any-treatment, including treatment aims or options, drug therapy and written information. The patient needs to be given an opportunity to ask questions and consider the treatment before signing their consent form.

Common side effects of chemotherapy

Haematological toxicity
- Anaemia—a reduction in the concentration of haemoglobin.
- Leucopaenia—a decrease in the number of circulating white blood cells.
- Thrombocytopaenia—a reduction in the number of platelets.

Bone marrow depression
Leucopaenia, thrombocytopaenia, anaemia. Myelosuppression usually occurs 7–14 days following administration. Patients will need to have their blood count checked if they notice any fever, infection, bruising, bleeding, sore mouth or being generally unwell.

Nausea and vomiting
- The use of modern anti-emetics has minimized this considerably.
- Patients are advised to take their anti-emetics regularly, particularly for 48 hours following treatment.
- Commonly used anti-emetics include: granisetron, ondansetron, cyclizine, prochlorperazine, domperidone, metoclopramide.

Taste changes
- Tends to occur if cyclophosphamide is given. It can happen almost immediately and patients are given a sweet to suck during treatment.

Reduced fertility
- Female—irregular periods, amenorrhoea, There is a risk of genetic damage to a fetus, so conception during chemotherapy and for two years afterwards should be avoided.
- Male—patients need to be informed that chemotherapy can make them infertile, and sperm banking can be arranged if required.

Renal impairment
- Some drugs can damage the kidneys if they are not fully excreted.
- Kidneys must be functioning well prior to treatment.

Hair loss
- Alopecia does not happen with all regimes of chemotherapy, but can be the most emotionally distressing aspect of treatment.

Newer treatment options

Research and developments in the field of molecular biology, genomics and proteomics has led to huge increases in knowledge and treatment options for all types of brain tumours.

Temozolomide

This is an alkylating agent derived from dacarbazine and is given orally. It is usually well tolerated and side effects are minimal, they include; occasional bone marrow suppression, nausea, lethargy. Clinical trials are still ongoing.

PCV

This has been used for some time as the main chemotherapy treatment for brain tumours. It consists of three drugs:

Procarbazine

This is taken orally and can occasionally have some side effects, such as nausea, vomiting, diarrhoea, rash, flu-like symptoms and sometimes dizziness. Side effects don't usually last very long and tolerance develops over a few days.

Patients should avoid eating certain foods whist taking procarbazine, these include cheese, yoghurt, sour cream, gravy, pickled herrings, broad bean pods, alcohol, chicken livers and bananas. Eating or drinking any of these may cause an allergic reaction and nausea.

CCNU

Given in Lomustine capsule form, may cause nausea and vomiting. Antiemetics are usually effective.

Vincristine

A vinca alkaloid derived from the South American periwinkle plant, Vinca rosae. Administered intravenously, the side effects often include hair loss, constipation, bone marrow suppression, muscle weakness and mild nausea and vomiting.

Carboplatin

Given as a third line agent when the tumour has progressed having used temozolomide and PCV. Given intravenously, side effects include bone marrow suppression, nausea, vomiting, electrolyte disturbances and peripheral neuropathy and may involve an overnight stay in hospital. Patients usually request carboplatin when all other therapy has failed. Response to this chemotherapy is often quite low, when administered as a third line agent.

Further developments

Current work is focusing on antibodies or inhibitory molecules that are designed to aim for specific molecular targets, for example, angiogenesis inhibitors, growth factor receptor inhibitors, and vascular targeting agents.

Future management may involve a combination of these therapies along with existing conventional cytotoxic treatments. There is interest also in the development of monoclonial antibodies, immunotoxins and gene therapies.

Gene therapy

Currently there is a randomized efficiency trial of the herpes simplex virus (HSV). This has been approved by the GTAC (Gene Therapy Advisory Committee). This therapy is only used to treat patients with recurrent malignant glioblastoma multiforme.

Controlled by DNA, human cell division generally stops when we are adults, but for some reason, some cells do not stop dividing resulting in tumours and cancer.

HSV has the same biological growth dividers as human cells, through manipulation, this growth divider is removed so that it can no longer replicate. The cancer cells contain the exact sequence that is missing in the virus, this is the vital component that allows the virus to reproduce. The virus is injected directly into the brain via a burr hole procedure. The active herpes virus will replicate faster than the cancer cells. Once the cancer cells are destroyed, the virus will not destroy normal brain tissue.

There is a large amount of screening and investigations that takes place prior to any patient being entered into trials. This particular trial is given over four cycles, stringent follow-up is provided.

Gliadel® implants

- Gliadel® wafers (carmustine-impregnated biodegradable wafers), are biodegradable polymers that contain 7.7mg of the drug carmustine (BCNU).
- The wafers are inserted into the surgical cavity at the end of the surgical procedure and the BCNU is released directly into the tumour.
- The wafers do not have to be removed and they slowly dissolve over the next two to three weeks releasing the chemotherapy drug directly to the surrounding cells, thereby overcoming the blood–brain barrier.
- They do not cause any myelosuppression or other systemic toxicity.
- These wafers are licensed for treatment of both primary and recurrent malignant gliomas.
- Gliadel® wafers have been shown to prolong survival time by around 20% in patients with malignant gliomas.

Further information for health professionals and the public

Cancer BACUP (2005) *Understanding brain tumours.* Cancer BACUP
Abrey, E.L. and Mason, W.P. (2003). *Brain tumors. FF Fast Facts.* Health Press Limited.

Cerebral abscess

Cerebral abscess occurs when bacteria or a fungal infection affects parts of the brain. As the infection develops, it becomes encapsulated and produces pressure symptoms with corresponding signs and symptoms of raised intracranial pressure. In younger children abscess formation is associated with congenital heart disease, but may develop at any age due to local pathology.

Contributory factors
- Acute frontal sinusitis.
- Severe ear infections.
- Dental infections.
- Skull fracture following penetrating injuries or surgical procedures.
- In many cases the source of the infection may never be isolated.
- Secondary sources of infection may be transmitted from lung (pneumonia), kidney (carcinoma, UTI), heart (bacterial endocarditis), HIV.

Incidence
In less developed countries, abscess formation may be caused from tuberculosis and gastrointestinal infections.

Symptoms
- Symptoms may develop insidiously or more acutely.
- Symptoms depend on the specific location of the abscess.
- Signs and symptoms of increased intracranial pressure—headache, vomiting, confusion, changes in level of consciousness, seizures.
- Focal neurological signs—hemiparesis, aphasia.
- Signs of infection—pyrexia and fatigue.

Diagnosis
- Blood cultures
- CT or MRI (with contrast), may demonstrate areas of inflammation, necrosis and empyema.
- Tissue biopsy to identify the infecting organism.
- Lumbar puncture is contraindicated if there are signs of papilloedema.

Pathophysiology
- Brain abscesses are usually of mixed organisms (often anaerobes).
- Fungi—*Cryptococcus, candida, aspergillius.*
- Bacterial—*streptococcus, pneumococcus, meningococcus,*
- HIV patients—*mycobacterium tuberculosis.*

TREATMENT
- Insertion of peripherally inserted central catheter (PICC) to facilitate aggressive intravenous antibiotic therapy.
- Anti-fungal medications.
- Symptomatic management of ↑ICP.
- Intensive care nursing and management.
- Dental clearance.
- Nasal sinus decompression.

Surgery may be indicated if:
- ↑ICP with acute neurological signs.
- Abscess does not respond to I.V drug therapy.
- Abscess ruptures.

Prognosis
- High mortality if diagnosis delayed.
- High level of disability.
- Depends on the location of the abscess.

Complications
- Meningitis.
- Seizures.
- Neurological dysfunction and long-term disability.
- Recurrence of infection.
- Antibiotic resistance.
- Side effects from antibiotics.

Hydrocephalus

Hydrocephalus occurs when too much CSF is produced, re-absorption is reduced or when it is prevented from circulating through the ventricular system resulting in raised intracranial pressure.

- Normal CSF production is 500ml/24h.
- Total CSF circulating volume is approx. 120–150ml (in adults).
- CSF is recycled 3 x daily.
- Increased CSF pressure within the ventricles reduces cerebral blood flow and increases ICP.

Types of hydrocephalus

- Communicating hydrocephalus: there is CSF flow through the ventricular system and the subarachnoid space. However, reabsorption is impaired e.g. sagittal sinus thrombosis involving the arachnoid villi.
- Non-communicating/obstructive hydrocephalus: occurs when there is blockage within the ventricular system preventing CSF flow, e.g. ependymomas or acoustic neuromas hypertension.
- Idiopathic intracranial hydrocephalus (IIH), previously referred to as benign intracranial hypertension (BIH), a syndrome where CSF volume is raised, but the pressure is normal. More common in females. May cause visual impairment, memory loss, ataxia and urinary incontinence (🕮 see p 252).

Aetiology

- Tumours—posterior fossa lesions, ependymoma.
- Cerebellar haemorrhage or infarction.
- Subarachnoid haemorrhage
- Head injury.
- Meningitis/encephalitis, exudate blocks the aqueduct of Sylvius.
- Genetic disorders—Dandy-Walker malformation, Arnold Chiari, aqueduct stenosis.
- Infection—toxoplasmosis.
- No underlying diagnoses in many cases.

Clinical features

- Signs and symptoms of ↑ ICP
- Headache, vomiting, papilloedema
- Reduced or loss of upward gaze, diplopia
- Changes in level of consciousness
- Blindness—damage to the optic nerves
- 'Sunsetting eyes'—in babies where the eyes appear to be pushed into a downward position.
- Dementia and poor concentration.
- Learning difficulties.

Diagnosis

- CT.
- MRI scan.
- Medical history.

Short-term management
- External ventricular drain or lumbar drain.
- Serial lumbar punctures (IIH).

Long -term management
- Ventricular peritoneal shunt or lumbar peritoneal shunt.
- Endoscopic 3rd ventriculoscopy—creation of a hole in the floor of the 3rd ventricle to drain the CSF into the basal cisterns.
- Acetazolamide—reduces the rate of CSF production, (patients often experience unpleasant side effects).
- Programmable or adjustable shunt valve—has variable settings that can be adjusted with an external magnet placed over the skin.

Dealing with shunts and shunt problems

Complications

Shunt infections

- Shunt infections are the commonest cause of shunt malfunction.
- Diagnosis is frequently difficult and multifaceted. Infection frequently results from contamination with coagulase-negative *Staphylococcus aureus* from the skin during surgery.
- Symptoms include fatigue, irritability, ↓ appetite, general aches and pains, mild infections, urinary tract infections.
- Blood and CSF cultures may be negative.

Management

- Routine laboratory tests including CRP and WCC.
- External ventricular drain for immediate relief of acute symptoms.
- Systemic antibiotics.
- Remove and revise shunt system.
- Prompt shunt revision normally leads to a complete and rapid recovery.

Over-drainage

- CSF drains from the ventricles more quickly than it is produced.
- Patient will complain of headaches (sometimes called a low pressure headache), dizziness (worse after sitting up from lying).
- Sudden over-drainage will cause the ventricles to collapse, tearing blood vessels away from the skull and causing a subdural haematoma.
- More gradual over-drainage reduces the ventricles to resemble small slits on CT scanning and interferes with shunt function.
- Both high- and low-pressure valves may cause over-drainage.

Management

- Remove and revise valve.
- Insert temporary external ventricular drain (see p 284).
- Changing valve to a different pressure is not always effective.

Under-drainage

- Blockage of the ventricular end of the catheter or shunt tubing with tissue, plugging the entry holes.
- Shunt breaks or becomes disconnected (some shunts are now manufactured as one system).
- In babies, enlarging head circumference, bulging fontanelles, seizures, prominent neck and head veins may indicate shunt malfunction.
- Symptoms vary from patient to patient. Parents or carers may be able to differentiate the symptoms from other illnesses.
- Often a gradual onset that can follow a minor illness such as a cold. Specific symptoms include: abdominal tenderness, pain or swelling around shunt site, increased irritability, disruptive or anti-social behaviour.
- Headache often worse in the morning before getting up.

- Blockage can be fatal, particularly when there is a delay in diagnosis or treatment.
- It is sometimes possible to revise portions of the shunt system.

Management
- Insert a temporary external ventricular drain to relieve the pressure.
- Intracranial pressure monitoring to assess best treatment options.
- Serial CT scanning.
- Remove and revise shunt.

Follow-up care
- Regular CT scans.
- Patient information and education of the symptoms and signs of shunt blockage.
- Access to specialist nurse to support and advise patients in the community.

Prognosis
- Rate of shunt blockages is highest in the first year after insertion.
- 50% of patients will need at least one shunt revision in the following 10-year period.

Spinal cord injury

Injuries to the vertebral column and spinal cord (SCI) may occur following accidents involving excessive forces resulting from acceleration–deceleration injuries:

- Hyperflexion—compression of the vertebral body with damage to posterior longitudinal ligaments and intravertebral discs.
- Hyperextension—fractures to posterior portion of vertebrae and damage to anterior longitudinal ligaments.
- Excessive rotation of the head—compression fractures, rupture to the posterior ligament and fracture/dislocation at the joint.
- Deformation of spinal vertebra and soft tissues.
- Axial loading—crush and compression injuries.

Causes of SCI

- Road traffic accidents.
- Sports injuries—diving, rugby.
- Domestic accidents—falls down stairs, trees, ladders.
- Accidents at work—penetrating injuries, crush injuries.

Injuries to the vertebral column

Fractures—may be simple, compression, or wedge fracture.

- Fracture without dislocation.
- Fracture/dislocation.
- Fracture with subluxation.

Damage to spinal cord

Injury to the spinal cord can have a devastating effect on the patient's independence and long-term quality of life.

High cervical cord injury above C-5, results in loss of diaphragmatic function and will require some level of respiratory support (📖 see p 356).

Cervical injury above C-8 affects intercostal muscle function. The loss of function may be permanent or temporary.

- Quadriplegia—involves one or more of the cervical segments and affects both legs, arms, bowel and bladder function.
- Paraplegia—involves the thoracic, lumbar or sacral regions resulting in loss of lower limb function, bowel and bladder function.
- Incomplete damage—preservation of some sensory or motor pathways (may be central, lateral, anterior or peripheral).
- Complete cord lesion—total loss of sensory and motor function.

The facts

- 15% of traumatic brain injury may also have a concomitant SCI
- 35% of SCI patients can have a concomitant TBI.
- Severity of TBI increases in proportion to the level of injury.
- Incidence of concomitant cervical spine and spinal injury is significant amongst patients with a GCS <14 and greatest in those patients with a GCS <8.
- Spinal precautions are necessary in any patient with GCS <15 until appropriate screening has been completed.

Diagnostic indicators

Where there is evidence of spinal trauma but cord involvement cannot be excluded, the diagnosis is of 'potential' SCI. Where definitive spinal clearance is impossible, the diagnosis is of 'uncleared SCI'.

Up to 10% of 'actual SCI' patients are missed or misdiagnosed during their initial admission.

Problems with accurate diagnosis

- Failure to identify different injury mechanisms, particularly in patients >55 years old.
- Failure to examine or screen thoroughly.
- Unable to access CT/MRI at appropriate time.
- Failure to recognize discrete SCI symptoms.
- Inappropriate spinal clearance.
- Unconscious patients.
- Sedation/alcohol or substance abuse.
- Multiple trauma.
- Existing neurological problems.

Key SCI indicators in unconscious patients include:

- Flaccid limbs/flaccid anal tone/lack of splinting at fracture sites.
- Diaphragmatic respiration (in higher lesions).
- Incontinence and priapism (in males).
- Hypotension (in the absence of fluid loss/organ failure/past history).
- Bradycardia (in higher lesions/absence of TBI).
- Absent, reduced or abnormal reflexes on testing (depends on level).
- The presence of spinal shock (complete loss of function below level of injury), can delay accurate assessment of neurological impairment for at least 6 weeks post-injury.

Spinal alignment and stabilization

Failure to maintain effective alignment of the spine following SCI or spinal surgery will cause further neurological deficits. Methods include:

- Cervical traction—application, care of tongs/halo vests, weights and pinsites.
- Cervical collars—sizing, fitting, maintenance, skin care, ICP hazard.
- It is essential to know how to measure and size a hard collar and be aware of the different manufacturers.

Initial management

- Patients with lesions >C-4 will require careful intubation and ventilation
- Lesions <C-4 may need some respiratory support and O_2 therapy.
- Hypotension and bradycardia should not be confused with TBI or hypovalaemia—avoid large volume fluid replacement.
- Immobilize the whole spine during any lateral transfers.
- Secondary survey—identify the sensory and motor level of the SCI.
- Note any signs of drug or alcohol—must not influence the assessment.

Further information for health professionals and the public

Manji, H. *et al.* (2006) *Oxford Handbook of Neurology.* Oxford University Press, Oxford.
Harrison, P. (2000) *Managing spinal injuries: critical care.* Spinal Injuries Association.

Emergency and acute care

Management according to SCI critical care bundle (Harrison, 2000)

Element 1 Referral to a nominated SCI centre should occur as soon as possible after diagnosis (i.e. within 24 hours).

- The rapid transfer of SCI to specialist units is the most effective method of reducing the effect and incidence of SCI complications.

Element 2 Prevention of secondary injuries due to inappropriate mechanical forces, hypoxia or circulatory insufficiency.

- Spinal protection must be maintained until the patient has regained consciousness sufficient for a full neurological assessment.
- Medical staff should make the decision to discontinue precautions.
- Surgical stabilization and mobilization of SCI patients should only be undertaken following consultation with SCI centre.
- Maintain spinal alignment throughout all turns, procedures, transfers.
- Use of a dynamic air mattress, even in static mode is contraindicated.
- TBIs—head of the bed can be elevated using a reverse Trandelenburg position—maximum 15° head-up bed angle.
- Maintain oxygen saturation at 100%. Monitor BP and pulse.
- Manage cervical traction/ halo/collars appropriately.
- Identify rises in ICP—establish that the collar has been sized and fitted correctly; loosen the collar, if it does not improve within 15 minutes, then it should be reapplied; a loosened collar acts as a 'flag' to alert staff to the possibility of an uncleared cervical spine.
- All staff should be competent in the recognition and recording of motor and sensory impairment due to SCI.

Element 3 Minimize incidence of DVT and pulmonary embolus (PE) formation

- Commence prophylactic anticoagulation within 24h of diagnosis.
- Apply properly sized thigh-length stockings or pneumatic compression.
- Work with therapy staff to provide twice daily range of passive limb movements, supported by regular turning and repositioning of limbs.
- Position lower limbs on pillows when patient is supine to encourage venous drainage. Monitor for unexpected pyrexia or limb swelling.

Element 4 Manage the impact of spinal shock.

- Loss of vasomotor tone throughout the paralysed areas provides the diagnostic observations of spinal shock (hypotension, bradycardia).
- Administer I.V fluids and vasoactive drugs judiciously.
- Monitor and act upon the trend of recorded observations rather than the numerical values alone.
- Monitor temperature—actual body temperature can be 10°C below normal due to influence of environmental temperature.

Element 5 Prevent gastric ulceration due to vagal overactivity and initial 'nil enterally' requirement.

- Perform risk assessment based on previous medical history.
- Commence prophylactic gastric protection within 24hrs.
- Assess patient for commencement of enteral feeding after 48hrs.
- Continue with gastric protection upon commencement of feeding.

Element 6 Prevent prolonged paralytic ileus and vomiting due to early commencement of enteral feeding.
- Patient must remain 'nil' enterally for at least first 48hrs.
- Monitor for return of peristalsis, monitor abdominal girth.
- Avoid passing NG tube unless indicated.
- Introduce enteral fluids gradually.
- Assess nutritional status, provide TPN if nutritionally compromised.

Element 7 Prevent over-distension of the rectum from constipation which can cause bowel perforation.
- Perform PR examination within 24 hours to establish sphincter status and presence of faeces.
- Daily digital removal of faeces in presence of flaccid sphincter.
- In presence of reflexive sphincter, introduce daily/alternate days of rectal stimulant and digital rectal stimulation.
- Introduce oral aperients and stool softeners only as advised by SCIC.
- Do not use large-volume enemas.

Element 8 Prevent pressure ulcer formation
- Implement 2–4-hourly turning regime or transfer to electric turning bed.
- Inspect all skin surfaces, collars, splints must be removed and inspected at least once daily.
- Avoid the use of foot splints unless prescribed.

Element 9 Improve ventilation and perfusion, promote postural drainage
- Regular turning mobilizes chest secretions, 2-hourly turning to a 30^0 position is the ideal standard.
- Oropharyngeal/tracheal suctioning in lesions >T6 can induce vasovagal stimulation sufficient to induce cardiac syncope. Monitor pulse and keep atropine easily accessible.
- Monitor for hypoxia, hypercapnia, respiratory fatigue and sleep apnoea.
- Monitor for abdominal distension which can splint diaphragm.

Element 10 Prevent bladder distension and agitate urine in the bladder to prevent sedimentation and catheter blockage.
- Catheterize on admission and change catheter every 4 weeks.
- If catheter blocks change catheter rather than flushing.
- Avoid use of antibiotics unless symptoms systematic.

Element 11 Prevent foot drop and upper limb and finger contracture which will delay and prevent meaningful rehabilitation.
- Unless contraindicated by other injuries, provide range of passive exercises twice daily, supported by regular repositioning.
- 'Block' feet to 90° resting angle using pillows.
- Elevate hands on pillow and observe for signs of gravitational oedema.

Element 12 Manage impact of spinal shock
- Monitor body temperature and respond to visible signs of hypothermia or pyrexia in non-paralysed areas, irrespective of core temperature.

Further information for health professionals and the public

Harrison, P. (2000) *Managing spinal injuries: critical care*. Spinal Injuries Association.

Long-term care and rehabilitation

Patients with SCI require a multidisciplinary approach to reduce their risk of developing complications and achieve their highest level of independence possible.

Transition from critical care to rehabilitation can be hugely stressful for the patient and represents relearning of all activities of daily living. The ultimate goal is to enable the patient to make the successful adjustment to living at home, ideally resuming previous occupations and family responsibilities.

Psychological and emotional support

Psychological management and support of the SCI patient should initially aim to inform and give some reassurance to the patient and their family.

Significant skill will be required to support the patient's psychological needs—helplessness, fear, anxiety, anger, changing body image.

The patient needs the team to be truthful and honest with their questions.

Autonomic dysreflexia

Autonomic dysreflexia (AD) is a potentially fatal complication for patients with an established SCI lesion above T6.

Presenting symptoms
- Severe hypertension.
- Bradycardia.
- Severe headache.
- Flushed or blotchy appearance of skin above level of lesion.
- Profuse sweating above level of lesion.
- Skin pallor below level of lesion.
- Nasal congestion.

Common causes
- Distended bladder—usually due to blocked catheter.
- Distended bowel—constipation or impaction.
- Pressure sores, burns.
- Urinary tract infection/renal or bladder calculi.
- Pregnancy.
- Deep vein thrombosis or pulmonary embolism.
- Ingrowing toenail/fracture below level of lesion.

Management
- Identify and eliminate cause of AD—reassure the patient.
- Remove noxious stimulus, e.g. re-catheterize, bladder washouts are contraindicated.
- Induce postural hypotension, sit up or tilt head of bed.
- Medication—glyceryl trinitrate or captopril.
- Referral to specialists, e.g. psychologists.

Bowel management
- Bowel care must be individualized to the patient.
- Manual evacuation (ME) is an accepted method of management for lesions below T12 level. Their bowels will not empty in a reflex response to rectal stimulants or suppositories.

- Patients with lesions above T12 are usually able to achieve good reflex bowel emptying without resorting to ME.

Bladder management
- Reduced bladder activity increases the incidence of sedimentation and tube blockage.
- Over-distension of the bladder causes overstretching of muscles and nerves within the bladder, reducing potential to recover normal reflexes.
- Frequent changes of position will agitate the bladder, reducing sedimentation and risk of infection.

Ventilator dependency
- Recent advances in medical technology allows SCI of >C3 to survive.
- Patients who are ventilator-dependent need a comprehensive care package to enable them to re-establish their independence.

Sexual dysfunction
- Affected by S2–S4 damage.
- Urologists can provide advice on specific problems and provide information and options.

Management of spasm
'Spasm is the manifestation of the body's innate protective withdrawal mechanism in response to locally perceived noxious stimulus' (Harrison, 2000). It presents as sudden, violent contractions of muscles below the level of the lesion.

With education, drugs, and physiotherapy, spasm may be used to the patient's advantage to facilitate standing, sitting transfers, pressure area care or bladder emptying.

Tissue viability
The prevention of pressure sores is given the highest priority in the rehabilitation pathway and patients will quickly learn to manage their own pressure areas.

The patient will be assessed for an appropriate wheelchair.

⚠ NB: Patients are particularly vulnerable when readmitted to general wards for treatment for other conditions.

Further information for health professionals and the public
Harrison, P. (2000) *Managing spinal injuries: critical care*. Spinal Injuries Association.

Grundy, D. and Swan, A. (2002) *ABC of spinal cord injuries*, 4th edn. London: BMJ Books.

Manji, H. *et al.* (2006) *Oxford Handbook of Neurology*. Oxford: Oxford University Press.

Degenerative spinal lesions and prolapsed intravertebral discs

- Degenerative spinal disorders are commonly associated with the normal effects of ageing. It is estimated that at least 30% of people over 30 years old will have some degree of disc space degeneration, although not all will be symptomatic.
- The discs between the vertebrae are composed of cartilage, fibrous tissue, and water. With age the discs weaken and eventually crack. Disc herniation occurs when the internal nucleus pulposus herniates through a tear in the disc, causing pressure against the nerve root. Inflammation and further compression occurs due to osteoarthritis and spinal stenosis.
- Other causes of degeneration may be infection, tumours, arthritis, movement and handling related episodes (bending, twisting posture) and congenital deformities.
- L4/5, S1 levels are the most common lumbar levels of occurrence. C5/6 and C6/7 are the most common sites for cervical disc lesions.
- Thoracic disc prolapse is rare.
- Degenerative spinal disease presents in three forms:
  - Mechanical spinal pain.
  - Radiculopathy—compression of nerve roots causing peripheral symptoms along the nerve—numbness, tingling, weakness.
  - Myelopathy—direct compression of the spinal cord.
  - Combination of both.

Symptoms
- Acute, sharp and/or chronic pain.
- Motor or sensory changes.
- Paraesthaesia.
- Reduced mobility and stiffness.
- Symptoms of central spinal cord compression include:
  - Motor and sensory loss.
  - Loss of bladder and bowel function.
  - Sexual dysfunction.

Diagnosis
- MRI scan.
- CT scan.
- Careful history—important to always treat the patient not the images.
- Complete neurological examination.

Treatment
- Depends on the severity of the condition.
- Bed rest for short periods only.
- Gentle mobilization.
- Physiotherapy—to improve flexibility and range of motion.
- Analgesia +/– muscle relaxants. Severe cases may respond to epidural injections of steroids and opiates.

Surgery

Indicated for patients with severe pain, neurological signs and symptoms and findings from radiological investigations that support the clinical symptoms.

Microdiscectomy

Minimally invasive technique to remove prolapsed disc material.

Fenestration

A window of bone is removed to allow easy access to the disc.

Laminectomy

More complex cases need a wider incision, removing the lamina and dividing the erector spinal muscle.

Anterior cervical discectomy and fusion

Anterior approach to remove disc fragments, followed by fusion of one or more levels with bone, plastic or metal.

Cervical lesions

The cervical region is particularly vulnerable to damage from trauma, degeneration and arthritic changes. Localized damage will cause nerve root compression, resulting in pain and muscle weakness. Disc prolapse can occur laterally affecting the local nerve root, commonly at C5/6, 6/7 levels or may centrally compress the spinal cord (□ see Neurological emergencies, p 148).

Contributory causes

- Spondylosis
- Osteoarthritis
- Osteoporosis
- Whiplash and hyperextension injuries

Signs and symptoms

Radiculopathy

Pain will be dermatonal, radiating down the area of skin supplied by the affected nerve root. The more rapid the progression the more compromised the spinal cord.

- Thumb—C6
- Middle finger—C7
- Little Finger—C8
- There is usually a history of mechanical neck pain
- The radicular pain becomes the predominant complaint

Myelopathy

Onset is usually insidious.

- Progressive loss of function is the primary complaint
- Clumsy and numb hands +/– gait and sphincter disturbances
- Hands usually worse than legs
- Not uncommonly asymptomatic
- The least common presentation
- Often spinal pain is not a feature

Examination and diagnosis

- CT scan—narrowing, lordosis, disc space and osteophyte protrusion, subluxation.
- MRI scan.
- Radiation—sensory loss, muscle weakness.
- Reflexes may be impaired in or absent in a radiculopathy but may be increased in patients with a myelopathy.
- Motor symptoms—difficulty walking.
- Pyramidal signs—increased tone, clonus and extensor plantar responses.
- Sphincter disturbance.

Management

- Surgical opinion for radiculopathy unresponsive to conservative management.
- Decompressive surgery.
- Simple analgesics +/– diazepam to relax the muscles.
- Physiotherapy (unlikely to be of benefit for myelopathy).
- Modify cervical posture.

Surgery
- Cervical microdiscectomy
- Cervical laminectomy
- Anterior cervical decompression and fusion
- Spinal fusion is the last resort—titanium alloy cage and integral anterior plate.
- Prosthetic disc replacement.

Myelopathies are classified according the degree of neurological deficits.

Table 9.4 Modified Frankel classification scale

Grade A	Complete motor and sensory involvement
Grade B	Complete motor involvement, some sensory sparing including sacral sparing
Grade C	Functionally useless motor sparing
Grade D	Functional motor sparing
Grade E	No neurological involvement

Post-operative management
Record vital signs and:
- Spinal observations—motor and sensory function, comparing with pre-op power, range, sensation.
- Observe wound for signs of excessive leakage.
- Monitor amount of drainage in wound drainage (usually removed 24hrs post-operatively.
- Provide adequate analgesia.
- Follow doctor's instructions regarding mobilization. Depending on level of pre-op disability, patients are encouraged to mobilize as soon as clinically stable.
- Sutures/clips removed 7–10 days.

NB: Some patients may experience transient swallowing difficulties immediately post-operatively, observe for signs of aspiration/penetration. Refer to SLT.

Lumbar lesions

Intravertebral disc prolapse is a major cause of acute and chronic back pain in the lumbar region. Lateral disc herniations will compress the nerve root exiting through the foramen below the affected level, e.g. L3/4 disc lesion will compress the L4 nerve roots. Occasionally discs will protrude centrally compressing the cauda equina (📖 see Chapter 6, p 146)

Contributory causes

Occupation
- Heavy lifting—engineering, ambulance service.
- Static postures—computer workers, telephonists, supermarket cashiers.
- Top-heavy postures—nurses, doctors, dentists.

Previous history
- Ankylosing spondylitis and other congenital malformations.
- Osteoarthritis.
- Osteoporosis.
- Smoking, alcohol and obesity.

Signs and symptoms

Radiculopathy—diagnostic feature.
- Sciatica.
- Leg pain much worse than back pain.
- Pain is worse if patient coughs or sneezes.
- Leg pain is exacerbated by exercise (spinal stenosis).
- Pain extends to the termination of the dermatome:
  - L4/5 toes
  - L5 S1 calf
  - L3/4 knee and shin
  - Myelopathy symptoms of epidemic proportions caused by compression of the spinal cord rather than a single nerve root.
- Often insidious onset.
- Restricted mobility.
- Progressive functional loss and muscle atrophy.
- Clumsiness and ataxia.

Examination
- Radiation—central/one leg/below knee.
- Parasthaesia.
- Dysasthaesia in a radicular distribution—sensory loss is dermatomal.
- True motor symptoms are uncommon—motor dysfunction is myotomal.
- Difficulty passing urine.
- Assess the site of pain and degree of movement.
- Straight leg raise—reproduces pressure on the spinal cord/nerve root.
  ⚠ Exclude possible alternative diagnosis—renal disease, aortic aneurysm, peripheral vascular disease, hip or knee osteoarthritis.

Management
- Conservative management.
- Many patients will experience low-grade continuous but tolerable pain that will occasionally intensify for a few days or more.
- Simple analgesia—applying heat to increase flexibility and range of motion, or ice packs to reduce inflammation.
- Non-steroidal, anti-inflammatory drugs and benzodiazepines.
- Bed rest, short period only followed by gentle mobilization.
- Physiotherapy and exercise—walking, swimming.
- Modifying activities to avoid heavy manual lifting.
- Alternative therapies—chiropractoric or osteopathy.

Surgery
- Laminectomy, discectomy, fenestration.
- Lumbar spinal fusion surgery.
- Artificial disc replacement—maintains normal movement in the lumbar spine, reducing incidence of stress either side of the original surgery.

Ideal neurosurgical patient
- Young.
- Short history.
- Leg pain predominates.
- Good signs.
- Unequivocal imaging.
- Positively motivated attitude.

Patients are reviewed pre-operatively to assess their degree of deficit and the level of improvement that might be expected post-operatively. It is important that the patient has realistic expectations of recovery as sustained nerve root damage is likely to leave the patient with some degree of disability that requires an intensive programme of physiotherapy and which might continue to restrict their mobility, lifestyle and return to normal functioning.

Post-operative management
Record vital signs and:
- Spinal observations—motor and sensory function (☐ see Chapter 3, p 61).
- Observe wound for signs of excessive leakage.
- Drain usually removed 24hrs post-op.
- Monitor urine output. If retention of urine is suspected, use bladder scanner to assess volume before performing residual catheterization.
- Sutures usually removed 7–10 days post-op.
- Most patients are encouraged to mobilize as soon clinical condition allows following anaesthetic. Patients should be taught to stand from lying, placing minimal strain on the wound.
- Patients should be advised to avoid long periods in a sitting position.
- Inform doctors if patient unable to pass urine—complete neurological examination should be performed.

Hind brain hernia (Arnold Chiari malformation)

- This is a condition in which the cerebellar tonsils herniate through the foramen magnum. There can be varying degrees of herniation, and they are graded according to Chiari 0—II classification, depending on how far down the upper cervical canal the tonsils herniate, and if it is further complicated by the presence of syringomyelia.
- The true incidence is not known, but MRI scanning indicates it is more common than previously recognized.
- Tends to affects females more than males.

Associations
- Hydrocephalus
- Spina bifida
- Tethered cord
- Intracranial tumours
- Intracranial haemorrhage
- Klippel Fiel syndrome
- Trauma
- Congenital malformations
- Prolonged childbirth, particularly forceps delivery can predispose towards hind brain herniation

Symptoms
- Can be asymptomatic
- Headaches
- Visual disturbances
- Neck pain
- Vertigo
- Neuropathic pain
- Tinnitus
- Sleep apnoea
- Ataxia, clumsiness and coordination difficulties
- Bulbar signs
- Neurological deficits—varying degrees

Diagnosis
- MRI scan
- CT scan
- Many are found incidentally in patients undergoing imaging for other conditions

Treatment
Surgical
- Cranial–cervical decompression.
- V-P shunt to relieve hydrocephalus.
- Un-tethering of the spinal cord.
- Excision of tumours.

Conservative

Close monitoring by a consultant neurosurgeon is usually advocated, where symptoms are stable and non-progressive and there is an absence of any underlying pathology.

Syringomyelia (hydromyelia, syringohydromyelia)

Syringomyelia is a rare, chronic, progressive degenerative condition affecting males more than females, occurring in approximately 8 in 100,000, predominantly younger people. The condition refers to a fluid-filled cavity which forms in the spinal cord, called a syrinx. The syrinx can be any size and length, and often has multiple loculated areas, presenting at any level of the spinal cord. As the syrinx expands, CSF flow is reduced allowing fluid to accumulate within the spinal cord resulting in compression and motor and sensory deficits.

Associations
- Hind brain herniation
- Spinal cord tumours
- Scar tissue
- Spinal cord trauma
- Arachnoiditis
- Meningitis
- Haemorrhage
- Hydrocephalus
- Tethered spinal cord
- Prolapsed cervical or thoracic disc
- Sometimes the cause is never discovered

Presentation
Patients may be asymptomatic and the syrinx can be an incidental finding following other investigations. Symptoms can vary, and may increase with coughing and/or sneezing:
- Headaches.
- Intermittent/constant limb pain/numbness/tingling.
- Intermittent/constant chest and/or back pain/numbness/tingling.
- Loss of proprioception.
- Weakness of a limb.
- Loss of function of a limb.
- Sensory dissociation, and loss of ability to differentiate hot and cold, especially in the hands.
- Dysfunctional bladder and bowels.

Diagnosis
MRI scan—shows the cavity or cavities in the spinal cord.

Treatment
The aim is to alleviate the symptoms, and prevent further deterioration. Sometimes a 'watchful wait' is used, in conjunction with medical supervision.

Surgery
- Craniocervical decompression for hind brain hernia.
- Decompression of cervical or thoracic disc.
- Syringo pleural/peritoneal shunt.

Conservative
Medication: gabapentin/pregabalin analgesia.

Further information for health professional and the public

Woodward S. (2006) Syringomyelia. *British Journal of Neuroscience Nursing*, 2(10): 505–506.

Neuroscience critical care

Head injury management

Over a million people suffer a head injury each year in the UK, 150,000 require hospital admission and over 4,000 require some level of neuro-surgical intervention. A small percentage of patients will die from their injuries, a larger number will suffer long-term disability. Early detection and timely intervention can minimize some of the complications.

National guidance has been issued to ensure that all patients suffering a head injury receive the optimum level of care. Five areas of management have been identified as priorities for care:

Prompt assessment in accident and emergency department

Patients must be assessed within 15 minutes of admission, focusing on exclusion of potential cervical or spinal injury and possible developing haematomas.

Patients that are likely to be discharged following a minor head injury should receive verbal and written advice regarding signs and symptoms of neurological deterioration or possible delayed complications.

Urgent neuroimaging

CT scanning is an essential diagnostic tool to identify early indicators of neurological deterioration. Risk factors include:
- GCS less than 13/15 on admission or less than 15/15, 2 hours after the injury.
- Depending on the clinical stability of the patient, the cervical spine should be scanned at the same time as the head.
- Signs of focal neurological deficits.
- Any signs of fractured skull, e.g. peri-orbital haematoma, CSF or blood leaking from the nose or ears.
- Epileptic-type seizures.
- Coagulopathy such as warfarin or aspirin can sometimes make patients more susceptible to developing haematomas.
- Repeated episodes of vomiting, can be an early sign of ↑ICP.
- Period of amnesia, particularly if the patient was over 65 years old.
- Mechanism of injury, particularly if the patient fell from a height.

Criteria for admission
- Patients should always be admitted for close monitoring if there are any delays in the assessment process, for example patients suspected of substance abuse, uncooperative or intoxication patients or if the CT scan is unavailable.
- Patients identified as being at particular risk of developing neurological complications should be observed and managed in an area where medical and nursing staff are competent to monitor, assess and recognize changes in the patient's neurological condition, referring them to neurosurgical specialist services as clinically indicated.
- Observation in hospital should be maintained if the CT scan identifies any suspicious or possible abnormalities.
- Any patient with a GCS less than 15 on their normal baseline recording.

Referral to a neurosurgical unit

With the advent of improved inter-hospital computer network links, referral to a neurosurgeon has significantly improved. Patients should be referred if:

- The GCS remains less than 8, excluding all other contributory causes of ↓conscious level.
- The patient continues to be confused.
- Any unexplained deterioration in GCS.
- Any focal neurological deterioration.
- Unexplained seizure activity.
- Suspicions of penetrating injury.
- CSF leak from ear or nose.

Inter-hospital transfers must be performed with staff who are competent, experienced, and if possible trained in the transfer of critically ill patients.

Management of patients with long-term disability

Following head injury many patients can experience complex physical, psychological and cognitive problems. Referral to specialist rehabilitation units and third sector agencies is essential to ensure that brain-injured patients achieve their optimum quality of life and improvement.

- Patients and carers must receive support, information and advice regarding the potential short- and long-term sequelae following head injury.
- Patients should be referred to a brain-injury team to facilitate continuity of care, access to services, enrolment on the brain injury pathway and good communication with primary carers.

Further information for health professionals and the public

National Institute for Health and Clinical Excellence (2007) *Head injury: triage, assessment, investigation and early management of head injury in infants, children and adults.* London: National Institute for Health and Clinical Excellence . Available at http://www.nice.org.uk/CG056

Basal skull fractures

Basal skull fractures are associated with severe brain injury from an assault or fall.

The fracture can extend from a linear fracture in the frontal/temporal region and involve the anterior and middle fossa.

These fractures may be further complicated by the involvement of the ethmoid and maxillary air sinuses in the frontal and temporal bones. Damage will allow air to leak in and blood or CSF to leak out. Identified as peri-orbital swelling (panda eyes), and bruising behind the ear (Battle's sign).

Signs and symptoms

CSF leakage may not be immediately obvious. The patient may complain of an unpleasant taste at the back of their mouth as CSF drips down the back of their oro-pharynx.

More commonly, CSF drips down the nose from the paranasal sinus, (rhinorrhoea) and is usually exacerbated when the patient leans or bends forwards.

CSF leaking out of the ear (otorrhoea), can be difficult to differentiate from blood, except that it will leave a yellow tinge encircling the blood left on the pillow or dressing.

If the CSF leakage is significant, the patient might also complain of headaches due to low ICP.

The identification and implications of clinical signs such as orbital hae-matomas, Battle's sign or cranial nerve damage, e.g. facial nerve or vestibulocochlear nerve with petrous bone fractures, are important to highlight the importance of close monitoring for potential signs of infection or secondary complications.

Complications
- Meningitis
- Cerebral abscess
- Aerocele
- Dural tear
- Cerebral vascular thrombosis and infarction
- Carotid cavernous fistula

Management

The majority of CSF leaks will heal spontaneously within a few days.

Surgery and a dural repair is only required if the leak persists or an aerocele becomes more symptomatic.

Long-term antibiotic cover is rarely prescribed, however, Pneumovax® II and meningococcal vaccine is usually recommended for confirmed CSF leaks.

Carotid cavernous fistula

An abnormal fistula that forms between the internal carotid artery and the venous cavernous sinus that allows arterial blood under pressure to be forced into the venous circulation.

Signs and symptoms include visual disturbances, pain behind the eye, proptosis of the eye and facial palsies due to pressure on the cranial nerves III, IV, VI, V.

Treatment options include detachable balloon catheterization and occlusion of the fistula.

Decompressive craniectomy

Decompressive craniectomy involves removing a large bone flap from part of the skull, allowing the brain space to expand through the decompression thereby reducing the intracranial pressure (ICP), improving cerebral blood flow, and improving cerebral perfusion pressure. Raised intracranial pressure is a frequent complication following severe acute head injuries resulting in significant mortality and morbidity. A range of treatment options are available, escalating incrementally with the severity of the injury and the response to specific interventions.

First-line treatments

- Elective ventilation, to control hypercapnia and hypoxia.
- Sedation to facilitate compliance with ventilation and reduce cerebral metabolism.
- Fluid management with isotonic saline to maintain cerebral perfusion pressure.
- Diuretic therapy—mannitol or furosemide to control acute ICP rises.
- Hypertonic saline is sometimes used as an alternative to treat cerebral oedema and control ICP by osmotically moving excess fluid from cerebral tissue into the blood.
- Maintenance of normothermia.
- External ventricular drain.

Second-line treatments

- Controlled hyperventilation—lowers intracranial pressure (ICP) by inducing a state of hypocapnia to effectively vasoconstrict the cerebral blood vessels and decrease cerebral blood volume. **Only justified in acute episodes**, e.g. a blown pupil, to buy time until other interventions can be instigated. Research studies have shown that unless closely monitored will cause ischaemia due to excessive vasoconstriction.
- Barbiturate therapy, e.g. thiopental.
- Decompressive craniectomy—recommended procedure for patients that have failed to respond to conventional measures and the ICP is consistently above 25mmHg or CPP is below 60mmHg.

Clinical indications

- Head injury
- Stroke
- Subarachnoid haemorrhage
- Encephalitis

Surgical options

Unilateral decompression for localized oedema with mid-line shift, for example from a direct coup injury.

Bilateral decompression is indicated for diffuse or generalized brain swelling. The decompression may be:
- Bicoronal bone flap.
- Bilateral frontal decompression extending through to posterior coronal suture.

In children with severe head injuries, decompressive craniectomy has already been established as a beneficial treatment.

In adults, whilst there is significant anecdotal evidence to support the surgical procedure, it is usually performed when all other treatment modalities and interventions have been ineffective.

The ICP (randomized controlled, international multicentre) 'Rescue' trial is still in the process of collecting data. The principle difference to conventional decompression is the extensive or wide decompression that is performed.

Whilst it has already been established that the procedure helps to manage ICP, reduce the length of stay in ITU and improves survival, there is unsufficient data to state whether it significantly improves morbidity and quality of life measures.

Nursing management

- Observe full head dressing for signs of haemorrhage and excess leakage (report to doctors for possible re-suturing).
- Head bandage usually replaced with smaller dressing after 24hrs.
- Avoid lying patient directly onto side of decompression.
- Monitor wound site for signs of inflammation/infection.
- Remove sutures 7–10 days following surgery.

NB: patients with a large bone defect may prefer to wear a bandage/scarf for cosmetic reasons until bone flap replaced.

Cranioplasty

The bone flap can be sterilized and stored until the patient has sufficiently clinically improved.

The patient's own bone or a titanium mesh plate can be custom fit to repair the defect.

Until the bone flap is replaced, patients need to be particularly vigilant and protect the soft decompressive area over the brain. This usually means wearing a crash helmet if they are prone to seizures or refraining from work or returning to school.

Many patients report significant physical, psychological, and cognitive improvements in their recovery once the bone flap has been replaced.

Further information for health professionals and the public

Jagannathan, J., Okonkwo, D. and Dumont, A.S. (2007) Outcome following decompressive craniectomy in children with severe traumatic brain injury; a 10-year single centre experience with long term follow-up. *Journal of Neurosurgery Paediatrics*, 106(40): 268-75.

RESCUEicp study http://www.rescueicp.com

Brain Trauma Foundation guidelines http://www.braintrauma.org.

Spinal clearance

Cervical spine clearance in trauma settings and in an accident and emergency department is always difficult (□ see Spinal cord injury, p 332). According to the advanced trauma and life support guidelines, the cervical spine should be immobilized using triple immobilization unless C-spine damage is excluded by specialists. Triple immobilization consists of:

- A hard collar
- Two sand bags or blocks either side of the head
- Strapping of the forehead and chin to the spinal board

Patients should be placed on an MRI-compatible spinal board during transfer from the trauma scene to the hospital. The patient should not be on the spinal board for more than 5 hours, to prevent the development of pressure sores, however triple immobilization should be maintained.

Primary survey

Plain X-rays—must include the lateral view showing the occiput C1 junction to upper border of the T1 vertebra.

Secondary survey

- Essential to have an anterior–posterior view of the cervical spine, showing the spinous process of C2 to T1 and an open mouth view of the odontoid process, revealing the entire odontoid process of C2 and the lateral mass of C1.
- If the X-rays are reported as normal and the trauma patient is alert, awake, has no alterations in their mental status, no neck pain and no distal neurological deficit, it is likely that the cervical spine is stable and doesn't require any further radiological studies.
- Whilst cervical spine clearance and management is the priority, it is important to remember to exclude fractures in the rest of the lumbar and thoracic spine by obtaining a good history, looking at the mechanism of injury and observing motor function. Maintain log rolling and spinal alignment until cleared.

A C-spine CT is required

- When there is a neurological deficit.
- If there are any suspicious areas on the X-ray that cannot exclude injury.
- Suspected lower cervical spinal injury which cannot be visualized on plain radiograph.
- C-Spine CT scan is routinely preformed in many centres:
  • In unconscious or intoxicated patients
  • If the C-spine X-rays are normal, but the patient continues to
  • complain of neck pain, flexion–extension radiological views can exclude any ligament injury.
- X-ray views with axial CT scan provides the safest, most efficient and cost effective method of excluding C-spine injury in polytrauma patient, including comatose patients.

An MRI is required
- Any suspicion of cervical spine injury.
- Any neurological deficit, ligamentous damage, acute disc prolapse or bleeding inside the spinal cord.
- Before any spinal surgical intervention.

C-spine immobilization must be maintained until the stability of the cervical spine has been confirmed by senior medical staff or the radiologist, or if there are any premorbid conditions that may complicate the diagnosis.

Intracranial pressure monitoring

Raised or increasing intracranial pressure is a major complication following severe brain injury. Accurate monitoring and measurement of ICP enables timely interventions to maintain cerebral oxygenation, perfusion and blood flow.

Normal ICP is between 5-15mmHg. ICP measurements recorded above 20mmHg indicate a raised ICP and demand urgent medical attention.

ICP monitoring is useful in a range of patients including:

- Trauma
- Brain tumours
- Subarachnoid haemorrhage
- Stroke
- Hydrocephalus
- Neurological infections

Types of ICP monitoring systems

- Intraventricular catheter records global cerebral pressures and allows CSF drainage to control pressure spikes and fluctuations.
- Subdural or epidural fibre optic catheters are inserted into the sudural space—prone to compression as brain swelling increases (can be tunnelled under the skin to reduce the risk of infection at the entry site).
- Fibre-optic 'bolted' system that records pressure directly from the cerebral tissues.

Complications

- Infection and meningitis
- Haemorrhage
- Focal neurological deficits
- Inaccurate placement of the catheter

Analysis of wave forms

Normal ICP is pulsatile due to intracranial arterial pulsation reflecting the cardiac and respiratory cycles. In head-injured patients it is more common to observe rises in baseline pressure, rather than waves of raised ICP. Continuous recordings display A, B and C waves that can be used to identify any changes from the baseline that indicate the need for treatment or clinical interventions.

If the bone flap has been surgically removed pressure readings will often be unreliable.

P1 (percussion wave)

This is the first sharp peak representing the arterial conduction of impulses from the intracerebral blood vessels and choroid plexus to the brain tissue and CSF.

P2 (tidal wave)

Elevated P2 is associated with increasing and sustained ICP and reflects decreasing levels of compliance and impaired autoregulation.

P3 (dicrotic wave)

Final waveform that follows the dicrotic notch.

ICP trends

A waves (plateau waves)

Clinically the most important because they indicate dangerously reduced intracranial compliance. Elevations in ICP that remain high (>50mmHg) for over 5–10 minutes despite exclusion of contributory factors is a very serious signs that demands urgent attention.

B waves

Most frequent type of pressure wave but of less adverse clinical significance. Rhythmical oscillations normally occur once or twice every minute, corresponding to fluctuations in the cerebral blood flow.

C waves

Small rapid oscillations normally occurring four to eight times a minute.

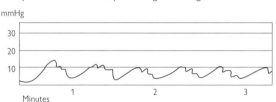

Fig. 10.1 A normal ICP waveform.

Changes in waveform may be affected by:
- Increasing ICP
- Cerebral vasospasm
- Elevation of the head position
- Severe hypoxia or hypercapnia
- Increased CSF volume
- Compression of jugular vein
- Removal of bone flap
- Hyperventilation reflected in the amplitude of P2

Nursing management
- Apply universal precautions when caring for entry site and catheter.
- The catheter is covered with an occlusive dressing that should be clean and dry (report signs of leakage to medical staff).
- Perform neurological assessment incorporating GCS assessment.
- Titrate nursing activities with ICP recordings.
- Record cerebral perfusion pressure: CPP = MAP – ICP
- CSF specimens as clinically indicated (often obtained daily by drs for MCS).
- Catheter transducer may require periodic recalibration.
- Observe waveform:
  - Dampened trace.
  - P1-P2-P3 waveforms, correlation with arterial pulse waveforms.
  - Occlusion of tubing with blood or debris.

Further information for health professionals and the public

AANN (2005) *Guide to the care of the patient with intracranial pressure monitoring*. The AANN reference series for clinical practice. Available at http://www.aann.org

ICU management of raised ICP/CPP

Cerebral perfusion pressure = mean arterial pressure – intracranial pressure (CPP = MAP – ICP).

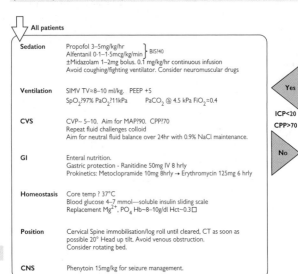

Sedation	Propofol 3–5mg/kg/hr Alfentanil 0·1–1·5mcg/kg/min } BIS?40 ±Midazolam 1–2mg bolus. 0·1 mg/kg/hr continuous infusion Avoid coughing/fighting ventilator. Consider neuromuscular drugs
Ventilation	SIMV TV≈8–10 ml/kg. PEEP +5 SpO₂?97% PaO₂?11kPa PaCO₂ @ 4·5 kPa FiO₂≈0·4
CVS	CVP~ 5–10. Aim for MAP?90. CPP?70 Repeat fluid challenges colloid Aim for neutral fluid balance over 24hr with 0·9% NaCl maintenance.
GI	Enteral nutrition. Gastric protection - Ranitidine 50mg IV 8 hrly Prokinetics: Metoclopramide 10mg 8hrly → Erythromycin 125mg 6 hrly
Homeostasis	Core temp ? 37°C Blood glucose 4–7 mmol—soluble insulin sliding scale Replacement Mg²⁺, PO₄ Hb~8–10g/dl Hct~0·3
Position	Cervical Spine immobilisation/log roll until cleared, CT as soon as possible 20° Head up tilt. Avoid venous obstruction. Consider rotating bed.
CNS	Phenytoin 15mg/kg for seizure management.

Yes
ICP<20
CPP>70
No

Consider surgical intervention

Repeat CT? Haematoma?
CSF drainage? Decompressive craniotomy

Barbiturate coma

Following consultation with senior clinician.
Options include Propofol 50–200mg bolus or 250mg thiopental boluses
upto 3–5g, supporting MAP with Fluids/Vasopressors. If favourable effect on ICP/CPP,
commence thiopental infusion 5mg/kg/hr (may need potassium replacement during
barbiturate infusion)
Risk of rebound Hyperkalaemia on cessation

Fig. 10.2 Managing raised intracranial hypertension. Cerebral perfusion pressure = mean arterial pressure – intracranial pressure (CPP = MAP–ICP).

❶ Consider ICP probe accuracy/drift

Consider a surgical intervention
Repeat CT? Cerebral haematoma?
CSF Drainage? Decompressive craniotomy

Haemodynamics
If fluid challenge→↑CVP then commence vasoconstrictor:
Noradrenaline: 0·1–1 mcg/kg/min
12 lead ECG—observe for arrythmias

Neuromuscular blockade
Atracurium 0·5 mg/kg/hr
Aim for BIS ? 40

Homeostasis
20%Mannitol 2ml/kg bolus 8hrly until plasma 320mosm/L
Bumetanide 0.5mg if balance>1L/24hrs
Core temp 35°C
High-dose Propofol? check triglycerides daily

CNS
EEG to exclude subclinical seizures (esp. if BIS↑)

No

ICP>25
CPP<70

Yes

Consider a surgical intervention
Repeat CT? Surgical lesion?
CSF drainage? Surgical decompression

Yes

ICP>25
CPP<70

No

Consider inducing state of hypothermia
Reduce Propofol, guided by BIS
Aggressive correction of diuresis and electrolytes

Fig. 10.2 (*Continued*)

Electrolyte disturbance

Neuroscience patients are particularly susceptible to electrolyte, metabolic and fluid balance disorders that in many cases are life-threatening, particularly if there are delays in diagnosis or appropriate treatment. Diagnosis is frequently complex but the nurse plays an important role in identifying essential elements and triggers related to disturbance and imbalance.

Hypernatraemia

- Serum Na >150
- Symptoms: thirst, vomiting, confusion and agitation, neuromuscular hyperactivity, coma.

Diabetes insipidus (DI)

Due to insufficient ADH resulting in large quantities of dilute urine and ↑ thirst. Two main types: neurogenic and nephrogenic.

Nephrogenic

Resistance to ADH receptors in the kidney
Causes: hypocalcaemia, chronic renal failure, drugs (lithium).

Neurogenic

Hypopituitary axis dysfunction
Causes: head injury, basal skull fractures, infections—meningitis, encephalitis, tumours and surgery damaging pituitary stalk or posterior portion of pituitary gland or stalk. Three types:

- Transient DI that resolves after 12–36 hours.
- Prolonged DI—weeks to permanent.
- Triphasic response with intermittent surges of DI.

Diagnosis

- Thirst.
- Low urine osmolarity (normal 500–800). DI 50–150 or SG <1.005
- Persistently high urine output >250ml/hr
- Normal or raised serum Na and osmolality
- Normal mineralocorticoid function

Treatment (acute)

- Strict fluid balance, SG urine 4-hrly, 6-hrly serum electrolytes and OSM
- IV fluid, base rate 100 ml/hr PLUS replacement ml for ml urine output with 0.9% NaCl.
- Be aware of post-op diuresis.
- If unmanageable—replacement desmopressin either SC or IM, 2 mcg or if VERY severe—vasopressin IV infusion 0.2 U per min and titrated.
  Thirst mechanism intact:
- Mild—keep up with losses, drink only to thirst.
- Severe—desmopressin titrated to response.
  Absent thirst mechanism:
- Risk of dehydration or fluid overload (accurate fluid chart, daily weigh, serial bloods).
- Desmopressin as needed.

Hyponatraemia

Two main causes in neurosurgery: SIADH and cerebral salt wasting (CSW).

Symptoms
- Headache, anorexia if drop gradual, secondary fluid overload.
- Sudden drop in Na leads to neuromuscular excitation and cerebral oedema—stupor, seizures, coma and death.

Treatment
- Rapid correction of hyponatraemia can lead to central pontine myelinosis—osmotic demyelination syndrome.
- Insidious onset flaccid quadriparesis, mental impairment, pseudobulbar palsy.

Cerebral salt wasting

Causes: head injury, intracerebral tumours, SAH, intracranial surgery. Important to differentiate from SIADH as treatments are different.

Diagnosis: loss of renal sodium, causes loss of water by osmotic effect. CSW patient is hypovolaemic whereas SIADH patient has hyponatraemia secondary to hyovoleamia. The mechanism remains unclear, but may be due to:
- Dopamine and sympathetic nervous system causing renal natriusis.
- A protein has been identified in plasma of acutely ill neurosurgical patients that inhibits sodium reabsorption in the proximal tubule.

Treatment
- Volume replacement and positive Na balance.
- Rehydration +/– oral Na replacement.
- Hypertonic saline and fludrocortisone (to promote salt and water retention).

SIADH

Causes: head inury, tumours, meningitis, malignancy, lung cancer, severe pain and hypotension, carbamazepine and thiazides, anaemia

Diagnosis: hyponatraemia, low serum OSM, high urinary Na (also in CSW), high serum OSM. Normal renal function and adrenal function. Water load test—20ml/kg up to 1.5l. Failure to excrete >65% in 4 hours or 80% in 5 hours = SIADH.

Treatment

Acute
- Mild and asymptomatic—fluid restriction 1L/day.
- Beware in SAH—risk of volume depletion and secondary vasospasm
- If severe use hypertonic NaCl +/– diuretics.

Chronic
- Long-term fluid restriction <2L daily.
- Demeclocycline—partial ADH antagonist.
- Furosemide and high sodium diet.

Metabolic disturbance

The pH of the body is affected by food, drink, medications and various disease processes. Body fluids are normally slightly alkaline (pH 7.35–7.45). To maintain a normal pH value, the body must continually compensate for excess acid or alkaline states by maintaining stable levels of hydrogen ions through the production of buffers from the respiratory and renal systems.

If there is a metabolic reason for the abnormal pH level, the body will try to use the respiratory system to compensate. If the underlying pathology is caused by the respiratory system, the kidneys will try to maintain the balance.

Metabolic acidosis—the body will try to raise the pH by blowing off extra CO_2. known as compensated metabolic acidosis. If the pH remains low, but the $PaCO_2$ is below 5.3Kpa, it is referred to as a partially compensated metabolic acidosis.

Respiratory system

The respiratory system is the major mechanism for eliminating excess carbon dioxide and carbonic acid from the body. Each exhalation reduces the amount of carbonic acid and carbon dioxide in the extracellular fluids. For every molecule of CO_2 exhaled by the lungs, a H+ ion is converted to water. CO_2 is the most important modulator of cerebral blood vessel calibre. There is a linear relationship between $PaCO_2$ and cerebral blood flow, as $PaCO_2$ rises, cerebral blood flow will increase by up to 15% for each KPa rise in $PaCO_2$.

Following acute brain trauma, controlled hyperventilation is used with caution for short periods to induce hypocapnia. However, excessive hyperventilation can produce a vasoconstriction of the blood vessels reducing cerebral blood flow and compromising CPP, leading to ischaemia and infarction. $PaCO_2$ should be maintained at the lower end of normal ranges, around 4.5kPa.

Metabolic acidosis—occurs when CO_2 tension and H+ ion concentration increases, for example during exercise or acute illness. This causes the pH to fall, stimulating the respiratory centre in the brain to breathe deeper and faster. This effectively decreases blood CO_2 concentration and increases pH, eventually compensating for the increased metabolic rate and returning blood gas levels to normal.

Renal system

The kidneys excrete excess hydrogen ions and reabsorb bicarbonate to maintain normal pH levels, but are not as effective as the respiratory system. It can take the kidneys several hours or even days to react to abnormal serum levels.

A metabolic acidosis will occur when:
- There is kidney failure, preventing them from producing bicarbonate (HCO_3), to act as a buffer.
- There is an increase in other acid producing by-products such as lactic acids caused by acute trauma.
- Additional acids are taken orally such as aspirin or tricyclic anti-depressants, acetazolamide.

A metabolic alkalosis will occasionally occur with:
- Severe vomiting episodes
- Large amounts of gastric aspirate
- Ingestion or administration of large amount of alkaline, e.g. antacid medication
- Diuretic therapy with loss of Na, K^+ and CL^+

Hyperglycaemia

In critical care patients the reduction of blood glucose levels below 7mmol/L is known to reduce the risk of infection, reduce lipolysis breakdown of fat, producing high levels of ketones in the blood, and reduce metabolic and calorific demands.

In the acute brain injured patient, hyperglycaemia is known to exacerbate cerebral ischaemia by increasing brain tissue acidosis, increases blood-brain permeability leading to ↑cerebral oedema and reduced blood flow.

Treatment
- A sliding scale soluble insulin regime to maintain blood glucose between 4–7mmol/L.
- Regular blood glucose monitoring.

Hypoglycaemia

Is equally detrimental to cerebral function as hyperglycaemia. Blood glucose levels less than 3mmol/L will cause seizures, unconsciousness and leads to permanent focal neurological damage.

Treatment
- 50ml of 50% glucose solution IV
- Hourly blood glucose monitoring

Other causes of metabolic disorders include:
- Diabetes insipidus
- Electrolyte imbalance
- Cerebral salt wasting (📖 see Electrolyte disturbance)

Further reading

Singer M., Webb A. (2005) *Oxford Handbook of Critical Care*. Oxford: Oxford University Press.

Brain tissue oxygen monitoring

Many routine interventions that we perform in critical care will impact on brain tissue oxygenation. The concept of solely using ICP monitoring and CPP calculation limits the ability to assess one of the most important parameters: oxygen (Bader *et al*, 2003).

Titration of fraction of inspired oxygen (FiO_2), partial pressure of carbon dioxide (PCO_2), CPP, ICP, Hb and body temperature, and the use of barbiturates can all affect oxygen delivery and consumption (Bader *et al*, 2003).

Inclusion of brain tissue oxygen monitoring along with ICP monitoring and CPP calculation and cardiovascular assessment will allow the practitioner to tailor the interventions to meet the needs of the patient. Brain tissue oxygen monitoring should be utilized as part of protocol-driven therapy in the ICU.

Interventions that impact oxygen delivery/consumption will be demonstrated by the brain tissue oxygen readings.

Outcome studies (Stiefel *et al*, 2005) have shown that incorporating tissue O_2 monitoring into patient management protocols that utilize the Brain Trauma Foundation Guidelines has led to a reduction in mortality. Licox has been accepted into routine management of patients that may be at risk of hypoxia developing secondary to their primary injury, e.g. TBI and SAH population.

Brain tissue oxygen may be monitored by using a catheter inserted through a single burr hole, directly into the white matter of the brain via a bolted or tunnelled system. Multiple parameters may be measured, including brain tissue oxygen ($PbtO_2$), intracranial pressure (ICP) and brain temperature.

The technology

The oxygen monitoring catheter works by Clark cell technology, containing two electrodes (a gold and a silver wire), in a semi-permeable membrane. Oxygen diffuses through the semi-permeable membrane, a charge is created and the monitor displays the brain tissue oxygenation as a partial pressure reading in mmHg.

Unlike jugular bulb monitoring, where a monitoring catheter is inserted directly into the internal jugular vein to give an oxygen saturation reading, the Licox catheter is inserted directly into the frontal white matter of the brain and gives information on the partial pressure reading of oxygen. The Licox monitor provides real time data for the bedside clinician to interpret and utilize to adjust their interventions accordingly.

Brain tissue oxygen readings

Normal brain tissue oxygen using the Licox system is in the range of 20–35mmHg.

Studies have shown that brain tissue oxygen readings below the critical threshold of 15mmHg are predictive of poor outcomes (Bader *et al*, 2003). The depth and duration of hypoxia will negatively impact on patient outcome (Valadka *et al*, 1998).

Safety considerations

The patient must have a blood clotting profile within normal parameters before this procedure may be undertaken by the neurosurgeon. The risks of the procedure are reported as similar to the insertion of an intraparenchymal ICP catheter (Lang *et al*, 2007). During insertion there may be some microtrauma caused and reliable brain tissue oxygen readings are available after a tissue stabilization time of 20 minutes, however, it may take up to 2 hours before the readings stabilize (Integra Neurosciences 2004). To avoid traumatic removal, the triple lumen bolted system must be removed by a neurosurgeon using a safe removal technique, i.e. loosen the compression cap, remove each catheter individually, then the introducer, then the bolt. The catheter is validated for a maximum of 5 days use.

References

Bader, M.K., Littlejohns, L. and March, K. (2003) Brain tissue oxygen monitoring in severe brain injury, 1: research and usefulness in critical care. *Critical Care Nurse*, 23(4): 17–27.

Integra NeuroSciences (2004) *Licox IMC directions for use*. Integra NeuroSciences. www.integra-ls.com

Lang, E.W., Mulvey, J.M., Mudaliar, Y., Dorsch, N.W.C. (2007) Direct cerebral oxygen monitoring—a systemic review of recent publications. *Neurosurgery Rev*, 30: 99–107.

Steifel, M.F., Spiotta, A., Gracias, V.H. *et al.* (2005) Reduced mortality rate in patients with severe traumatic brain injury treated with brain tissue oxygen monitoring. *Journal of Neurosurgery*, 103: 805–11.

Valadka, A.B., Gopinath, S.P., Contant, C.F. *et al.* (1998) Relationship of brain tissue pO_2 to outcome after severe head injury. *Critical Care Medicine*, 26: 1576–81.

Jugular bulb venous oxygen saturation monitoring

Oximetry probe-tipped catheters are now available to insert directly into blood vessels to estimate the percentage O_2 saturation of haemaglobin contained in red blood cells. Since virtually all the blood from the brain drains into the internal jugular veins, an oximeter probe placed in the internal jugular vein with its tip lying in the jugular bulb will measure the saturation of blood returning from the brain. As such, it allows us to draw conclusions about the extraction of oxygen by the brain, when compared with the arterial (or peripheral pulse oximetry) saturation.

Clinical uses

Cerebral ischaemia and hypoxia is a frequent complication following any brain injury including trauma, stroke, haemorhage or infection. Early diagnosis and prompt, appropriate intervention such as management of raised intracranial pressure, can help to reduce the level of neurodisability.

Monitoring of systemic (arterial) blood pressure and oxygenation are now relatively easy, but how readily the values reflect what is happening to the supply of oxygenated blood to injured brain tissue is difficult to assess. A monitor that tells us how much oxygen is being extracted by the whole brain, a 'global' measurement, might be useful to determine adequacy of supply at the arterial end.

Why is measuring SJO_2 useful?

The Fick equation describes the relationship between cerebral blood flow (CBF), arterial (CaO_2) and venous (CJO_2) oxygen content and cerebral metabolic rate of oxygen extraction ($CMRO_2$).

$$CMRO_2 = CBF \times (CAO2 - CJO_2)$$

Essentially, the amount of oxygen used by the brain equals that delivered to the brain (arterial) minus that leaving the brain (venous).

Arterial and venous oxygen content are the amount of oxygen that the red blood cells are able to carry. This is directly related to the saturation of haemoglobin, which we measure by oximetry. We can therefore see that SJO_2 is dependent on SAO_2, $CMRO_2$ and CBF.

Interpretation

The normal levels for SjO_2 is 50–60%. Venous saturations recorded below 50% are associated with poor long-term prognosis.

Low values
- Increased O_2 extraction due to systemic arterial hypoxia.
- Low CBF due to hypotension or raised intracranial pressure.
- Increased cerebral metabolic requirements, e.g. pyrexia, seizures.

Increased value
- Hyperaemia (increased CBF)
- Poor oxygen extraction, e.g. infarcted tissue
- Cessation of CBF (blood in jugular bulb no longer contains desaturated blood returning from the brain)

Limitations

- Migration of the catheter from the jugular venous bulb. Position of the catheter in the vein affects data reliability, since the facial veins drain into the internal jugular vein below the jugular venous bulb.
- Venous obstruction, infection and any sequelae associated with intravenous cannulation.
- Data produces a global rather than localized measure of ischaemia, as the whole venous return is analysed.
- Limited availability in many neuroscience intensive care units.
- Still largely used as a research tool.

Transcranial doppler

Transcranial doppler (TCD) uses ultrasound to measure the velocity of blood moving through the basal (large, conducting) cerebral blood vessels. The technique involves an ultrasound beam at a known frequency (from a hand-held or headset-fixed probe) passing through a 'window' of thin bone in the skull and directed onto these blood vessels.

Some of these sound waves will hit moving red cells in the blood vessel and be reflected back to the probe. Depending on how fast the red cells are moving and in which direction there will be a shift in the frequency of this reflected beam (Doppler shift).

The blood vessels can be 'mapped out' at different depths from the surface by an experienced operator, and the velocity data obtained and used to draw conclusions about cerebral blood flow and vessel diameter.

TCD is used to identify ischaemia (inadequate blood flow) or hyperaemia (excessive flow) following cerebral haemorrhage, thrombosis or trauma.

Where changes in cerebral blood flow are detected early enough, a proactive approach to treatment may prevent further deterioration. Complications and response to treatment can be monitored by serial or continuous examination.

Clinical applications
- Subarachnoid haemorrhage to detect the presence or degree of vasospasm
- Arterial venous malformations
- Emboli detection and ischaemic strokes
- Particularly beneficial during thrombolysis
- Peri-operative monitoring during neurosurgical/vascular procedures
- Potential for non-invasively estimating intracranial pressure
- Diagnosing intracerebral circulatory arrest

Common problems
- Difficulty obtaining and maintaining a good signal
- Interpretation of data
- Identifying artefacts from surrounding blood vessels

Although it is a non-invasive technique that can readily be used at the bedside, equipment costs and personnel training mean it is only available in a few specialist units across the UK. The therapeutic benefits of TCD are still being explored.

EEG in ICU

EEG (📖 see p 102) monitoring can be continuous or intermittent using either standard recording equipment or specialized cerebral function monitors.

Recording conditions in ICU are usually suboptimal. Biological and/or external artefacts can contaminate recordings.

It is important to distinguish EEG abnormalities from the effects of sedation and anaesthesia.

Status epilepticus

- Diagnostic EEG required in suspected convulsive status—need to exclude pseudostatus and investigate other possible causes of reduced level of consciousness.
- EEG monitoring essential to guide intravenous therapy and ensure all epileptic discharges are controlled.
- Continue monitoring as clinical signs of ongoing seizure activity may be subtle.

Non-convulsive status epilepticus

- EEG shows continuous or virtually continuous paroxysmal epileptiform activity.
- EEG improvement is simultaneous with clinical response to anticonvulsant medication.
- Diagnosis difficult in severe symptomatic epilepsies and patients with acute cerebral damage.

Encephalitis

- Diffuse slow activity
- EEG findings are consistent with depth of coma
- Florid epileptiform discharges may be seen
- Focal repetitive periodic discharges in herpes simplex encephalitis, subacute sclerosing panencephalitis and Creutzfeldt–Jakob disease.
- Triphasic waves over one or both temporal lobes—common in herpes simplex encephalitis.
- In terminal states, complexes on an iso-electric background may be indistinguishable from burst-suppression.

Prognosis after cardiac arrest

- Presence of continuous EEG activity within first 4 hours indicates a good recovery.
- Recovery of continuous activity after 48 hours indicates poor prognosis.
- Burst suppression pattern indicates poor prognosis.

Coma

- Depth of coma is defined clinically, according to reactivity and can be quantified by EEG monitoring.
- Reactivity may be intermittent, therefore monitoring of arousal with EEG can give more reliable results.

- Non-convulsive status epilepticus may be shown, giving an explanation of patient's obtunded state.
- Sleep pattern integrity is a useful predictor of favourable prognosis in coma.
- Alpha coma seen after cardio/respiratory arrest is a poor prognostic feature.

Metabolic and toxic encephalopathy

- EEG always abnormal
- Diffuse slow activity
- Runs of broad triphasic waves seen in severe metabolic encephalopathy.
- Typical changes are slowing, loss of reactivity and eventual EEG silence in irreversible cases.
- Sepsis-based encephalopathy monitored by severity scores based on EEG features.

Head injury

- Control of raised intracranial pressure and adequate cerebral perfusion, aided by monitoring of EEG.
- EEG assists management of sedation in ventilated patients following head injury.
- EEG monitoring is a useful adjunct for the detection of new or progressive mass lesions in acute head injury.
- Poor prognosis implied by unreactive alpha, burst suppression pattern and periodic bursts of epileptiform activity.

Reactivity and arousal

- EEG reactivity more prognostically useful than predominant frequency.
- Arousal patterns in the EEG of comatose patients vary enormously.
- Prolonged responses associated with clinical change may mimic epileptic seizures.
- Measurement of muscle and movement artefact confirm arousal of patient.

Drug changes

- Agents that affect the EEG are major sedatives, analgesics and muscle relaxants.
- Increased beta activity seen with sedative drugs, hypnotics and anti-epileptics.
- Slowing of EEG activity is seen with overt sedation and medication intoxication.
- Drug withdrawal can induce abnormalities, including epileptiform abnormalities.

Ventilation

The indications for commencing mechanical ventilation support are predominantly due to respiratory failure caused by the patient's inability to maintain their own ventilation or adequate oxygenation.

Many neurological conditions including disease and trauma adversely affect a patient's ventilation and oxygenation, resulting in hypercapnia, respiratory acidosis and hypoxia leading to further neurological impairment.

Some patients will require long-term or ongoing ventilation either in a hospital environment or at home.

Acute respiratory insufficiency

- Respiratory failure due to overwhelming demands on respiratory muscles, e.g. status asthmaticus, acute respiratory distress syndrome (ARDS), pneumonia, chronic obstructive pulmonary disease (COPD), congenital heart disease, severe shock and blood loss, bronchospasm.
- Depressed respiratory drive—patients have reduced respirations due to poor tidal volumes and/or respiratory rate, e.g. alcohol, narcotics, poisons, cervical fractures above level of C3, head injury, hypoxic brain injury.
- Mechanical respiratory failure increasing the work of breathing, e.g. flail chest, tension pneumothorax, electrolyte imbalance.

Indications for mechanical ventilation support

- GCS ≤8
- Loss of protective mechanisms, i.e. cough or gag reflex
- Cheyne-Stokes or ataxic respiratory pattern
- Hypoxia: PaO_2<9 on air, PaO_2 <12 on O_2. Oxygen saturation <95%
- Hypocarbia <4.5kPa
- Peripheral neuromuscular disease e.g. Guillian–Barré, myasthenia gravis
- Control of ↑intracranial pressure
- Elective ventilation—status epilepticus, inter-hospital or department transfer, e.g. CT/MRI scan

Modes of ventilation

The mode of ventilation will vary depending on the underlying clinical condition, their level of consciousness and the results from arterial blood gases. Ventilation may be:

- **Volume support**—provides a single, pre-set controlled tidal volume on each respiration breath. It is important to monitor airway pressures to reduce the risk of complications.
- **Pressure control ventilation**—breathing is time triggered by a preset respiratory rate on spontaneous inspired breaths. The delivered volume will vary according to lung compliance, making the work of breathing easier for patients. Particularly useful for patients with severe ARDS who benefit from high peak inspiratory pressures.
- **CMV/IPPV**—continuous mandatory or intermittent positive pressure ventilation (the traditional means of ventilation). The respiratory rate, minute and tidal volumes are preset and the ventilator delivers these values irrespective of what the patient may be trying to do. Rarely used

except in theatre or acute neurosurgical units as it requires continuous use of muscle relaxants.

- **SIMV**—synchronized intermittent mandatory ventilation ranges. One of the most useful ventilator patterns as it allows spontaneous breathing supplemented by triggered mandatory breaths from the ventilator. Frequently used during the weaning process and is used in conjunction with CPAP and PEEP.
- **BIPAP**—biphasic positive airway pressure, sometimes called airway pressure release, combines two different levels of pressure, a higher one during inspiration and a lower pressure during expiration, that makes the work of breathing easier and more natural for the patient.
- **CPAP or PEEP**—continuous positive airways pressure is used for spontaneous breathing or positive end expiratory pressure is applied during mechanical ventilation. In both cases there is a valve on the expiratory side of the patient's ventilation system that makes the alveolar pressure greater than atmospheric pressure, enabling the lungs to be kept at a greater than normal volume throughout the respiratory cycle and rendering more alveoli available for gas exchange.
- *End-tidal CO_2 measurement is recognized as an important parameter within neuro-critical care. It can be used to identify excess hyper- or hypoventilation and reduced pulmonary perfusion.*

Hyperventilation

The use of hyperventilation to control raised intracranial pressure is largely contraindicated. Reduction of $PaCO_2$ to <3.5kPa effectively induces cerebral vasoconstriction but may also cause cerebral ischaemia and exacerbate existing cerebral damage.

The adequacy of ventilator therapy must be continuously assessed via:
- General observation of the patient
- Observation of respiratory pattern
- Chest auscultation for altered breath sounds
- Observation of normal cardiovascular parameters
- Monitoring of urine output
- Ventilator observations (tidal volume, expired volume, peak airway pressures, plateau pressure, respiratory rate, end expiratory pressure)
- Pulse oximetry
- Observation of tracheal secretions—amount, consistency, colour
- End tidal CO_2 monitoring
- Regular arterial blood gas sampling

Sedation/analgesia/paralysing agents

Adequate sedation is essential to ensure the patient is kept comfortable, pain-free and unaware of unpleasant and painful procedures and interventions such as endotracheal intubation, mechanical ventilation, and insertion of invasive lines.

For the neuro patient, sedatives and opiod analgeasia help to reduce cerebral metabolic rate, improve cerebral perfusion and reduce the likelihood of cerebral ischaemia.

Sedation

Benzodiazepines are sedative drugs that reduce anxiety and promote amnesia. They are normally used in combination with opiates to ensure that the patient has little recall of events and strengthen the effects of the analgesia. Individual patient response is variable but can adversely affect the cardiovascular system by decreasing blood pressure and cardiac output.

Midazolam, etomidate

Short-acting sedative–hypnotic drugs, frequently used as an induction agent. The use of etomidate as a continuous infusion is associated with increased mortality resulting from adrenal suppression. Bolus doses are effective at reducing acute bursts of ICP without inducing hypotension.

Propofol

Has a quick onset, but brief duration of action. Usually administered as a continuous infusion, the dose is titrated to optimise the effect. In the neuroscience environment it has the additional benefit of decreasing ICP and cerebral metabolism and has anticonvulsant properties.

Thiopental

A barbiturate that is used to manage intractable raised ICP that has proved unresponsive to conventional measures. It effectively decreases cerebral metabolism, oxygen demand and cerebral blood flow, lowering ICP. The drug has a much longer half-life than conventional analgesia which can make assessment of brainstem death difficult and protracted.

Side effects include respiratory complications, hypotension and renal impairment.

Analgesia

Patients requiring ventilation support will frequently suffer from painful underlying problems and in addition will need to endure various painful procedures.

Alfentanil, fentanyl, Remifentanil—short-acting analgesics, mainly delivered as a continuous infusion.

There are many documented complications associated with inadequate pain relief from hormone-related stress responses to decreased respiratory function and ICU psychosis.

Side effects may include nausea, vomiting, drowsiness, decreased gut motility, urinary retention, constipation, and bradycardia.

The dose must be carefully titrated to avoid effects of hypotension that can have devastating effects on cerebral perfusion.

Morphine in particular can induce pinpoint pupils that could mask any underlying changing neurology.

Neuromuscular blocking agents

Administered within critical care areas to relax skeletal muscles prior to endotracheal intubation, surgical procedures, relieve laryngeal spasm or maintain synchronization and compliance with ventilation.

Specific drugs can have a depolarizing or non-depolarizing action.

- Depolarizing agents—binds with the receptor site at the neuromuscular junction preventing neuromuscular transmission, e.g:
  - Suxamethonium (succinylcholine) is used during anaesthetic induction because of its rapid onset but short-acting qualities. However, is known to produce an acute rise in ICP and therefore may be contraindicated in patients with acute head injury.
    May cause bradycardia due to stimulation of sino-atrial (SA) node.
- Non-polarizing drugs—competes with acetylcholine at the receptor sites at the motor end plates, e.g. atracurium, vecuronium bromide, have a longer-lasting effect and are therefore used for the maintance of and compliance with mechanical ventilation.
- It is essential to maintain effective sedation and analgesia alongside muscle relaxants.
- Should be used with bispectral index (BIS) or cerebral function monitor (CFM) monitoring to ensure adequate sedation.
- Paralysing agents may mask underlying seizure activity.
- Naloxone will reverse the effects of opiates.

General management measures

- The dose of sedation must be titrated against a recognized sedation scoring tool, to ensure patients aren't under- or over-sedated and to rationalize on high cost of many of the sedative medications.
- 'Sedation holds' are commonly used in general critical care areas to assess the need for continued sedation, however, for patients with acute brain injury, this practice is frequently contraindicated as it increases ICP.
- Bolus doses of sedatives should be administered prior to painful procedures such as suctioning, change of position etc, to avoid 'spikes' in ICP.

Further information for health professionals and the public

Sasada, M. and Smith, S. (2003) *Drugs in anaesthesia and intensive care*, 3rd edn. Oxford: Oxford Medical Publications.

Arterial blood gas analysis

Arterial blood gas analysis (ABGs), is an essential monitoring tool for any patient that requires intensive monitoring of their PaO_2, $PaCO_2$ and acid-base levels in the blood.

Patients with significant brain injury are particularly sensitive to a rise in CO_2. Hypercapnia acts as a vasodilator to cerebral blood vessels, thereby exacerbating existing or developing raised intracranial pressure. Serial arterial blood gas analyses enable:

- Titration of the ventilation settings to optimise oxygenation.
- Control of CO_2 to decrease cerebral blood flow and reduce intracranial pressure.

Arterial blood is defined according to its acidity and base. A pH of 7.4 is considered the equilibrium point. Normal arterial blood has a pH range of 7.35–7.45, so is slightly alkaline. When the pH of the blood falls below 7.35, the patient is in acidosis. When the pH of blood rises above 7.45, the patient is in alkalosis.

An arterial blood gas determines the pH and the partial pressure of carbon dioxide and oxygen in arterial blood ($PaCO_2$ and PaO_2). The pH, PaO_2 and $PaCO_2$ are directly measured and are used to calculate other information such as O_2 saturation, bicarbonate levels and base excess.

The following results may be found on a blood gas report:

ABG Report	
pH, H+	measure H+ ion concentration
HCO_3, BE	measure amount of base (acid buffer)
PaO_2, $PaCO_2$	measure partial pressure of gases

NB: Saturation of Hb with oxygen (SaO_2) may also appear as a percentage. The following are normal values for these measurements.

- Arterial pH: 7.35–7.45 (low value indicates acidosis).
- Arterial H+: –40nmol/L. (High value indicates acidosis.)

NB: the pH scale is an inverse scale of hydrogen ion concentration—the higher the H+ concentration the lower is the pH.

- HCO_3 24–28mmol/l
- Base –2 to +2
- PaO_2 >11.3–14kPa
- $PaCO_2$ 4.7–6kPa
- SaO_2 >95%

To convert from kPa to mmHg multiply by 7.502 and from mmHg to kPa divide by 0.133.

There are some important rules to follow that can make the analysis of blood samples more systematic and enable consistent interpretation. This five-step approach is utilized in most critical care areas.

Step 1

- Take note of the PaO_2 measurement and determine whether it is normal, decreased, or increased from the baseline.

- A low value could indicate that the oxygen level needs to be increased.
- A higher value is a good indication the inspired oxygen concentration (FiO_2) needs to be reduced or the ventilator settings adjusted.
- Levels below 8kPa indicate respiratory failure, providing the $PaCO_2$ is relatively normal.

Step 2
- Assess the pH (or H+) levels—is the patient in a state of acidosis or alkalosis?

Step 3
- Look at the $PaCO_2$ and compare it with the pH; if they are moving in opposite directions, the pH imbalance is most likely caused by a respiratory problem.

Step 4
- What is the HCO_3 or base excess (BE) measurement? Compare it with the pH and if they are moving in the same direction, the imbalance is probably metabolic in origin.

Step 5
- Compare the $PaCO_2$ with the HCO_3 (or BE), if they are moving in the same direction, one system is trying to compensate for the other. If they are moving in opposite directions the patient has problems of a respiratory and metabolic nature.

Tracheostomy

A tracheostomy is an artificial airway inserted through the anterior wall of the trachea that bypasses the body's natural protective mechanisms.

Clinical indications

- Acute upper airway obstruction—neoplasm, anaphylaxis, facial trauma.
- Long-term mechanical ventilation.
- Posterior fossa injury or surgery and upper cervical spine injury.
- Chronic respiratory disease.
- Excessive secretions with recurrent aspiration.
- Poor or absent bulbar function.
- Management of obstructive sleep apnoea.

Insertion

- Surgical tracheostomy, inserted in theatre. Indicated for patients with anatomical difficulties (short neck, obesity) coagulopathy.
- Percutaneous tracheostomy, inserted at the bedside.

Types of tube

- Single lumen tubes—often the first tube inserted.
- Double lumen tube—maybe fenestrated or unfenestrated.

Good practice guidance

- The use of double cannulated tubes is recommended for general ward areas, to ensure good tube cleanliness and patency.
- Essential equipment is checked and recorded at least daily:
  - Rebreathe bag or ambu bag with oxygen tubing
  - Oxygen and suction equipment
  - Humidification equipment
  - Spare tracheostomy (same size and one size smaller)
  - Suction equipment, suction catheters, Yankeur sucker
  - Sterile water
  - Sterile gloves, apron and eye protection
  - Cuff pressure manometer—check cuff pressure at least once per shift maintaining a pressure between 15–20mmHg

Humidification

- All patients with a tracheostomy should receive some form of humidification even if not receiving O_2 therapy:
  - Heated humidification
  - Heat–moisture exchanger (HME)
  - Buchanan bib
- Sterile water should be used in the humidification systems. Oxygen therapy must be prescribed clearly stating the percentage, duration and delivery system.
- Distilled water and saline reservoirs in humidification systems have been shown to be a source of infection.

Cleaning inner tubes

- Brushes should not used on plastic tubes.
- Inner tubes should be cleaned with warm water and air-dried prior to reinsertion.
- The inner tube should be removed at least once every 4 hours or as frequently as the patient's clinical condition demands, i.e. dependent on the quantity and type of sputum produced.
- Regular multidisciplinary team meetings should re-evaluate the ongoing need for the tube

Stoma care

- The wound is cleaned with warm normal saline using non-fibre shredding gauze to remove exudate or secretions.
- Stoma dressings are indicated based on clinical need, a non-adhesive dressing is recommended.
- Tapes should be changed at least every 24 hours or when soiled.
- The tension of the tapes should be assessed to ensure two fingers can slide between the tapes and neck comfortably.
- An airtight dressing is placed over the stoma when the tube is removed to prevent air leakage and promote wound healing.

Tube management

- Recommended tube changes are dependent upon the type of tube used, however a maximum of 28 days is advised.
- Tube changes are performed by two practitioners deemed to be competent.

Nutrition

A formal swallowing assessment is undertaken with involvement of the dietitian and SLT.

Communication

- Patients with a tracheostomy have complex communication problems and require a multidisciplinary approach to address their needs.
- Consideration must be given to the psychological impact resulting from the loss of their voice.
- Nursing documentation must include the following information:
  - Type of tracheostomy   Stoma care
  - Size of tube   Date to be changed
  - Date of insertion   Oxygen requirements
  - Method of humidification   Date of removal

Weaning and decannulation

- The process of weaning and decannulation is a multiprofessional one with clear rationales identified in the decision-making process.
- Weaning may be considered when there is a strong, spontaneous cough reflex, the patient is able to cope with their own secretions and their O_2 requirement is less than <40%.

Suctioning

Tracheal or endotracheal suctioning is performed to remove excessive secretions and maintain patency of the tube. In a patient with raised intracranial pressure, the procedure can provoke a transient intracranial hypertension and should be performed with care.

Specific management

- Ideally perform suction when ICP is below 20mmHg and CPP >50mmHg.
- Bolus doses of analgesia/sedation prior to suctioning may reduce sudden spikes of hypertension.
- Consider pre-oxygenation prior to suctioning, dependent upon the patient's clinical needs.
- Suctioning should last no longer than 10–15 seconds at a time. Allow at least 2 minutes in between each suction pass.

General measures

- Set suction pressure below 16 kPa/120mmHg in adults.
- Catheters should be single use, soft-tipped and multi-eyed.
- The catheter diameter should be less than half the internal diameter of the tube to allow airflow around the side of the catheter.

  Catheter size = (tube size–2) × 2

- Closed-circuit suctioning is preferable and should be used on all ventilated and high-flow O_2 patients (PEEP is maintained improving oxygen saturation during suction.)
- Suction is only applied during withdrawal of the catheter.
- The instillation of saline should not be used.
- Open suctioning is performed as a sterile technique.

Brainstem death

Diagnosis

The Code of Practice for confirming brainstem death has been recognized in the UK since 1983. The 1998 Code of Practice for the Diagnosis of Brainstem Death gives guidelines for the identification and management of potential organ and tissue donors.

Exclusions

All reversible causes of unconsciousness must be excluded including:
- All sedative drugs, hypnotics, muscle relaxants, poisons or alcohol
- Hypothermia—temperature must be above $35°C$
- Abnormal electrolyte or acid-base values
- Metabolic disorders—hyperglycaemia
- Endocrine abnormalities

Pre-conditions

There is a clinical diagnosis that would indicate irremediable brainstem damage of known aetiology.

Any sedation that has previously been administered, particularly barbiturates, must be at a subtherapeutic level that would not render the patient unconscious.

Primary hypothermia as a cause of unconsciousness must be excluded.

The patient is dependent on mechanical ventilation support for oxygenation.

Patient is completely unresponsive to any kind of stimulus.

Clinical testing

Testing must be completed by two senior doctors who have been qualified a minimum of 5 years and have been involved with the patient's care.

Members of the transplant team must not be involved with the brainstem death tests.

Two formal tests are performed on two separate occasions. The time interval can be a matter of a few minutes or several hours.

Although death is not pronounced until the second set of tests has been completed, the legal time of death is after the first set of tests.
- Absence of brain stem reflexes:
  - Negative pupillary light reflex response
  - Absent corneal reflex—(cranial nerves V and VII), tested with a wisp of cotton wool across the cornea
  - Absent vestibular–ocular reflex (cranial nerve VIII). Caloric test involves injection of ice cold water into the external auditory canal whilst observing for a conjugate lateral eye movement towards the affected side (ensuring that the ear is clean from blood, wax etc.)
  - Absent gag and cough reflex (cranial nerves IX and X). Stimulated with a suction catheter against the sides of the pharynx and by agitating the endotracheal tube
  - Absent oculocephalic reflex (doll's eye movement), assessed by rotating the head rapidly to one side and observing if the eyes move in the same direction as the head (contra-indicated for known or suspected cervical spine injury)

- Absent motor reflexes—response to deep painful stimulus
- The apnoea test assesses the anoxic drive stimulus in the respiratory centre in the medulla:
  - Pre-oxygenate with 100% O_2 for 10 minutes prior to commencement of tests (some units will administer 5% CO_2 in oxygen for 5 minutes)
  - Avoid hypoxia by diffusing O_2 via a catheter directly into the lungs until the test is completed
  - Disconnect the patient from the ventilator to allow the $PaCO_2$ to increase above 6.65kPa—observe for any signs of respiration
  - Reconnect the patient to the ventilator

Physiological testing

Cerebral angiography fulfils the same function if TCD is not available.

In the past, EEG's and Isotope blood flow studies were used to confirm brainstem death diagnosis.

Transcranial doppler ultrasound will confirm the absence of adequate blood flow to the brain, but is rarely indicated.

Ongoing management

The patient should be referred to the donor transplant coordination team (DTC) as soon as sedation is discontinued—this is an ideal 'referral trigger' for informing the DTC's of a potential donor.

The patient and their family will require all intensive care support from the nursing team until a decision has been reached by the patient's family regarding organ donation or discontinuation of treatment.

The local coroner must be notified when there is any trauma, violence, unexplained or suspicious circumstances.

Further information for health professionals and the public

Baron L, Shemie SD, Teitelbaum J, Deig CJ. (2006) Brief review; history, concept and controversies in the neurological determination of death. *Canadian Journal of Anesthesia*, 53: 602–8. Available at http://www.cjajca.org/cgi/content/full/53/6/602

Department of Health (1983) *Cadaveric organs for transplantation—a code of practice including the diagnosis of brain death*. London: Department of Health.

Department of Health (1998) *A code of practice for the diagnosis of brainstem death*. London: Department of Health.

Organ donation

Current situation
- Indications for transplantation are broadening and future demand for organs is likely to continue to increase.
- There is a large disparity between supply and demand of organs for transplantation
- Fewer patients are becoming brainstem dead largely due to improved screening, improved treatment options and improved road safety measures.
- Government initiatives—Organs for Transplant (2008).

Who can be an organ donor?
- Any intensive care patient who has been confirmed brainstem dead.
- Any patient on the intensive care unit or in the emergency department who is having treatment withdrawn due to futility.
- A dying patient with a proven diagnosis.
- A patient who is either:
  - Registered on the Organ Donor Register or carries a card.
  - Expressed a wish written or verbally to donate their organs in the event of their death.
- A dying patient whose relatives or carers have no objection to donation.

Which organs can be donated?
- Heart
- Lungs
- Liver
- Kidneys
- Pancreas
- Small bowel

Tissues that can be donated
- Bone
- Skin
- Corneas
- Tendons
- Ligaments
- Veins and heart valves

Who cannot be an organ donor?
- Patients with HIV
- Patient with actual or suspected CJD

Other possible contraindications
- Systemic infection
- Excessive trauma
- Multisystem autoimmune diseases
- CJD risk factors
- Infectious disease risk factors

- Malignancy
- Disease of unknown aetiology
- Haemodilution
- Degenerative neurological diseases

Sources of organs for transplantation

Living related, unrelated or altruistic donation.

Solid organ donation → cadaveric (heart beating or non-heart beating)

1. Heart beating donor

The patient is declared brainstem dead. If consent is given the DTC will evaluate the patient as a potential donor. The patient will be taken to theatre while still ventilated.

2. Controlled non-heart beating donor

The patient is identified as a potential donor following discussion and agreement between the doctors and patient's family that ongoing care is futile. The family is approached by the DTC and if consent is given, the patient is evaluated as a potential donor. The patient's ventilation is discontinued and if the patient's heart stops within a stated period of time, surgery for donation may then proceed.

Nursing management

Organ and tissue donation is part of 'end of life' care and the dignity and care of the patient is paramount throughout the pathway.

The nurse has an important role in identifying and referring potential donors. All impending brainstem dead patients and all patients who are going to have treatment withdrawn due to futility, should be referred to the transplant coordination team.

Following consent and assessment for suitability the priority is to support the donor until the appropriate surgical teams can be assembled.

The management of the organ donor is almost identical to any other patient nursed in the critical care unit, however the focus changes to identifying and treating common complications that arise in the period after brainstem death has been diagnosed and prior to organ retrieval.

Families often find the next few hours very difficult and need a lot of support from the nursing team as it can take several hours to coordinate the various transplant teams

The transplant teams will identify particular targets and parameters including:

- MAP 70–80mmHg—using fluids and vasoactive drugs to prevent hypotension. (The DTC may ask to change from noradrenaline to vasopressin to maintain blood pressure).
- PaO_2 >10kPA, with the lowest possible FiO_2 to avoid hypoxia
- CVP >10–12. Identify and treat developing coagulopathy.
- Chest X-ray and echocardiogram.
- Identification of arrhythmias—12-lead ECG recording and report.
- Urine output >1ml/kg/hr—monitor and treat any electrolyte imbalance
- Monitor for signs of diabetes insipidus—urine and serum osmolarity.
- Monitor blood glucose levels and treat hyperglycaemia.
- Maintain normothermia.

- Routine bloods will be requested by the donor coordinator that will include:
  - Arterial blood gas
  - Clinical chemistry inc. amylase
  - Liver function tests
  - Full blood count and blood grouping
  - Hormone levels (thyroid function), toxicology, virology, DNA tissue typing to be organized by the DTC
- Confirm with medical staff that the patient has been discussed with the coroner.

Neurorehabilitation

Definition of rehabilitation

Rehabilitation is defined as an educational process that enables an individual to regain optimum physical, psychological and social functioning and maximize independence. The patient is central to the rehabilitation process throughout and rehabilitation is achieved by the patient, rather than something that is done to a patient by healthcare professionals.

Rehabilitation requires a goal-directed approach and an integrated interdisciplinary approach.

Rehabilitation is part of a continuum of care that is to be considered in terms of primary, secondary and tertiary healthcare, rather than occurring in a particular place, so there is no need to wait for a patient to be transferred to a rehabilitation unit and it can begin as soon as the patient is medically stable.

Rehabilitation commences at the time of injury or incident and continues until maximum recovery has been achieved (up to 2 years and beyond).

The major aim of rehabilitation is to ensure that the level of recovery achieved is maximized and then maintained after discharge from the rehabilitation service.

Rehabilitation models

Commonly used models in rehabilitation are based on a medical model with the focus on functional ability. Other models include:
- Activities of living model
- Self-care model

Holistic health

Holistic health involves a patient-centred approach wherein the individual needs of the patient are the central focus.

Approaches to rehabilitation

During rehabilitation, the patient's goals may be achieved by:
- Improving their level of physical and psychosocial functioning
- Learning new skills or strategies to adapt to residual disability
- Adapting the patient's environment to reduce the impact of disability on functioning

Principles of rehabilitation

- Rehabilitation journey commences at the time of injury or incident
- The road to and within rehabilitation is not simple
- Patient's attitude must be one of accepting rehabilitation
- For maximum effect, rehabilitation needs to take place in a conducive environment
- Rehabilitation needs to be dynamic
- Rehabilitation is a positive process
- Correct timing for rehabilitation is imperative
- In rehabilitation we need to face harsh realities, hope is essential but false hope is destructive
- Honesty is imperative
- Accurate documentation and record keeping are essential

Further information for health professionals and the public

Barnes, M.P. and Ward, A.B. (2005). *Oxford Handbook of Rehabilitation Medicine*. Oxford: Oxford University Press.
Jester, R. (2007). *Advancing practice in rehabilitation nursing*. Oxford: Blackwell Publishing.

Rehabilitation nursing

Rehabilitation nursing entails specialist practice committed to improving the quality of life for individuals with a disability or chronic illness. It involves helping the patient to achieve maximum independence.

Rehabilitation nurses require commitment to the speciality, a holistic approach to care and a positive attitude.

Rehabilitation nursing applies principles of rehabilitation in a variety of clinical settings.

Nurses at the centre of the rehabilitation team

Nursing personnel are with the patient 24 hours a day and may be the only member of the team to have insight into the patient's level of functioning throughout a 24-hour period. Nurses are able to observe patients during the evenings and when they are socializing, thereby developing valuable insight into the patient's:
- behaviour during social interaction
- concentration
- attention and memory

when not under direct supervision from a therapist.

The nurse shares responsibility for the patient's physical and psychosocial, spiritual and cultural needs with other members of the team, but the nurse is the only member of the team that can ensure that therapy continues outside of timetabled therapy sessions, which is vital to reinforce and maximize the adaptation occurring in the brain.

Creating an environment conducive to rehabilitation

It is important that nurses control the rehabilitation environment for the patient, particularly if the patient is confused (📖 see p 157):
- Minimize noise and external distractions
- Provide aids to orientation, e.g. clocks
- Ensure adequate lighting
- Ensure the environment is free of obstructions and accessible
- Provide familiar pictures in the environment, e.g. family photos

Nurse-led aspects of care

Rehabilitation nursing can often prove challenging and takes some getting used to.
- Nurses need to take a step back from 'doing for' the patient and allow them to care for themselves as much as possible, which may be much more time-consuming.
- It is tempting to 'help' the patient, but this may not be helpful in the long run.

Nurses work as part of an interdisciplinary team and there is often overlap between the roles of different disciplines. Respect for the roles and contribution of individual team members is essential, but there are some aspects of care that are nurse-led, including:
- Bladder and bowel care
- Skin care
- Nutrition, e.g. PEG feeds
- Tracheostomy care

- Seizure management
- Pain assessment and management
- Risk assessment and behavioural assessment
- Advocacy
- Discharge coordination

Nurses are also instrumental in assisting the patient to re-establish their identity, ensuring that a 'normal routine' is maintained wherever possible, e.g.

- Helping patients to dress in their usual clothes daily, rather than wear night-clothes
- Helping patients to apply make-up

Consent and mental capacity

Nurses may be required to advocate for a patient who does not have the mental capacity to consent to care (☐ see the discussion of the Mental Capacity Act on p 446). Gaining consent from patients who have sustained a brain injury can often be problematic. If no advance directives have been established prior to the patient entering rehabilitation then all health professionals must always act in the patient's best interests.

Confidentiality and autonomy has to be protected and while it may be helpful to have family support, with the patient's consent, not all patients want their family members to have access to their medical details.

Further information for health professionals and the public

Jester, R. (2007). *Advancing practice in rehabilitiation nursing.* Oxford: Blackwell Publishing.

Rehabilitation outcomes

It is important to consider outcomes that affect quality of everyday life and consider both objective and subjective features to enable the measurement to be more complete and more useful. There is no clear agreement as to how to measure outcome. The majority of outcome measures are professionally directed.

The rehabilitation outcome is determined by a number of factors:
• Age of patient
• Gender of patient
• Past experience
• Premorbid personality
• Psyche, anxiety level and emotional status
• Environmental factors
• Support services within immediate environment
• The actual injury/incident
• Readiness for rehabilitation
• Access to services
• Socio-economic status of patient

Health professionals need to focus on the outcomes, rather than on the processes alone. Rehabilitation outcomes must be documented and achieved outcomes compared with expected outcomes. Variations need to be justified in terms of the patient's level of function and the prescribed programme.

Early referral to rehabilitation services is recommended. Should there be delay in admission of the patient to a rehabilitation unit, the rehabilitation team may recommend aspects of preventive rehabilitation that can be introduced to the patient's routine.

Generic outcome measures

A number of outcome measures are used to determine patient progress and final outcome, regardless of presenting condition:
• Barthel Index
• Functional Independence Measure
• Functional Independence Measure + Functional Assessment Measure
• Glasgow Outcome Score

Specific outcome measures

Other outcome measures are specific to patients with certain neurological disorders, e.g.:
• The modified Rankin Scale (stroke)
• Stroke Impact Scale

Self-care versus functional independence

Self-care is a holistic concept that entails physical, psychosocial and emotional well-being.

Self-care is an important consideration in quality of life measures and managing chronic conditions.

Functional independence relates mainly to the adaptation to or recovery from physical disability. Patient outcome measures used to measure functional ability include the Barthel Index and FIM+FAM (📕 see Chapter 3).

Self-care implies the need to accept responsibility for managing oneself and attend to aspects of care independently. Where this is not possible various levels of assistance or intervention may be required.

Further information for health professionals and the public

British Society of Rehabilitation Medicine (2000). *Measurement of outcome in rehabilitation—basket of measures.* Available at http://www.bsrm.co.uk/ClinicalGuidance/ClinicalGuidance.htm

Barnes, M.P. and Ward, A.B. (2005) *Oxford Handbook of Rehabilitation Medicine*. Oxford: Oxford University Press

Quality of life

What is quality of life?

Quality of life (QoL) identifies a person's interpretation of their response to health issues occurring within their life. It is the person's perception of their experience of physical, psychological, and social well-being within a particular community. It may be expressed in terms of their level of happiness or satisfaction with life.

QoL domains

There are numerous categories/domains used for measuring QoL:
• Physical functioning
• Psychological well-being
• Social interaction
• Employment
• Happiness
• Pain
• Medication
• Sleep
• Eating
• Holidays
Some measurement tools use all or a selection of domains within the questionnaire

Importance of QoL in rehabilitation

QoL is an important goal in rehabilitation:
• QoL domains are inherent within rehabilitation practice
• Rehabilitation is the penultimate stage of the patient's recovery
• The patient may need to adjust to a new lifestyle
• The patient/family may need to adjust to patient's new role in family/ society
• Factors influencing QoL outcomes include:
  • Cognitive ability
  • Coping strategies
  • Positive/negative mood

QoL outcome measures

There are a number of QoL measures. These include numerous items related to QoL. A patient rates their own ability or a carer rates the person's ability, against each item. The scores are then aggregated to produce a result.

To obtain a holistic overview of the patients QoL it is possible to use a generic QoL measure and a more specific measure, e.g. multiple sclerosis, Parkinson's disease

Generic measures

Generic measures can be used for most patient groups. Examples of generic health related QoL measures include:
• World Health Organization Quality of Life Scale (WHOQOL)
• Quality-adjusted life years (QALYs)
• Nottingham Health Profile

- Short Form 36 (SF-36)
- The Sickness Impact Profile
- General Health Questionnaire (GHQ-60)

Disease-specific measures

There are few disease-specific measures. Research is currently being undertaken for QoL measures for neurological patients in particular multiple sclerosis (e.g. MusiQoL-Multiple Sclerosis International Quality of Life Questionnaire; QoLIBRI-Quality of life in brain injury) and TBI.

It is possible to utilize more than one measure but this raises the possibility of repetition.

Further information for health professionals and the public

Bowling, A. (2005) *Measuring health. A review of quality of life measurement scales,* 3rd edn. Open University Press.

Rehabilitation settings

Only a small proportion of people who would benefit from rehabilitation, gain access to rehabilitation services.

Nurses must be able to apply principles of rehabilitation as rehabilitation can be undertaken in all settings.

The term 'rehabilitation without walls' describes the need for rehabilitative intervention to take place as and when required. Rehabilitation should be included in all settings, pre-hospital, acute, subacute and intermediate and in the home environment, in order to meet the needs of the patient. Appropriate rehabilitation will reduce costs, maintain quality of life, realize patient outcomes and eliminate the need for readmission.

Rehabilitation can take place in a number of primary, secondary and tertiary settings.

Community-based services

Early discharge to home and community-based rehabilitation has improved patient outcome and satisfaction.

Acute hospitals

Rehabilitation in acute hospitals includes the prevention of halitosis, dental caries, gastric ulcers, contractures, foot drop, deep vein thrombosis and constipation.

It is essential to position patients correctly from day one and to prevent complications that will hinder recovery and prolong rehabilitation, e.g.:
- Muscle loss
- Spasticity
- Contractures
- Pain

Tertiary services

These include acute rehabilitation services, intermediate care services and outpatient services.

The rehabilitation team

Team structure and input will depend on the needs of the particular patient and each is responsible and accountable for their practice.

Team members

The rehabilitation team includes:
- Patient and family
- Nurse
- Doctor
- Physiotherapist
- Occupational therapist
- Speech and language therapist (SLT)
- Neuropsychologist
- Dietician
- Social services

Tips for successful teams

- Maintain central focus on patient and family
- Respect for each other
- Minimize territoriality
- Use common documentation, which includes entries from all team members (reduces duplication and promotes shared responsibility)
- Effective communication via multidisciplinary team meetings, case conferences
- Outcomes-based care
- Evidence-based practice
- Team decisions
- Sense of humour, patience, tolerance
- Celebrate achievements

Multidisciplinary versus interdisciplinary teams

Multidisciplinary teams

- Each team member sets own discipline-related goals—no joint goal-setting.
- Team members work within own professional boundary—no cross-boundary working
- Minimal role for patient

Interdisciplinary teams

- These teams are most suited to rehabilitation settings.
- Care is patient-centred—fits with strategy outlined in the national service framework for long-term conditions (Department of Health, 2005).
- Teams have common goals and there is flexible cross-boundary working.
- Joint decision-making regarding rehabilitation goals.
- Each team member makes a unique contribution to the patient's outcome.
  All interdisciplinary team members are involved in the following activities:
- Multidisciplinary team (MDT) meetings and case conferences
- Chairing MDT meetings
- Named key worker
- Shared responsibility for patient management
- Joint decision-making
- Joint goal planning
- Implementing agreed plans
- Family and/or significant other communication and support
- Discharge planning

Reference

Department of Health (2005) *National service framework for long-term conditions*. London: Department of Health.

Patient and family

The patient is the focus of the team. Family and carers may be involved in the development of the rehabilitation programme, particularly with regard to discharge planning, with the consent of the patient.

Family relationships are an important consideration in rehabilitation. It is advisable that the patient and family are referred to social services and a psychologist.

Carers play an important role within rehabilitation. It is essential to involve carers in the rehabilitation process as soon as possible. Discharge planning undertaken without the input of proposed carers is seldom effective. Family and carer education is essential.

Empowerment and motivation

It is essential that the patient and family are encouraged to achieve maximum independence. The patient should be encouraged to take responsibility for their own health and future lifestyle. This is not always possible and this responsibility may devolve to a family carer. Support for the family and patient is essential.

Maintaining motivation is essential to effective rehabilitation. Valuing the individual, setting realistic achievable goals and praising small achievements will aid the patient's motivation.

The patient and family may express anger, anxiety, loss of interest, and signs of depression. It may be necessary to seek professional help where symptoms persist.

Patients often feel worthless and have poor self-esteem—needs to be recognized and control given back to the patient.

Where anger is expressed, nurses should:
- Be empathetic, but establish appropriate boundaries for acceptable behaviour
- Utilize de-escalation techniques
- Be aware of potential triggers
- Be aware of breakaway techniques if their personal safety is threatened

Empowerment

Empowerment enables the patient to make decisions, if they are able to leave, take control of own life and goals, to help themselves maximize QoL. The patient is given skills, opportunities and permission to take back control of their own life again.

The rehabilitation process involves a partnership between patient and health professionals. Empowering patients means shifting the balance of power to patient from professional.

Good communication is required to empower aphasic patients and for their voice to be heard—advocacy is important here.

Some patients do not want to be empowered—respect this—at some stages during the rehab process they may want to simply be cared for and do not have the mental strength to make necessary decisions. Professionals then need to act in the patient's best interest at all times.

Ways of empowering
- Be aware that patient might feel powerless/vulnerable
- Give control back to patient and family
- Involve patient in goal-setting/planning
- Respect patient wishes at all times
- Offer choice—what patient normally prefers
- Ensure environment facilitates patient wishes, e.g. peace and quiet

Further information for health professionals and the public

Davis, S. and O'Connor, S. (1999) *Rehabilitation nursing: foundations for practice.* Edinburgh: Bailliere Tindall

Physiotherapist

The physiotherapist attends to mobility and movement disorders, assists patients in coming to terms with major physical (muscle function, power, tone), behavioural and emotional changes, and inspires confidence and motivation to take them through the rehabilitation process

Aims of physiotherapy
- Improve patient positioning—functional position and neutral alignments
- Improve neuromuscular coordination, e.g. sitting balance and head control
- Increase muscle power and range of movement—active and passive exercises
- Improve functional abilities, e.g. transfers
- Improve general fitness and exercise tolerance
- Assess for mobility aids
- Prevent and treat infection—chest physiotherapy
- Promote continence—pelvic floor exercises and continence work
- Ultimately to achieve functional independence

Presenting problems
- Mobility and movement disorders
- Posture
- Gait
- Balance
- Walking
- Motor deficits
- Muscle wasting
- Transferring

Role of physiotherapist
- Involved in multidisciplinary team decisions and planning.
- Assesses and implements treatment programmes relating to motor disorders
- Provides person-centred management
- Acts as key worker
- Involved in various education programmes for personnel, patients and carers

Intervention
- Comprehensive assessment of movement, function and posture of patients with complex neurological presentations in order to plan treatment and predict outcome:
  - Assess for 24-hour postural control systems
  - Assess and review appropriate seating
  - Assess for and prescribe appropriate equipment to aid mobility, stabilize joints, and maintain range
  - Assess pain and work with MDT to try relieving it using positioning, handling, movement, and electrical stimulation

- Facilitate the return of normal movement after injury to prevent compensatory activity/abnormal patterning and therefore maximize function
- Re-educate balance and movement in lying, sitting, standing and walking
- Re-educate, practice and ensure safety of practical techniques, e.g. getting in/out of bed, using the toilet, getting in/out of a car
- Mobilize muscles and joints to maintain/improve range of movement.
- Splint limbs (serial casting) to maintain and/or increase range of movement in conjunction with the use of botulinum toxin
- Provide and modify exercises to strengthen muscles/maintain joint range and improve function while in the unit and at home
- Monitor and reassess patients' progress, incorporating the use of appropriate outcome measures
- Work with patients with challenging behaviour, who are unable to understand the rehabilitation process—modifying approach and content of treatment as necessary
- Participate in the decision-making process concerning the use of medication and botulinum toxin
- Liaise with other medical staff concerning patients ongoing care, for example surgeons regarding the need for tendoachilles lengthening in order to improve rehabilitation potential
- Liaise and work with carers/relatives during rehabilitation and the discharge process to ensure patient and carer safety and maximize patient function
- Refer to orthotics department as appropriate for specialist aids to help maintain joint range/support joints to improve function.
- Refer to Social Services and other external agencies to facilitate successful discharge and ongoing rehab in the community
- Liaise with community rehabilitation teams
- Maintain accurate records

Tips for nurses
- Success is rarely achieved by one health professional in isolation and techniques need to be reinforced by nurses on the wards. The brain has to relearn patterns of functional movement—neuroplasticity—so positioning etc. must be put into practice 24 hours a day.
- Refer to physiotherapy early in patient's management
- Ask for assistance from physiotherapist

Acknowledgements
Ms S. Billing, Senior Physiotherapist, Plym Neurorehabilitaton Unit, Plymouth Teaching Primary Care Trust

Occupational therapist

The occupational therapist aims to utilize specialist knowledge and expertise to maximize patient skill, independence and limit disability.

Aims of occupational therapy

- Assess functional abilities
- Help patient regain maximum function in activities of living (AL)
- Help patient and family adjust and adapt to new circumstances
- Prevent deformity and provide splints
- Provide aids and appliances
- Help patient resettle into own home
- Assists patient with social skills, leisure activities, work and study skills

Role of OT

- Involved in multidisciplinary team decisions and planning.
- Provides person-centred management.
- Treats physical, cognitive, perceptual and psychological problems throughout the patient's rehabilitation journey.
- Assesses and helps with cognitive and perceptual problems, e.g. loss of executive skills, neglect
- Act as key worker
- Involved in various education programmes for personnel, patients, and carers

Presenting problems:

- Altered cognitive functioning
- Altered perception and neglect/hemi-inattention
- Physical deficit
- Poor seating balance
- Emotional lability
- Inability to perform activities of living
- Safety in home/kitchen

Interventions:

- Assesses patient physical, cognitive, perceptual, and emotional well being.
- Works with individuals or groups
- Assists patient to learn or relearn tasks related to basic AL such as self-care and instrumental AL that enable the patient to live in the community, e.g. care of others, care of pets, community mobility
- Attention to safety/risk in the home environment
- Arranges home visits and graded discharge
- Assists with use of adaptive equipment
- Designs special equipment, e.g. splints
- Works with team regarding splinting programme
- Plans programmes related to executive functions
- Trains patient to use adaptive equipment, e.g. computer technology
- Recommends adjustments to be made in home environment
- Assesses patient ability to utilize transport/drive
- Liaises with community rehabilitation teams and physiotherapists
- Maintains accurate records

Tips for nurses
- Seek advice from an OT early in a patient's management
- Ask for help if your patients have these kinds of problems

Top tips for managing neglect

1. Differentiate neglect from visual problems
To tell the difference between neglect and a visual field defect, draw a straight line on a piece of paper and ask the patient to mark the mid-point.

If they mark the middle of the line then their problems are related to visual field defects. If they mark one-quarter of the way along the line then their problems are due to altered perception (neglect). For these patients half of the world does not exist—it isn't that they just don't see what is there—it just isn't there according to what their brain perceives.

2. Keep everything directly in front of patient
There is no point putting bed tables and lockers on the affected side of a patient with neglect—they will never know they are there. Keep everything in the midline, directly in front of them or slightly over towards their unaffected side.

3. Turn the plate one-quarter turn
Patients with neglect will often only eat half the food on a plate in front of them—they do not perceive the other half to be there.

Teach the patient to turn the plate one-quarter turn after each mouthful, then when they have turned it four times and there is no food left, they will know they have eaten it all!

4. Support affected limbs
How many times have you seen a stroke patient with their arm fallen down the side of their wheelchair, possibly even getting trapped between the arm of the chair and the wheel?

Patients with neglect will not realize that this has happened because they do not perceive their arm to exist—so make sure that limbs are well supported at all times.

Speech and language therapist

Aim of service

Provides detailed and individualized assessment/diagnosis, treatment and management of patients with varied and complex needs and backgrounds within the multidisciplinary team (MDT).

Role of the SLT

- Optimise the patient's communication potential
- Perform detailed assessment of patient's communication and swallowing abilities
- Support and educate family/carers, MDT
- Liaise with outside agencies, e.g. social services, residential/nursing homes, the police and solicitors, regarding the impact of the person's communication impairment.
- Establish capacity of a patient to make fundamental decisions around their care and future needs.
- Key worker
- Training and participation in the use of goal setting, outcome measures (FIM+FAM), multidisciplinary team meetings and educational activities.

Presenting problems

- **Aphasia/dysphasia:** acquired language impairment
- **Dysarthria:** disturbance in muscular control of the speech mechanisms
- **Apraxia of speech:** impaired motor programming and coordination of speech muscles
- **Dysphagia:** swallowing difficulties, including tracheostomy
- **Cognitive communication impairment:** impaired communication resulting from combination of linguistic and cognitive deficits

Intervention

- Tailored to the person.
- Takes place in one-to-one sessions, group/joint sessions, and in combination with other team members/therapists, where appropriate.
- Aims to treat high-priority patients at least daily.
- Arranges weekly speech and language therapy groups.
- Can be directed at the level of impairment, disability, participation and psychosocial adjustment—often simultaneously.
- Is strictly goal-led, with a strong focus placed on enabling the person to set their own goals wherever possible.
- Establishes safe oral intake and effective verbal communication where possible.
- Aims to establish sufficient insight into their difficulties in order to have effective intervention, whilst enabling the person to communicate their needs and feelings effectively.
- Educate the person and significant others about the nature of the difficulty and how to compensate for lost skills.
- Make referrals for videofluoroscopy assessments and to other departments where necessary, e.g. ear nose and throat.

- Responsible for identifying the need for alternative means of communication (communication aids) and referring to the appropriate centres for assessment e.g. 'lightwriter'.

Acknowledgement

Ms K. Searle, Senior Speech and Language Therapist, Plym Neurorehabilitation Unit, Plymouth Teaching Primary Care Trust. Devon England.

Neuropsychologist

A clinical neuropsychologist is usually a qualified clinical psychologist who has undertaken postgraduate professional training in neuropsychology

Role

As a resource for the application of specialist psychological knowledge, skills and expertise. The level and scope of the role will depend on the training and experience of the neuropsychologist and the service context, e.g. inpatient, outpatient or community-based.

Presenting problems

- Neuropsychological impairment: perceptual, language, communication, attention and information processing, memory, reasoning and executive abilities
- Behaviour
- Concurrent medical conditions: other injury or trauma, pre-existing illness or disability
- Medication: sedatives, anticonvulsants, anti-psychotics, antidepressants
- Pain control: mental and emotional distraction, pain control medication
- Mood and emotion: reactive anxiety, depression
- Mental health issues: premorbid anxiety, low mood, psychosis, drugs and alcohol use

Intervention

- Detailed assessment of cognitive functioning to define neuropsychological impairment
- Working with the MDT to evaluate the impact of these impairments on behaviour, mood, emotion and functional daily activities
- Design and implement individually directed cognitive rehabilitation, psychological intervention and management programmes
- Working with individuals and families to facilitate support and understanding, adjustment and coping with the consequences of changes in abilities and function
- Key worker
- Training and education, implementation of national guidelines

Acknowledgement

Ms M. Smith, Consultant Clinical Neuropsychologist, Southampton University Hospitals Trust.

Dietitian and nutrition services

The dietitian attends to the energy and fluid requirements of the patient.

Presenting problems

- Malnutrition
- Weight loss
- Weight gain
  Responsibilities include:
- Monitoring kilojoule intake
- Recommendations regarding kilojoule intake and the types of feeding
- Preparation of appropriate diet

Aims of dietetics

- Liaise with SLT and diet cooks
- Advise re: special diets and kilojoule intake
- Ensure adequate kilojoule intake, regardless of route of feeding
- Calculate enteral feed requirements
- Liaise with nurses re patient feeding and nutrition regime
- Advise re weight loss and diet
- Education of patient and family/carers

Intervention

- Monitor weight/BMI
- Adjust intake to level of activity
- Promote healthy eating lifestyle
- Manage medical problems such as:
  - Diabetes mellitus
  - Raised cholesterol
  - Gastrointestinal problems

Tips for nurses

- Monitor weight loss/gain at regular intervals
- Note alteration in bowel function related to diet, e.g. constipation/ diarrhoea
- Refer to dietitian early in patient's management

Social Services

Social Services attend to the social care needs of the patient. to assist people to achieve their full potential within the family, community and society.

Responsibilities include:
- Finances
- Placement
- Housing
- Adapted living
- Care packages
- Grants
- Vulnerable patients

Aims of social services

- Intervene early following early referral to plan discharge. Many arrangements required may take time to sort out
- Effective liaison between health and social care services (quality requirement in the National Service Framework 2005)
- Establish community care packages and sort funding arrangements
- Liaise with local authority re housing
- Advise re grants for adaptations etc. to living space
- Arrange meals on wheels service
- Advise on benefits
- Liaise with employers—social services are knowledgeable about disability and employment law and discrimination etc.
- Help with travelling
- Recreation for disabled
- Protection of vulnerable adults

Intervention

- Advice/counselling of patient/carer/family
- Negotiate on behalf of patient
- Ensure patient has capacity to make decisions
- Patient may require assistance regarding power of attorney, guardianship etc.

Neuroplasticity

What is neuroplasticity?

The ability of the brain to alter and reorganize its 'structure and function in response to experience' and learning by establishing new neural connections. The brain is thus enabled to reorganize alternate neural pathways. This development occurs as a result of axonal sprouting, whereby undamaged neurons continue to develop nerve endings to reconnect with other nerve endings. These interconnections enable neurons to compensate for injury and changes in the environment. Neuroplasticity, as a process of remodelling, occurs throughout life. Previously it was believed that the brain was 'hard-wired', i.e. unable to alter or change function in the event of injury or illness. The current thinking is that the brain is 'soft wired', i.e. it can adapt to changes in its environment

Ensuring optimum conditions for neuroplasticity

- Prevent neuronal cell damage, e.g. raised intracranial pressure, cerebral oedema
- Ensure conducive environment
- Enable appropriate stimulation of patient to establish 'connections'
- Utilise goal directed experiential therapeutic programmes
- Use positive sustained reinforcement
- Ensure consistency in learning and mental training
- Thought processes, attention, learning and memory are important considerations
- Attempt to encourage use of long-term memory

The rehabilitation process

The management of the patient needs to occur using a systematic, logical sequence (📖 see Fig. 11.1).

The process is a cyclical process in that one is able to return to any stage of the process during the rehabilitation of the patient. Documentation occurs throughout the process.

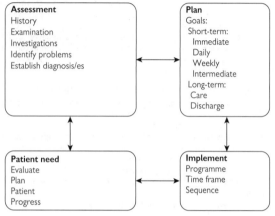

Assessment
History
Examination
Investigations
Identify problems
Establish diagnosis/es

Plan
Goals:
Short-term:
　Immediate
　Daily
　Weekly
　Intermediate
Long-term:
　Care
　Discharge

Patient need
Evaluate
Plan
Patient
Progress

Implement
Programme
Time frame
Sequence

Fig. 11.1 The rehabilitation process.

Assessment

Assessment of the patient takes place at various stages. Comprehensive assessment is performed prior to admission and on admission to the rehabilitation centre. Assessment of progress and recovery is undertaken throughout rehabilitation, depending on the needs of the patient.

Pre admission assessment

This assessment is undertaken by one, or preferably two of the rehabilitation team, often including medical consultant

Purpose of the assessment

- To determine whether the patient meets the criteria for entry to and will benefit from rehabilitation. Different centres use various criteria for patient selection, e.g:
  - Age of patient
  - Medical diagnosis
  - Medical stability
  - Readiness for rehabilitation
  - Appropriateness for rehabilitation programme on offer
  - Level of consciousness
  - Current deficits
  - Cognitive level of patient
- To assess and ensure patient's medical stability
- To assess risk in order to prepare for admission

After assessment, the patient is presented to the team. It is a team decision as to whether the patient will be admitted.

Assessment on admission

Assessment is undertaken on admission, usually by allocated key worker.

Purpose of the assessment

- To determine current status of patient
- Risk assessment, e.g. moving and handling, pressure areas
- Form basis for care planning and developing rehabilitation programme
- Baseline against which to assess outcomes
- Assess appropriate aids and appliances, e.g. wheelchair, feeding, toileting

Performing the assessment

Due to fatigue it may be necessary to complete assessment over a few days. On completion a rehabilitation plan is compiled. The patient's case is then presented at the weekly case conference.

Content of assessment

General assessment

- Patient's condition—past medical history and presenting complaint
- General health history
- History of the injury/illness and progress to date
- Sequelae of the injury/incident, e.g epilepsy
- Current medication
- Presenting problems

- Review relevant investigations, e.g. MRI, bloods
- May include specific functional assessment baseline measures e.g Barthel Index/FAM

Needs/activities of living assessment (depending on framework used)

Problem-related assessment

More detailed assessment of specific problems may be required, e.g.

- Swallowing
- Pain
- Sensory function
- Cognition
- Mood (anxiety/depression/emotional lability)
- Challenging behaviour
- Family roles/needs

Tips for assessment

Determine the following:

- Level of understanding of patient
- Level of motivation of patient to recover function
- Assess individual patient need on weekly basis
- Assess level of independence regarding each appropriate need/AL
- Assess level of independence in performance of functions
- Safety when performing function
- Posture when performing function
- Correct completion of activity
- Effort needed to complete function
- Assess level of assistance required to meet need, e.g.:
  - Perform independently
  - Requires prompt/guidance only
  - Requires assistance of one or two people
  - Requires use of assistive devices/aids

Document findings and level of intervention required

Planning

On completion of the assessment it is necessary to plan the patient's programme. Planning and scheduling of the programme is undertaken at regular intervals throughout the programme, preferably on a weekly or two-weekly basis.

Planning the programme

Establish a weekly programme:

- Programme needs to be practical and pragmatic.
- Schedule activities to combine basic maintenance, interspersed with specialist activities and training.
- Allow time for rest, sleep, and recreation.
- Where possible, tasks within sessions can be integrated.
- Adjust according to the needs of the patient.
- Schedule the programme to avoid confusion and exhaustion.

Tips for planning the programme

- Involve the patient and family in decision-making
- Develop a daily schedule with the patient
- Maintain the daily schedule
- Enable patient to undertake as much activity as possible
- Ensure patient feels safe whilst undertaking activity
- Encourage independence
- Praise achievements

Depending on the patient's circumstances it may be necessary to alter the plan at other times. This needs to be documented in the patient's notes and reported at the interdisciplinary team meeting.

Goal-setting

From the outset it is important to set realistic short-term, intermediate and long-term goals at regular intervals. The goals set must be:
• Structured
• Measurable
• Achievable
• Realistic
• Appropriate time frame
  Setting appropriate rehabilitation goals leads to:
• Facilitating, enabling and empowering patients to achieve and maximize their potential
• Maximizing self-determination, restoration of function and optimising lifestyle choices
• Ensuring adequate physical, psychological, behavioural and social functioning to enable the patient to return to the family, community, previous leisure activities and gainful employment, where possible
• Enabling the patient to return to their level of function by preventing complications (misuse and disuse phenomena), modifying the effects of disability and increasing independence
• Maximizing the participation of the patient in the social setting
• Minimizing the pain and distress experienced by the patient
• Minimizing the distress of and stress on the patient's family and carers
• Maximizing the patient's independence within their personal environment
• Helping people manage long-term problems

Appropriate goals

Nurses must ensure that goals are:
• Acceptable to the patient
• Meaningful to patient (patient-centred)
• Interdisciplinary and set with patient involvement
• Set immediate, intermediate and long-term goals
• Communicated or written in language patient understands
• Related to patient's quality of life rather than disability and physical recovery
• Written in positive way to motivate patient and ensure persistent effort to achieve them

If patient feels that the rehabilitation programme is aimed at goals they want to achieve, they will be more motivated and empowered to achieve them.

Unrealistic goals

Setting unrealistic goals may cause false hope, raise expectations, result in the patient or family not accepting the final patient outcome. Unrealistic goals will lead to frustration and demotivate the team, patient and family, whereas realistic goal-setting will encourage goal attainment.

Consider

• Patient involvement in goal-setting
• Team roles in goal-setting

- Vocabulary used
- Proposed intervention to achieve goals
- Holding regular goal-setting and review meetings

Further information for health professionals and the public

Davis, S. and O'Connor, S. (1999) *Rehabilitation nursing: foundations for practice*. Edinburgh: Bailliere Tindall.

Importance of correct positioning

Objective
- Maintain body alignment
- Maintain joint flexibility
- Prevent disuse or misuse phenomena
- Encourage well-being
- Enhance mobility, hygiene
- Maintain independence
- Maintain skin integrity
- Prevent aspiration
  May be affected by:
- Altered level of consciousness
- Neurological deficit, e.g. paresis, paralysis, hemiplegia, quadriplegia,
- Low mood and depression
- Physical deficit
- Fatigue

Problems relating to position change
- Poor body alignment and posture
- Altered respiratory function due to poor chest expansion
- Inability to maintain clear airway
- Poor peripheral circulation/oedema
- Pressure sores
- Altered skin integrity
- Contractures
- Deep vein thrombosis
- Increased/decreased muscle strength or tone
- Limited physical ability
- Tiredness
- Decreased level of independence

Intervention may include
- Monitor patient's position whilst recumbent, sitting in chair and whilst mobile
- Maintain hygiene
- Maintain airway and respiratory function
- Prevent aspiration by correct positioning
- Ensure safety of patient and carers during position change
- Encourage patient to participate actively in position change
- Educate patient and carers
- Maintain correct position
- Maintain normal body alignment/posture/position where possible
- Encourage patient to maintain correct position at all times
- Maintain skin integrity and prevent pressure sores
- Use of aids and assistive devices
- When appropriate utilize splints.
- Work with physiotherapist and occupational therapist
- Provide written plan for correct positioning
- Record and report any issues relating to positioning

Sexual health needs

Refers to patient's sexual health, not merely the act of sexual intercourse. An area of neurorehabilitation that is often neglected.

May be affected by:

- Altered body image
- Poor self-esteem
- Low mood and depression
- Feelings of being damaged/incomplete
- Physical deficit
- Fatigue

Problems relating to sexual functioning

- Limited physical ability
- Tiredness
- Increased sexual activity
- Inappropriate sexual activity (for time, place, and situation)
- Decreased/increased libido
- Impotence
- Vaginal dryness
- Loss of inhibitions
- Unwanted pregnancy

Interventions may include

- Assist patient to identify sexual health needs
- Honest, appropriate discussion with patient, family, and partner
- Listening to patient, family or partner's perception and views on sexual health
- Maintain professional relationship with patient
- Monitor overt sexual behaviour
- Introduce diversional therapy
- Behaviour modification if aberrant sexual behaviour
- Advice from family planning service
- Referral to sex/relationship therapist
- Involvement of current partner in decision-making/problem resolution
- Ensure appropriate environment
- Ensure sufficient rest and sleep
- Use of lubricants
- Provide written information

Tips for partners

- Encourage patient and family to talk about relationship issues
- Secure emotional relationships lead to physical relationship
- Spouse/partner needs support to maintain emotional bond

Tips for nurse

- Be open and listen
- Allow opportunity for patient to discuss sexual health
- Allow patient, family or partner to set pace of progress of discussion
- Avoid showing signs of embarrassment
- Utilize drawings and models to explain concepts
- Ensure adequate training to advise regarding sexual health
- Discuss with interdisciplinary team

Psychological/emotional considerations

Problems relating to psychological/emotional needs

- Grief and bereavement
- Feelings of loss
- Facing transition and loss—adaptation
- Altered intellectual capacity
- Anxiety
- Depression:
  - Patient may experience natural reactive depression due to their clinical condition
  - Patient may also be depressed due to neurochemical changes in the brain, e.g. to serotonin levels, or due to structural change
- Altered mood/affect
- Anger, aggression, and challenging behaviour
- Lack of insight
- Lack of self-concept
- Loss of inhibitions
- Loss of self-control
- Emotional lability
- Loss of capacity

Intervention may include

- Monitor psychological/emotional status of patient
- Monitor behaviour/sleep patterns
- Introduce behaviour/sleep chart
- Referral to psychologist/neuropsychologist/psychiatrist
- Ensure patient is within calm, conducive therapeutic environment
- If patient is clinically depressed, they may require antidepressants
- Use of appropriate medication
- Grief counselling
- Referral to community resources

Strategies for managing challenging behavior in clinical practice

- Where possible, gather relevant information regarding potential influences
- Careful observation to identify triggers of behaviour and reactions or responses of others
- Reduce environmental noise and 'busyness'
- Ensure adequate rest periods
- Pace activities and visitors
- Know what patient's interests are in order to engage their attention
- Keep information simple and use appropriate communication methods
- Avoid trying to correct or argue with someone who is confused and/or confabulating as this can precipitate conflict, and sometimes aggression
- Use subtle diversion/distraction towards another topic/action
- If possible change environmental stimuli which trigger behaviour
- If necessary, orientate and tell the person who you are each time you have contact

- Do not suddenly engage in a task/activity without warning and explanation
- If the person is safe, it is sometimes better to 'ignore' the behaviour and just keep them under distant observation
- Do not inadvertently encourage behaviours that may become troublesome if they persist, with reactions that may be interpreted as positive social responses
- Agree an approach or strategy between staff and family
- Educate everyone who has contact with the person to maximize consistency of approaches and keep this updated
- Refer to neuropsychologist for specific behaviour techniques

Social and cultural considerations

Problems relating to social and cultural needs
- Altered communication, interpersonal skills and behaviour
- Loss of inhibitions
- Inappropriate behavior in social situations
- Isolation
- Acquisition of inappropriate social practices, e.g. use of recreational drugs or alcohol
- Inability to perform culture-related practices such as hygiene, cooking, cleaning, and prayer
  Intervention may include:
- Assess patients spiritual and cultural needs
- Monitor social interaction
- Encourage visits from family, friends, colleagues
- Encourage appropriate interaction with visitors
- Enable patient to continue with religious or cultural practices
- Introduce programme of social interaction as soon as possible, e.g group sessions, eating in dining room, sitting in communal lounge
- Referral to psychologist/neuropsychologist
- Referral to community resources
- Referral to social services

Vocational/educational considerations
Problems relating to vocational/educational needs
- Inability to return to previous education/vocation
- Physical deficits
- Cognitive/emotional deficits
- Lack of independence
- Lack of transport

Intervention may include
- Appropriate assessment for return to education/vocation/work
- Work assessment
- Facilitated return to work where possible
- Phased return to work where appropriate
- Refer to social services/educational resources as appropriate
- Monitor return to education/work
- May need to undergo further training
- Consider career change
- Support patient throughout process

Further information for health professionals and the public
Davis, S. and O'Connor, S. (1999) *Rehabilitation nursing: foundations for practice*. Edinburgh: Bailliere Tindall.

Health promotion

Throughout the patient's rehabilitation it is imperative to promote health and achieve a positive alteration in the patient's lifestyle with as little disruption as possible.

Tips for health promotion

- Introduce primary prevention programmes, developed for the local environment, into schools, churches, social clubs, rehabilitation centres, etc.
- Promoting health and preventing disease involves the community, patient and significant others in active health promotion programmes
- Promote a healthy lifestyle
- Prevent further injuries or accidents, particularly where the patient has had a traumatic brain injury or suffered a stroke for example
- When deciding on topics to include in programme allow patient choice
- Encourage active participation in programme
- Progress within programme determined by patient ability
- Use all teaching opportunities

Topics for health promotion

Possible topics could include:
- Safety in the home
- Prevention of strokes and falls
- Drink and driving campaigns
- Reducing alcohol/recreational drug consumption
- Safety in sport
- Nutritional intake and diet
- Stress or anger management
- Safe weapon policies
- Stopping smoking
- Lifestyle choices

Living with chronic illness

Chronic illness or a long term condition is defined as the presence of a health problem affecting a person's physical, psychosocial or mental well-being that persists for more than 12 months. A chronic condition is not curable but can be effectively managed in a primary care setting.

People over 60 years often have more than one chronic condition.

Risk factors for chronic conditions

Lessening risk factors will aid the management of chronic conditions:
- Smoking
- Obesity
- Cognitive deficit
- Altered mobility/immobility/inactivity

Self-management is key to managing chronic illness. Self-management involves patients learning to become active participants in their own health and social care.

Taking control

A patient with a chronic condition needs to accept responsibility and take control of their health and life. Depending on the level of cognitive functioning and any presenting neurological deficits, patients may require input from significant others to manage their health. The focus of life should be on living rather than on the chronic condition. The process of taking control involves self-management.

Benefits of self-management

↑ psychological well-being
↓ pain
↓ depression
↑ quality of life
↓ further disability
↓ admission to hospital
↓ visits to health professionals
↓ dependency on social services

Recovery of function or adaptation to a change in lifestyle may take several months or years.

Ensure that the patient maintains the level of function achieved during rehabilitation.

It is extremely difficult to predict final patient outcome.

Coping strategies for patients with chronic conditions

- On first diagnosis patient may demonstrate shock, denial, anger or grief and fear of the unknown.
- Be well-informed about the condition. Use reliable sources for information. Ask the health professionals
- Establish a trusting relationship with health professionals and make them partners in management
- Establish a team including experts. A case manager, care package, visits from the district nursing services of GP practice may need to be arranged for the patient

- Arrange for your care to be coordinated or do it yourself
- Invest in yourself. Make 'me' time. Perform a radical change to your lifestyle. Stop smoking, control obesity, introduce physical exercise. Be positive and enjoy living
- Involve family and friends in this new lifestyle. It is healthier for all
- Establish care plan for management in the community
- Manage medications effectively
- Manage symptoms appropriately, e.g. fatigue
- Stay fit. Encourage patient to attend to tasks within the home (activities of daily living and instrumental activities of daily living) as part of an exercise regimen, where possible
- Be aware of psychological changes such as depression. Seek assistance.
- Encourage socialization
- Join a support group. There are numerous local or national community organizations such as:
  - HEADWAY (National Head Injuries Association),
  - CBIRT (Children's Brain Injury Trust).
  - MS Society
  - Stroke Association
  - Check whether these organizations are available in the area
- Discuss life choices regarding death and dying, when appropriate
- Take control
- Be positive and assist the patient and family to face the challenges that are presented within their daily lives, leisure pursuit, educational and vocational needs

Initiatives to promote self management

A number of government lead initiatives have been introduced to empower people with chronic conditions.
- Development of the Expert Patient (📖 see p 23)
- Introduction of Medicine Management to improve health and reduce wastage
- Amended role of pharmacist
- Introduction of polyclinics
- Introduction of protocol-based care

Tips for managing chronic illness for patients and nurses

- Display a positive attitude
- Maintain a daily schedule
- Enable patient to be as active/independent as possible
- Schedule rest periods if necessary
- Involve others in patient's daily schedule
- Exhibit calmness, patience and tolerance
- Utilize community resources
- Get involved in community activities
- Maintain interest in recreational activities

- Take time out
- Utilize respite care
- Maintain your sense of humour
- Seek assistance when required
- Refer patient to community services

Further information for health professionals and the public

Department of Health (2001) *The expert patient: a new approach to chronic disease management for the 21st century*. London: Department of Health.

Warren Grant Magnuson Clinical Center, National Institute of Health (1996) *Coping with chronic illness*. Patient information publications. Bethesda. USA: Warren Grant Magnuson Clinical Center, National Institute of Health.

Gadgets and gizmos (aids and appliances)

Numerous appliances and aids are available for patients who have undergone a period of rehabilitation and recovery. The rehabilitation team will recommend assistive devices or aids appropriate to each patient's needs.

Aids and appliances are available for most aspects of patient management. The salient issue is whether these aids and/or appliances are necessary.

When recommending aids it is important to consider:

- Why is the aid being supplied/purchased?
- The level of independence/function of the patient
- Will the aid encourage or discourage independence
- For how long will the aid be needed?
- The aid may assist in the short term but is it appropriate for the patient's long term recovery and independence?

Advice regarding aids:

- Should a patient wish to buy or use a particular device this should be discussed with the appropriate therapist or knowledgeable person.
- If possible the patient should borrow or hire the aid/equipment prior to purchase to assess appropriateness.
- The majority of aids are expensive and therefore it is essential to ensure the patient understands the reason for the aid and that the patient will use the aid that is purchased.

Where to acquire/buy aids

- Whilst in the rehabilitation unit appropriate aids will be provided by the relevant therapist.
- On discharge it may be necessary for the patient to continue using an aid.
- An assessment will be completed by the physiotherapist, occupational therapist, nursing personnel and social services to decide on payment for the aids.
- Depending on the outcome the aid may be purchased in full or in part by the health services or social services or it may be necessary for the patient to purchase the aid.
- OT service/NHS direct or via the Internet patients can locate details of suppliers in the local area.
- Voluntary organizations or charitable organizations may also assist with the purchase or loan of equipment.

If a patient is visiting a relative and needs to have access to a piece of equipment for a short period of time, these may be borrowed from the local Red Cross Society.

Caution

Aids and appliances must undergo regular safety checks.

Further information for health professionals and the public

The Department of Health http://www.dh.gov.uk
Headway http://www.headway.org.uk
The Spinal Injuries Association http://www.spinal.co.uk
The Stroke Association http://www.stroke.org.uk
The Association of Rehabilitation Nurses http://www.rehabnurse.org
The World Health Organisation http://www.who.int.com
Sexual Health Network http://www.sexualhealth.com

Legal and ethical issues

Stem cell research

A stem cell is an undifferentiated cell that has the potential to be manipulated and caused to develop into any human cell, such as a neuron. Stem cell research is being carried out in the hope that one day it will help treat or prevent a variety of long term neurological conditions, such as:

- Motor neuron disease (MND)
- Stroke
- Spinal cord injury
- Alzheimer's disease
- Parkinson's disease

The supply of stem cells is not infinite and this has led to calls for development of human/animal hybrid stem cells as an alternative. More recently stem cells have been harvested from specially grown human embryos (which are created in a lab and then killed during the process). This practice is not supported by pro-life groups because destruction of the embryo for cells prevents it from become a viable human being.

While the majority of nurses are unlikely to be directly involved in the research or treatment of patients with stem cells, an awareness of the issues is necessary as patients may ask about these treatments.

Sources of stem cells

Fetal and embryonic stem cells

To date, most stem cells have been sourced from an aborted fetus and this has resulted in a number of ethical concerns, particularly in relation to the harvesting of the fetus. The collection of cells from an aborted fetus is closely regulated to avoid the potential problems and reduce people's concerns that:

- Undue pressure is being put on women or their decision has been heavily influenced to have an abortion simply to produce stem cells.
- Women may become pregnant with the intention of creating an embryo for stem cell research (perhaps if a family member is suffering from a neurodegenerative condition).
- The process involves destruction of a human embryo that could develop into a healthy individual.
- The process is the 'slippery slope' towards couples choosing the sex and other characteristics of their child.
- Certain religions argue that it devalues life and is akin to murder.

Adult stem cells

Stem cells can be collected from adults, but their use is more limited. They are also difficult to isolate and collect. It may be an advantage to collect adult stem cells from a patient for treatment as this would reduce the risk of rejection of the implanted cells.

Other potential sources of stem cells

- Menstrual blood
- Baby teeth
- Amniotic fluid
- Umbilical cord blood

Human Embryology and Fertilisation Bill 2007–08

This updated bill is currently progressing through parliament before being accepted into law. While the bill covers all aspects of embryo research and IVF, it has sparked great debate over the inclusion for the first time of sections permitting the development and use of human/animal hybrid stem cells for research purposes. Researchers believe that this is necessary as there are insufficient stem cells available from other sources.

These hybrid stem cells will be created from an animal egg (probably cow) from which all the DNA has been removed. An adult stem cell will then be injected into the egg and stem cell lines will be produced.

Many concerns have been raised about the use of human/animal hybrid stem cells, primarily because of fears born out of ignorance, but these stem cells are to be used purely for laboratory research and will never be used directly on humans.

Further information for health professionals and the public

Human Embryology and Fertilisation Bill (2007–08) http://www.publications.parliament.uk/pa/pabills.2007/08

Genetic testing—reproductive choices

Couples may choose not to have a test in pregnancy or not to have children at all, if they know one or both partners carry a faulty gene.

Prenatal testing

A test may be available during pregnancy (chorionic villus sampling and amniocentesis) which enables a couple to find out whether or not the fetus is affected and enable them to make decisions about whether or not to continue with the pregnancy.

Pre-implantation genetic diagnosis

This involves using fertility treatment to create an embryo for a couple. Before the embryo is placed in the uterus, a cell is removed from each embryo to determine the ones unaffected by the particular malformation or disease, these are then placed in the uterus.

This is a complex, time-consuming and expensive procedure, but is available to some couples who cannot accept the possibility of terminating an affected pregnancy.

Genetic testing, disclosure, and decision-making

The genetic contribution to neurological disorders and the testing available varies.

Types of inheritance

Autosomal dominant inheritance, e.g. Huntington disease

An individual needs to inherit only one faulty copy of a dominant gene to be affected. There is a 1:2 chance (50%) that each child of an affected individual will inherit the faulty gene.

Autosomal recessive inheritance, e.g. spinal muscular atrophy (SMA)

An individual needs to inherit a faulty copy of the gene from both parents to be affected. There is a 1:4 chance (25%) that each child of carrier parents will inherit two faulty copies of the gene.

X linked recessive inheritance e.g. Duchenne muscular dystrophy (DMD)

The faulty copy of a gene is only carried on the X chromosome. A woman has two X chromosomes (XX) and a man has one X and one Y chromosome (XY). The condition will usually only manifest in males. Women can be carriers of the genetic condition but will not be affected.

Genetic counselling

- A person with a close (usually 1st or 2nd degree) relative with a genetic neurological condition can be referred for genetic counselling.
- Genetic counselling may involve:
  - taking a full family history and drawing a family tree
  - confirmation of diagnosis in the family
  - discussion of risks and facts about the genetic condition and inheritance
  - options available for managing the risk
  - identification of psychosocial needs
  - discussion of reproductive options
  - discussion of genetic testing and its implications

Genetic testing

For some neurological conditions (where the faulty gene is known) genetic testing is possible. There are three categories of genetic test.

Carrier test

Once a faulty recessive gene has been identified, relatives may wish to know if they are carriers. This type of testing is mainly used by those making decisions about having children.

Diagnostic test

A person who is symptomatic may have testing as part of their management in order to make a diagnosis.

Predictive test

Once a faulty gene has been identified in a late-onset condition; a person requesting the test may not have symptoms. All predictive tests are undertaken following genetic counselling on several occasions to discuss the long-term implications of the test result.

Ethical dilemmas in genetic testing

Genetic testing in particular raises many ethical questions for individuals, families, and clinicians.

Decision-making and disclosure

- Making the decision to have a genetic test is a serious undertaking and impacts on many aspects of that person's life.
- Disclosure of the result to other people has huge implications, e.g. discrimination by insurance companies or discrimination at work.
- Occasionally a person requests a genetic test because of pressure from a third party, e.g. their employer.

Confidentiality in families

- The genetic results may have implications for other family members. Sometimes a person may refuse to share the genetic test results with other relatives, thereby denying information to others and raising a difficult dilemma for the genetic specialists involved.
- A family member may refuse to be tested even though this may benefit their children. Testing the children anyway would disclose the parent's results, but occasionally there is no other option.

Testing in children

- Genetic testing is only offered to children in early onset conditions, for example DMD, Charcot–Marie–Tooth, SMA.
- Genetic testing is not usually offered for late-onset conditions with no prophylactic treatment such as Huntington disease (<18 years of age).

Privacy, confidentiality, and disclosure of information

Importance

- Respecting the confidentiality of patient data is a strong prima facie duty.
- It helps to foster and preserve the trust between patients and professionals.
- It is required by the Nursing and Midwifery Council (NMC)—see, for example, the NMC's (2008) *Standard of conduct, performance and ethics* and *Guidelines on records and record keeping*—failure to comply may lead to removal from the Register.
- It is part of the common law of equity—if information is given in confidence then generally it is a reasonable expectation that it will be kept confidential.
- It is part of the duty of care—nurses who breach confidentiality without reasonable cause are liable through the tort of negligence.
- A duty of confidentiality is usually stated or implied in contracts of employment.
- It is recognized in statute—e.g. Article 8 of the Human Rights Act 1998 states that every person has a 'right to respect for private and family life'; also in The Data Protection Act 1998.

Circumstances when patient confidentiality can be breached

- When the patient consents—the duty is owed to the patient and it is in their power to decide if disclosures should be made.
- In the best interests of the patient:
  - For example, health professionals sharing information in an emergency that, if information is not passed on, would lead to the patient suffering harm.
  - The information should be limited to that which is necessary to protect the patient. Although professionals often routinely share information this should be with the consent (implied or express) of the patient.
  - Where a patient refuses to allow information to be shared, they should be made aware of the implications of their decision, their choice should be documented and, unless the breach falls into one or more of the other categories here, respected.
- Under a court order—ask to see the order.
- Where there are statutory duties to disclose:
  - For example Public Health (Control of Diseases) Act 1984; the Road Traffic Act 1988 (as amended by the Traffic Act 1991); the Prevention of Terrorism Act 2000; section 60 of the Health and Social Care Act 2001.
- In the public interest—one court case (*W v Egdell* [1990] CA Ch 359) has suggested the following issues for consideration:
  - The risk should be real, immediate and serious.
  - The risk should be substantially reduced by disclosure.

- Disclosure is the only way to reduce the risk.
- The disclosure is limited to that which is reasonably necessary.
- The damage to the public's trust by beaching confidentiality is outweighed by the likely damage to the public interest if confidentiality is respected.
- To protect a child or other vulnerable clients (The Children Act, 1989); the child's welfare is paramount.
- If unsure, seek legal advice.

Caldicott principles of disclosure of patient-identifiable information

- Justify the purpose.
- Do not use patient-identifiable information unless it is absolutely necessary.
- Use the minimum necessary patient identifiable information.
- Access to patient-identifiable information should be on a strict 'need-to-know' basis.
- Everyone with access to patient-identifiable information should be aware of his or her responsibilities.
- Understand and comply with the law—if unsure, get legal advice.

Further information for health professionals and the public

Department of Health (1999). *Caldicott Guardians.* http://www.dh.gov.uk/en/Publicationsandstatistics/Lettersandcirculars/Healthservicecirculars/DH_4004311

Human Rights Act (1998) http://www.justice.gov.uk/guidance/humanrights.htm

NMC (2008) *Nursing and Midwifery Council. The code. Standards of conduct, performance and ethics for nurses and midwives.* http://www.nmc-uk.org

Access to healthcare records

Importance

It is good practice to write records in collaboration with patients: this promotes trust and communication

Access to records—the Data Protection Act 1998 (DPA)

- The DPA gives 'data subjects' (i.e. an individual who is the subject of personal data, such as a patient) certain formal rights of access:
  - To be informed as to whether personal data is processed.
  - To be given a description of the data held, the purposes for which it is processed, and knowledge of the persons to whom it may be disclosed.
  - To be given a copy of the information constituting the data— copies should be in a legible form and with an explanation of any unintelligible terms.
  - To be given information on the sources of the data.
  - To have errors about them contained in the records corrected.
- For a patient to gain formal access to their records they must put their request in writing to the organization that holds the records (i.e. PCT or GP practice). The responsible manager has 40 days to respond.

Access to a record by a data subject is restricted

- When access would be likely to cause serious harm to the physical or mental health of the data subject.
- When to give access would reveal the identity of a third person (unless the third person has given consent to the disclosure). This exception does not apply if the third person is a health professional who has been involved in the care of the person (unless serious harm to that health professional's physical or mental health is likely to be caused by giving access).

Access to records—the Freedom of Information Act 2000 (FOI)

In addition to the DPA, the Freedom of Information Act, 2000 (FOI) requires that all public bodies (including the NHS and GP practices) produce a publication scheme giving details of all information routinely published by the organization. Certain data is exempt from this legislation, including personal data. Data subjects who wish to gain access to their records should follow the DPA.

Who can seek access to health records?

- Any competent person (including a competent child/young person) can apply for access to their personal records
- A person with parental responsibility for a child—where there is more than one person with parental responsibility, each person may apply separately—it should be noted, however, that a competent child/young person has a right to confidentiality

- Where a person is incapable of managing their affairs, a person appointed by a court may have access to information they require to discharge their duties
- A third party when authorized by the data subject—check for proof of authorization and contact data subject if unsure. NB family, friends and carers do not have a right of access unless the patient has specifically stated.
- The executor or administrator of a deceased person's estate may apply under the Access to Health Records Act 1990.

Further information for health professionals and the public

Department of Health *Electronic social care record* (ESCR). http://www.dh.gov.uk

Research ethics

Why research is important

High-quality research is essential for the development of clinical practice if it is to meet the needs of patients. Part of the research process is to ensure that it is ethically robust and strikes a balance between any risks and benefits. Nurses and other health professionals have a vital role in making sure that this standard is met, both as investigators and as advocates for patients.

Core principles that should underpin the conduct of ethical research

The most significant piece of international guidance on the ethics of research is the Declaration of Helsinki. First developed in 1964 by the World Medical Association (WMA), amended in 2004; is a recognized benchmark against which studies are measured identifying core principles on which research involving human participants can be judged ethically; including (WMA, 2004):

- It is the duty of the health professional to promote and safeguard the health of the people. The health professional's knowledge and conscience are dedicated to the fulfilment of this duty.
- Considerations related to the individual's well-being should take precedence over the interests of science and society.
- It is the duty of the health professional in medical research to protect the life, health, privacy, and dignity of the human subject.
- Medical research must conform to generally accepted scientific principles, be based on a thorough knowledge of the scientific literature, other relevant sources of information, and on adequate laboratory and, where appropriate, animal experimentation.
- Medical research should only be conducted if the importance of the objective outweighs the inherent risks and burdens to the subject.
- The right of research subjects to safeguard their integrity must always be respected. Every precaution should be taken to respect their privacy, the confidentiality of the patient's information and to minimize the impact of the study on the subject's physical and mental integrity.
- Each potential subject must be informed of the aims, methods, sources of funding, any possible conflicts of interest, institutional affiliations of the researcher, the anticipated benefits/potential risks of the study, and any discomfort it may entail. The subject should be informed of the right to abstain from participation in the study or to withdraw consent to participate without reprisal. Subsequently, the person responsible for conducting the research should obtain the subject's freely given informed consent, preferably in writing. If the consent cannot be obtained in writing, the non-written consent must be formally documented and witnessed.
- For a research subject who is mentally incapable of giving consent or is a legally incompetent minor, the investigator must obtain informed consent from the legally authorized representative in accordance with applicable law (sections 30–34 of the Mental Capacity Act 2005 or section 51 of the Adults with Incapacity Act). These groups should not

be included in research unless the research is necessary to promote their needs and the research cannot instead be performed on legally competent persons.

The above principles are reflected in the Nursing and Midwifery Council's advice on research and audit (NMC 2006) and the development of legislation—the Mental Capacity Act, 2005 (sections 30–34), the Adults with Incapacity Act, 2000 (section 51), the Human Tissue Act, 2004 and the Medicines for Human Use Regulations, 2004.

NHS research governance

The responsibility for giving ethical approval to research involving NHS patients, staff or resources lies with Local Research Committees (LRECs) and Multi-centre Research Ethics Committees (MRECs), coordinated by the National Research Ethics Service (part of the National Patient Safety Agency), The LREC/MRECs consider a range of factors when reviewing a research proposal (Herring, 2006: p. 618):

- That there are adequate arrangements to ensure the full consent of all participants or where the participants are incompetent to consent that the legal requirements are met (including information that is given).
- That the legal requirements are met.
- The study has scientific validity and will not cause harm or discomfort.
- The arrangements for recruitment are adequate (representation in terms of gender, age, ethnicity) and do not mislead.
- The arrangements for care and protection of participants are adequate (including ongoing care of participants on completion of research).
- That the participants' right of confidentiality is protected and the impact of the research on the wider community is considered.

Further information for health professionals and the public

Department of Health website on Research and Development http://www.dh.gov.uk/PolicyAndGuidance/ResearchAndDevelopment/fs/en. Accessed 13 December 2007.

National Research Ethics Service http://www.nres.npsa.nhs.uk. Accessed 13 December 2007.

Nursing and Midwifery Council (NMC) (2006) A–Z advice sheet: research and audit. Available at http://www.nmc-uk.org. Accessed 13 December 2007.

Office for Public Sector Information. The Human Tissue Act 2004 http://www.opsi.gov.uk/acts/acts2004/20040030.htm. Accessed 13 December 2007.

Office for Public Sector Information. Medicines for Human Use (Clinical Trials) Regulations 2004 http://www.opsi.gov.uk/si/si2004/20041031.htm. Accessed 13 December 2007.

Office for Public Sector Information. The Mental Capacity Act 2005 http://www.opsi.gov.uk/acts/acts2005/20050009.htm. Accessed 13 December 2007.

Office for Public Sector Information. The Adults with Incapacity (Scotland) Act 2000. Accessed 13 December 2007. www.opsi.gov.uk/legislation/scotland/acts2000/as

World Medical Association (2004) Declaration of Helsinki. Available at http://www.wma.net/e/policy/b3.htm. Accessed 13 December 2007.

Informed consent and mental capacity

Definition of consent

Voluntary agreement with (or refusal of) an action proposed by another. It is a continuous process, rather than a one-off act—it relates to all aspects of care. Seeking, and respecting, consent is fundamental to nursing practice because it:

- Recognizes the intrinsic value of patients.
- Fosters patient trust and confidence in health care professionals.
- Ensures the propriety of the act: protecting the professional from criminal charges civil claims or allegations of professional misconduct.

Necessary elements of valid consent

Valid consent must incorporate all of the following elements. It must be:

- Voluntary—i.e. given without undue pressure or coercion
- Reasonably informed—i.e. the person giving consent must have an understanding of:
  - The nature of the act proposed and its associated benefits and risks
  - Alternatives to the proposed act (including 'doing nothing')
  - The associated benefits and risks of the alternatives
- Made by a competent person—i.e. someone with mental capacity to:
  - Understand the information and weigh up the possible options
  - Competency is function-specific: an individual may have the capacity to take some healthcare decisions but may lack the capacity to decide about other, more complex matters
  - All adults (>16 years old) are presumed to be competent but that presumption can be questioned and refuted

Format of consent

The professional providing the care, treatment or investigation should seek consent. The format in which consent is given varies depending on the seriousness of the act. It can be:

- Implied consent
- Express verbal consent (for minor procedures, such as venepuncture)
- Express written consent (for more serious procedures)

Consent forms

Written consent forms are used as prompts and because of their evidential value: they act as a record providing evidence in case of future disputes.

Emergencies

Where consent is unobtainable, provide life-saving treatment if it is not known to be contrary to the expressed wishes of a competent patient (e.g. an advance decision).

Patients lacking capacity

Legislation is now in place to ensure that adults who lack capacity receive appropriate care—Mental Capacity Act 2005; Adults with Incapacity (Scotland) Act 2000—and is based on core principles:

- Assume a person has capacity unless demonstrated otherwise—age, appearance, diagnosis or behaviour do not in themselves establish a lack of capacity.

- Do not treat people as incapable of making a decision until all practicable steps have been taken to help them.
- A person should not be treated as incapable of making a decision simply because it appears unwise.
- Always do things, or make decisions, for people without capacity in their best interests. Remember that best interests are wider than best medical interests and should take into account the person's beliefs and values.
- Before taking action, consider whether the outcome could be achieved in a less restrictive way.

The above legislation provides defined ways in which the care of clients lacking capacity may be managed:

- A person may, whilst competent, appoint someone to make decisions on their behalf in the event that they become mentally incompetent. This is called a Lasting Power of Attorney in England and Wales and a Welfare Attorney in Scotland.
- If a person is already incompetent and lacks a Lasting Power of Attorney (or Welfare Attorney in Scotland), they may apply to the Court of Protection in England and Wales (or the Sherriff's Court in Scotland). Such an application may be for a one-off order to cover a single decision or, when a series of decisions are likely to be needed and a one-off order insufficient, then the Court of Protection may appoint a deputy in England and Wales (a Welfare Guardian in Scotland) to manage the financial and welfare needs of the individual.
- The Mental Capacity Act 2005 enables people lacking capacity who have no family or friends with whom it would be practicable to consult: Independent Mental Capacity Advocates (IMCAs). IMCAs should be consulted when decisions are being made about serious medical treatment or significant changes to the provision of care (e.g. moving care homes).
- In addition to the above, a competent person may make an advance decision refusing specific medical treatment in the event that they become incapacitated. The advance decision must be clear about which treatment it applies to, it must be in writing and witnessed if it applies to life-sustaining treatment. Treatment can be provided if there is doubt that the advance decision is invalid.

Further information for health professionals and the public

Ministry of Justice. *The Code of Practice for the Mental Capacity Act 2005* http://www.justice.gov.uk/guidance/mca-code-of-practice.htm. Accessed 13 December 2007.

Office for Public Sector Information. *The Mental Capacity Act 2005* http://www.opsi.gov.uk/acts/acts2005/20050009.htm. Accessed 13 December 2007.

Office for Public Sector Information. *The Adults with Incapacity (Scotland) Act 2000*. www.opsi.gov.uk/legislation/scotland/acts2000. Accessed 13 December 2007.

End of life care (EOL)

The 'End of Life' pathway enables patients with an advanced, progressive, incurable illness to live as well as possible until they die. It allows the supportive and palliative care needs of both patient and family to be identified and met throughout the last phase of life and into bereavement. Recent guidelines published by the Department of Health (2007), attempt to break down the prevailing 'live for ever' mindset by the public and health professionals that opposes the normality of death and dying, often hindering the wishes of patients who wish to die with the minimum of pain, in a place that they choose.

The guidance applies to:

- Adults with advanced, progressive, incurable illness (e.g. advanced cancer, heart failure, COPD, stroke, chronic neurological conditions, dementia).
- Care given in all settings (e.g. home, acute hospital, ambulance, residential/care homes, nursing homes, hospice, community hospitals, prison or other institutions).
- Care given in the last year(s) of life.
- Patients, carers and family members (including bereavement care).

The document identified the need to ensure that palliative care is seen as everyone's business, as part of good-quality general care and not just a specialist area of care associated with complex cases. It sets out key challenges that have to be addressed through local discussion and arrangements.

General principles

- Patients should be given the opportunity to discuss treatment options and plan their end of life care.
- Nurses and other health professionals must work together to provide skilled detection and management of symptoms, particularly adequate pain control.
- Patients should be treated with dignity and respect at all times.
- Support should be given to family and friends so that they are not overwhelmed by the burden of caring.
- All patients (regardless of diagnosis) should have access to appropriate services including, palliative care, hospice beds, bereavement services, spiritual care and access to information.
- Support should be made available for loved ones after bereavement.
- A single care coordinator is required to act as the end of life service provider with the authority to broker and assure care and support to patients and families.
- Training and education on EOL should be part of the core curriculum, professional continual professional development. Key skills include communication, palliative care and advance planning.
- Funding must be ring-fenced to support the provision of care from pooled budgets across health and social services to enable joint commissioning and investment.

Advance decisions

- A competent person may make an advance decision refusing specific medical treatment in the event that they become incapacitated. The advance decision must be clear about which treatment it applies to, it must be in writing and witnessed if it applies to life-sustaining treatment. Nurses and other health professionals must abide by a valid advance decision.

Withdrawing and withholding treatment

- Competent patients can decide for themselves what is in their best interests and whether to refuse or stop treatment.
- Requests for artificial nutrition and hydration (ANH) from mentally competent patients should be complied with when nourishment cannot be provided in other ways.
- Patients and their families cannot insist upon clinically inappropriate treatment: care should be based on the individual's best interests. Where treatment is, or would be, futile then it may be withdrawn or withheld (including ANH).

Euthanasia

Some patients with devastating, debilitating, and progressively deteriorating illness consider voluntary euthanasia in an attempt to achieve a 'dignified death', at a time when they feel that continuation of life is futile. Some patients have applied to the courts to gain permission to end their lives. When unsuccessful, a number of patients have obtained help from clinics in other countries, particularly Switzerland and the Netherlands.

Physician-assisted suicide

Refers to doctors whose actions directly cause or contribute to the patient's death in order to relieve their suffering, however,

- Procuring, assisting, aiding, abetting, or counselling someone to commit suicide is illegal and punishable by up to 14 years imprisonment under the Suicide Act, 1961.
- Deliberately killing someone through a positive act (such as administering a drug) with the primary intention to cause death is murder, punishable by life imprisonment.

Further information for health professionals and the public

Department of Health http://www.dh.gov.uk/nhs/endoflife

Economics and rationing of healthcare

Economics of health care

Health care is the single largest area of UK government expenditure: in the 2007–2008 budget, £105 billion was allocated for health care out of a total managed expenditure of £589 billion (HM Treasury, 2007). Although healthcare receives a large amount of funding, decisions on which work to undertake within the allocated budget have to be made every day and there are inevitably winners and losers. Decisions are made at macro, meso and micro levels:

- *Macro:* i.e. at governmental level (e.g. allocation of the social budget to different government departments and allocation within the different departments)
- *Meso:* i.e. at an organizational level (e.g. which services to fund)
- *Micro:* i.e. at an individual level (e.g. nurses and other clinicians deciding which patients to see and what care to provide)

Law

The NHS Act of 1977 sets out the obligations of the Government to provide health care services. Section three of the Act places a duty on the Secretary of State for Health (and, through him/her, healthcare organizations) to provide such services 'as he considers necessary to meet all reasonable requirements'. This includes:

(a) Hospital accommodation
(b) Other accommodation for the purpose of any service provided under this Act
(c) Medical, dental, nursing and ambulance services
(d) Such other facilities for the care of expectant and nursing mothers and young children as he considers are appropriate as part of the health service
(e) Such facilities for the prevention of illness, the care of persons suffering from illness and the after-care of persons who have suffered from illness as he considers are appropriate as part of the health service
(f) Such other services as are required for the diagnosis and treatment of illness

The Act does not require the Government to meet all healthcare demands. This has been recognized in subsequent case law (e.g. *R v Secretary of State for Social Services* ex p. Hincks [1980] 1 BMLR, *R v Cambridge Health Authority*, ex p. B [1995] 2 All ER and *R v North West Lancashire Health Authority*, ex p. A and others [1999] Lloyd's Rep Med 399).

Rather, the Secretary of State, health authorities and healthcare providers must make decisions that are based on reasonable and fair procedures and grounds.

Framework for ethical health care rationing (after Daniels 2000; Pencheon *et al.* 2001)

There are several recognized frameworks that can be applied to facilitate rationing and prioritization of services. QALY (quality-assurance life years), is recognized both nationally and internationally as a useful measure to evaluate high-cost interventions, for example making the drug trastuzumab readily available for women with breast cancer and balancing cost with long-term effectiveness.

The following framework provides an outline of steps for the fair allocation of scarce healthcare resources.

- Choose interventions that are known to be beneficial on the basis of evidence of effectiveness and minimize the use of marginally beneficial interventions (inefficiency is immoral).
- Decisions regarding the use of new technologies and interventions (and their rationales) must be publicly accessible.
- Advocate for one's own patients, but avoid manipulating the system to gain an unfair advantage for them (be aware of the bigger picture).
- Resolve conflicting claims for scarce resources on the basis of morally relevant criteria such as need and benefit, using publicly defensible procedures (ideally incorporating meaningful public involvement).
- The rationales for decisions should aim to provide a reasonable explanation of how the organization should provide value for money in meeting the diverse needs of its population under reasonable resource constraints.
- There should be a publicly accessible mechanism for challenging decisions, including the opportunity for revision in light of new evidence or arguments.
- Inform service users of the impact of cost constraints on interventions, but do so in a sensitive way.
- Seek resolution of unacceptable shortages, utilizing professional associations (e.g. the RCN): nurses must recognize that they have a political role to play and should be contributing to the different stages of the commissioning process (LNNM 2007):
  - Setting the strategic framework underpinning commissioning.
  - The strategic and operational planning of different services.
  - Purchasing activities and monitoring and evaluation of services.

Further information for health professionals and the public

Daniels, N. (2000) Accountability for reasonableness in private and public health insurance. In Coulter, A. and Ham, C. (eds) *The global challenge of health care rationing*. Buckingham: Open University Press

HM Treasury (2007) *Comprehensive spending review: where taxpayers' money is spent*. http://www.pbrscr07.treasury.gov.uk/page_08.html. Accessed 12 November 2007.

LNNM (London Network for Nurses and Midwives) (2007) http://www.lnnm.co.uk/publications/primarycaretoolkit.pdf. Accessed 12 November 2007.

Pencheon, D. *et al.* (2001) *Oxford Handbook of Public Health Ethics*. Oxford: Oxford University Press.

Walker, S. and Rosser, R. (1993) *Quality of life assessment*. 2nd edn, New York: Springer.

Record keeping

Importance

Good record keeping is an essential part of professional nursing practice. It promotes continuity of care (through accurate communication), acts as a means to demonstrate the quality and complexity of nursing and provides a resource if nurses are called to account at a later date (⚠ in the courts' eyes, if it wasn't recorded, it didn't happen).

What counts as a record?

Any permanent form of data recorded about a client or patient. This includes both paper and electronically stored information.

General principles for good record keeping

Records should be:
- Legible
- Written in black permanent ink (if handwritten)
- Contemporaneous
- Include the date and time the information was recorded
- Signed with printed name and designation clearly stated
- Clear, comprehensive and focused on the provision of accurate, objective, factual and relevant information relating to the client's diagnosis/needs and care/treatment
- Written in collaboration with patients

Records should not:
- Contain offensive remarks or jokes
- Contain ambiguous, unclear language or abbreviations
- Be altered except to make corrections to inaccurate information (any alterations should be clearly marked as such and signed/dated)

Details to include when making entries to patient records

- Information on which you have based your decision—the problems/needs presented by the patient/client; relevant information on past history (including health, medication, family and social history); test results and examination findings.
- Impressions of the current situation—priorities for care/treatment.
- Action plan—as negotiated with the patient/client (may include referrals made, prescriptions given, tests undertaken).
- Information shared and advice given—concerns/worries of the patient/client or their family/carers; health advice given to the patient; contact information (including out-of-hours services); plans for follow-up/next consultation.
- Other essential information—including details of correspondence with others.

Storage of records

- Do not leave records unattended.
- When not in use, store all files and portable equipment (e.g. laptops and personal digital assistants) under lock and key.
- If the records are patient or parent/child held, then reinforce the need to keep the information secure to the patient or parent/child.

Electronic records
- Do not leave a terminal unattended and signed-in.
- Never share passwords.
- Regularly change passwords and avoid using short or obvious ones.
- Clear the screen of one patient's information before seeing another patient.
- Use password-protected screensavers to prevent casual viewing of patient records by others.

Manual records
- Store files closed and in a logical order.
- Use a tracking system to monitor the whereabouts of files.
- Return files as soon as they are no longer needed.

Retention of records
- The Department of Health suggests that the length of time a record is retained should depend on the type of record and its continuing importance but provides the following guidance as minimum retention periods:
  - Children and young people: until 25th birthday, or 26th if young person was 17 at time of conclusion of treatment; or 8 years after patients death, if death occurred before 18th birthday.
  - Maternity (including midwifery and obstetric): 25 years.
  - Mentally disordered patients: 20 years after no further treatment; or 8 years after patient's death.
  - Oncology: 8 years after conclusion of treatment.
  - General: 8 years after conclusion of treatment.
  - GP records: 10 years after conclusion of treatment.

Destruction of records should be through a secure process.

Further information for health professionals and the public

Department of Health *Patient confidentiality and access to health records.* Available at http://www. dh.gov.uk

Complementary therapies

Introduction to complementary therapies

Complementary and alternative medicine therapies (CAM) are becoming more widely used throughout the UK and the rest of the world. There is concern that many of the therapies lack an evidence base and yet remain popular among patients and the public. It is estimated that in the UK around 2 million people are using a range of complementary therapies on a regular basis (Watkins, 1997). There is also growing interest among nurses in developing skills in complementary therapies for use in practice as well as research.

In 2000 the House of Lords Select Committee on Science and Technology produced a report on Complementary and Alternative Medicine. This report acknowledged the growth in CAM use in the UK and sought to identify, among other issues, the evidence base for the therapies considered and whether research was being carried out. The report identified that very little high-quality CAM research existed and recommended that government resources be put towards efforts to build up an evidence base for CAM with the same rigour required of conventional medicine.

The House of Lords Select Committee (2000) classified complementary therapies into three separate categories. Group 1 therapies, often referred to as the big 5 (acupuncture, chiropractic, herbal medicine, homeopathy, and osteopathy) were deemed to be the most organized professions and already have a substantial amount of research supporting their effectiveness. Group 2 therapies (e.g. Bach flower remedies, aromatherapy, massage, and reflexology) were less professionally organized, but clearly complemented conventional medicine. Group 3 (e.g. iridology, kinesiology, crystal therapy) therapies were those which could not be supported due to the lack of convincing evidence of efficacy.

This chapter addresses the most widely accessed therapies as well as those for which there is some evidence of effectiveness for neurological conditions.

References

House of Lords Select Committee on Science and Technology (2000) *Complementary and alternative medicine*. London: The Stationery Office.
Watkins, A. (1997) *Mind–body medicine: a clinician's guide to psychoneuroimmunulogy*. Edinburgh: Churchill Livingstone.

Homeopathy

Homeopathy is a therapy that uses highly diluted substances to treat symptoms. The substances, if administered without being diluted, would normally cause the same symptoms that the homeopath is attempting to treat.

This is based on the principle of 'like cures like'.

Following an extensive consultation and interview, homeopaths use two types of remedies:
* Constitutional (to treat the whole person, based on their personality)
* Symptomatic relief

Theories of mechanism of action

When homeopathic remedies have been analysed, it is often impossible to detect any trace of the original substance remaining and therefore critics have argued that it cannot work because there is no active ingredient in the preparation.

Homeopaths believe, however, that serial dilution leads to a more powerful remedy.

Evidence

Homeopathy has been subjected to numerous randomized controlled trials, but results are mostly inconclusive, conflicting or negative.

It is likely to be beneficial in relieving chronic fatigue syndrome, but has not been shown to be beneficial in studies using this treatment for headache or stroke.

Advice for patients

* Check with GP or neurologist prior to commencing therapy.
* There is no compulsory regulation for homeopaths; some homeopaths are medically qualified and the GP may be able to refer to an NHS homeopathic practitioner, or patients may seek private homeopathic treatment.
* Unlikely to cause any harm, but little published evidence of benefit.
* May be helpful in relieving some symptoms.
* Find a qualified/registered practitioner through professional body websites, e.g. http://www.trusthomeopathy.org.

Further information for health professionals and the public

Ernst, E. *et al.* (eds) (2008) *Oxford Handbook of Complementary Medicine*. Oxford: Oxford University Press.

Herbal medicine

Herbal medicine involves the medicinal use of preparations made from plant material.

Theories of mechanism of action

Many plants contain pharmacologically active ingredients and many well-known conventional drugs are derived from plants, e.g. digoxin from digitalis (foxglove) or aspirin from salix (willow tree).

Many people think that because these are natural substances, they cannot be harmful, but as they contain active ingredients that cause an effect, side effects can also occur and some preparations can interact with prescription medication, e.g. St John's wort with prescribed antidepressants.

Evidence

There is evidence of effectiveness from systematic reviews and randomized controlled trials (RCTs) for a number of conditions for specific herbal preparations. e.g.:
- Butterbur—migraine prophylaxis
- Cannabis—pain and spasticity in MS
- Capsicum (chilli)—neuropathic pain, back pain
- Devil's claw—back pain
- Ginkgo—dementia and cognitive impairment
- St John's wort—depression

Advice for patients

- Check with GP or neurologist prior to commencing therapy—it is important to tell medical practitioner because of potential interaction with prescription drugs, potential contraindications and potential adverse events associated with the respective plants.
- May be helpful in relieving some symptoms
- Find a qualified/registered practitioner through professional body websites, e.g. http://www.rchm.co.uk; http://www.herbalmedicine.org.uk

Further information for health professionals and the public

Ernst, E. *et al.* (eds) (2008) *Oxford Handbook of Complementary Medicine*. Oxford: Oxford University Press.

Acupuncture

Acupuncture involves placing extremely fine needles into the skin at specific points all over the body. Placement of the needles depends on the condition being treated.

Theories of mechanism of action

In traditional Chinese medicine it is believed that health and illness is controlled by a balance of Yin and Yang forces within the body and the flow of life-force (Qi/Chi) within a number of energy channels 'meridians'. Where there is a blockage to the flow of Qi ill health can result.

Acupuncture needles are placed through the skin along these meridians and manipulated by a twisting motion, to stimulate the flow of Qi, until a sensation of De-Qi is felt by the patient.

'Western' medical acupuncture is based on physiological concepts and focuses on pain relief.

Evidence

There is evidence that acupuncture is likely to be beneficial for a number of conditions, e.g.:
- Neck and back pain
- Nausea and vomiting associated with chemotherapy
- Anxiety

While studies in other neurological conditions have been undertaken, the evidence is not conclusive due to the small number of studies available, methodological weakness in the studies or because studies have produced conflicting results, e.g.
- Memory loss in Alzheimer's disease
- Reduction of seizure frequency and duration in epilepsy
- Headache and migraine
- MS
- PD
- Stroke

Advice for patients

- Check with GP or neurologist prior to commencing therapy
- GP may be able to refer for NHS treatment.
- May be helpful in relieving some symptoms, especially pain.
- The therapy is generally low-risk if administered by a suitably qualified practitioner, but bleeding may occur at insertion sites and it is contraindicated in patients with bleeding disorders
- Find a qualified/registered practitioner through professional body websites, e.g. British Acupuncture Council http://www.acupuncture. org.uk

Further information for health professionals and the public

Ernst, E. et al. (eds) (2008) *Oxford Handbook of Complementary Medicine*. Oxford: Oxford University Press.

Hypnotherapy

Hypnotherapy involves inducing a deeply relaxed trance-like state, in which the subconscious mind is open to suggestion.

Theories of mechanism of action

It is believed that the hypnotic state induced enables the patient to gain control over their emotions and behaviour. Patients are also able to gain control over some physiological functions during this state of intense relaxation.

Evidence

There is evidence that hypnotherapy is likely to be effective for a number of conditions, e.g.:
- Headaches
- Pain control (e.g. post-op and chronic pain)
- Anxiety
- Chemotherapy-induced nausea and vomiting

There is no conclusive evidence of effectiveness for other neurological conditions, although there have been some trials, for example in epilepsy and stroke rehab.

Advice for patients

- Check with GP or neurologist prior to commencing therapy
- GP may be able to refer for NHS treatment.
- May be helpful in relieving some symptoms, especially pain.
- The therapy is safe when undertaken by a suitably trained hypnotherapist, although recalling painful memories may be distressing for some patients.
- Find a qualified/registered practitioner through professional body websites, e.g. Hypnotherapy Association, http://www.thehypnotherapyassociation.co.uk; or the National Council for Hypnotherapy, http://www.hypnotherapists.org.uk/.

Further information for health professionals and the public

Ernst, E. et al. (eds) (2008) *Oxford Handbook of Complementary Medicine*. Oxford: Oxford University Press.

Osteopathy

Osteopathy is a manipulative therapy involving manipulation of both soft tissues and joints.

Theories of mechanism of action

It is believed that misalignment of bones and joints can be improved through manipulation and that this in turn will result in improvement of the flow of blood and lymph throughout the body.

Evidence

There is evidence that osteopathy is likely to benefit:

- Acute back pain
- Shoulder pain

There is no conclusive evidence of effectiveness for neurological conditions, although there have been some trials, for example in fibromyalgia.

Advice for patients

- Check with GP or neurologist prior to commencing therapy.
- Osteopathy teaching institutions often run clinics where treatment is provided by senior students under supervision. This may be a cheaper option than a qualified private practitioner.
- May be helpful in relieving some symptoms, especially pain relief.
- The therapy is relatively safe when undertaken by a suitably trained practitioner, but should be avoided if there are any degenerative bone conditions e.g. osteoporosis, bone tumours (especially of the spine).
- Find a qualified/registered practitioner through professional body websites, e.g. General Osteopathic Council, http://www.osteopathy.org.uk or the British Osteopathic Association http://www.osteopathy.org.

Further information for health professionals and the public

Ernst, E. *et al.* (eds) (2008) *Oxford Handbook of Complementary Medicine.* Oxford: Oxford University Press.

Chiropractic

Like osteopathy, chiropractic is a manipulative therapy involving manipulation, mainly of the spine, in order to influence the body's function. It is used mainly to treat musculo-skeletal problems

Theories of mechanism of action

It is believed that misalignment (subluxation) of the bones of the spine can disrupt the flow of vital life-force and result in ill-health. Chiropractic aims to realign the bones to improve symptoms.

Evidence

There is clear evidence of the effectiveness of chiropractic for back pain

It may also be helpful for some other neurological conditions, but there is currently insufficient or conflicting evidence on which to make a definitive judgement, e.g.:

- Migraine
- Headaches
- Whiplash injuries

Advice for patients

- Check with GP or neurologist prior to commencing therapy
- Chiropractic teaching institutions often run clinics where treatment is provided by senior students under supervision. This may be a cheaper option than a qualified private practitioner.
- May be helpful in relieving some symptoms, especially pain.
- Mild, transient adverse events are common, but serious complications (stroke or arterial dissection) are rare; chiropractic treatment should be avoided if there are any degenerative bone conditions, e.g. osteoporosis, bone tumours (especially of the spine), spinal degenerative conditions or inflammatory processes.
- Find a qualified/registered practitioner through professional body websites, e.g. General Chiropractic Council, http://www.gcc-uk.org or the British Chiropractic Association, http://www.chiropractic-uk.co.uk.

Further information for health professionals and the public

Ernst, E. et al. (eds) (2008) *Oxford Handbook of Complementary Medicine*. Oxford: Oxford University Press.

Reflexology

Reflexology applies pressure to different areas of the feet and sometimes hands that are thought to 'link' to organs and parts of the body.

Theories of mechanism of action

Many patients use reflexology and anecdotally report finding it beneficial. Speculation about possible mechanism of action includes:

- Links through nervous system directly
- Stimulates production of endorphins
- Induces relaxation
- Works through energy channels 'meridians' similar to acupuncture
- Placebo effect and human therapeutic relationship

Evidence

Little research evidence for neurological conditions is available. There is some evidence of effectiveness for MS. One study (Siev-Nier *et al.*, 2003) found reduced spasticity and improved bladder and bowel function in MS after reflexology.

Advice for patients

- Check with GP or neurologist prior to commencing therapy.
- Unlikely to cause any harm, but little published evidence of benefit.
- May be helpful in relieving stress and possibly some symptoms.
- Find a qualified/registered practitioner through professional body websites, e.g. Association of Reflexologists http://www.aor.org.uk.

Reference

Siev-Ner, I., Gamus, D., Lerner-Geva, L. and Achiron, A. (2003) Reflexology treatment relieves symptoms of multiple sclerosis: a randomised controlled study. *Multiple Sclerosis*, 9: 356-61.

Further information for health professionals and the public

Ernst, E. *et al.* (eds) (2008) *Oxford Handbook of Complementary Medicine*. Oxford: Oxford University Press.

Mackereth, P. and Tiran, D. (2002) *Clinical reflexology: a guide for health professionals*. Edinburgh: Churchill Livingstone.

Aromatherapy

Aromatherapy uses diluted essential oils derived from a variety of plants. These are often applied to the skin within a base oil during a massage treatment.

Oils may be inhaled by adding a few drops of the essential oil to bath water or simply inhaled from a small bowl or aromatherapy burner.

Theories of mechanism of action

It is believed that the olfactory stimulation from the essential oils influences the brain.

Evidence

There is some evidence of benefit or likely benefit for some conditions:
- Improved quality of life in palliative care
- Anxiety
- Back pain

There is little evidence of effectiveness for other neurological conditions, although there have been some trials, for example in dementias. Patients with Alzheimer's disease show an improved sense of well-being, but few other changes are noted.

Advice for patients

- Few serious harmful effects are documented, but aromatherapy is contraindicated in epilepsy.
- Check with GP or neurologist prior to commencing therapy.
- May be helpful in relieving some symptoms, especially pain relief and within palliative care settings.
- The therapy is safe when undertaken by a suitably trained aromatherapist, although some patients may have an allergic reaction to some essential oils and the oils should never be ingested.
- Find a qualified/registered practitioner through professional body websites, e.g. Aromatherapy Council, http://www.aromatherapycouncil.co.uk.

Further information for health professionals and the public

Ernst, E. *et al.* (eds) (2008) *Oxford Handbook of Complementary Medicine.* Oxford: Oxford University Press.

Massage

Massage involves applying pressure and manipulation to the soft tissues covering the body. Oil is usually applied to reduce friction between the therapist's hands and the patient's skin and reduce any discomfort.

Theories of mechanism of action

Massage results in increased flow of blood and lymph around the body, releases muscular tension and induces relaxation.

Evidence

There is evidence of benefit or likely benefit for a number of conditions:

- Anxiety
- Back and musculo-skeletal pain
- Depression
- Constipation (using abdominal massage)

While studies in neurological conditions have been undertaken and the therapy may be beneficial, the evidence is not conclusive due to the small number of studies available, methodological weakness in the studies or because studies have produced conflicting results, e.g.:

- Alzheimer's disease and other dementias
- Tension headaches
- Migraine
- MS (anxiety symptoms)
- Pain and anxiety following stroke
- HIV/AIDS

Advice for patients

- Check with GP or neurologist prior to commencing therapy.
- May be helpful in relieving some symptoms, especially pain, anxiety, and constipation.
- The therapy is safe when undertaken by a suitably trained massage practitioner.
- Some patients may experience a reaction to the oils used.
- Massage is contraindicated if the patient has a skin condition or wounds and in deep-vein thrombosis.
- Find a qualified/registered practitioner through professional body websites e.g. Massage Therapy UK, http://www.massagetherapy.co.uk.

Further information for health professionals and the public

Ernst, E. *et al.* (eds) (2008) *Oxford Handbook of Complementary Medicine*. Oxford: Oxford University Press.

Guided imagery

Imagery is a mind–body therapy in which the patient is guided through a series of imagined visual images. Patients may feel a deep relaxed, focused state, which may in turn influence the physical functioning of the body.

Theories of mechanism of action

Imagery works on the premise that the mind can influence the physical function of the body. The brain is stimulated by the patient being asked to visualize a mental image, e.g. to picture the body free of the condition from which they are suffering, which then can have a direct effect on both the endocrine and nervous systems.

Evidence

There is some evidence of effectiveness for a number of conditions:
- Anxiety and depression linked to cancer
- Post-operative pain
- Fibromyalgia

While studies in other neurological conditions have been undertaken and the therapy may be beneficial, the evidence is less conclusive due to methodological weakness in the studies or because studies have produced conflicting results, e.g.:
- HIV/AIDS
- Chronic back pain
- Headache
- MS
- Neuropathic pain
- Stroke
- Sleep quality in critical care

Advice for patients

- Check with GP or neurologist prior to commencing therapy.
- GP may be able to refer to an NHS group providing guided imagery.
- May be helpful in relieving some symptoms.
- The therapy is safe when undertaken by a suitably trained practitioner alongside conventional treatment.
- Guided imagery is contraindicated if the patient has significant mental health problems as they may become increasingly psychotic.
- Find a qualified/registered practitioner

Further information for health professionals and the public

Ernst, E. et al. (eds) (2008) *Oxford Handbook of Complementary Medicine*. Oxford: Oxford University Press.

Paediatric neuroscience care

Anatomical characteristics of children

Introduction

When caring for children with a neurological problem it is important for the nurse to be aware of the physical changes which occur from infant-hood to adolescence. By the time children reach adolescence they are considered to have similar physical attributes as fully grown adults. This section will focus on some of the general anatomical features of children, particularly those aspects which should be considered when managing hypoxia, hypotension and raised intracranial pressure (RICP).

The upper respiratory tract

Both infants and small children have relatively low oxygen reserves and high oxygen requirements, therefore infants and young children have increased respiratory rates to meet the demand of their relatively high metabolism.

Children who are neurologically compromised (e.g. as a result of head injury) are particularly susceptible to a sudden depletion of blood oxygen levels (because of the risk of secondary brain injury), and this is further compounded by several anatomical characteristics which increase the risk of airway obstruction:

- Their head is large in proportion to their body size and causes the head to flex forward in the supine position.
- They have small airways which are more susceptible to oedema and swelling.
- The tongue is also relatively large and can potentially obstruct the airway in the unconscious infant.
- Infants tend to nose-breathe until 6 months old; therefore anything that causes nasal obstruction (e.g. secretions and nasogastric tubes) will affect their ability to breathe.

As infants grow their head becomes smaller (in relation to the size of the thorax) and their airways also increase in size and the danger of airway obstruction is reduced. The mechanics of children's breathing changes throughout physical development. The infant has a pliable, cartilaginous rib cage and the diaphragm is the main muscle of respiration. In older children the rib cage is rigid and the diaphragm and intercostal muscles are involved in the mechanics of breathing.

The circulatory system

The size of the heart is relatively small in young children and to provide an adequate cardiac output they have a rapid heart rate. Therefore, epi-sodes of hypotension or bradycardia in a neurologically compromised child should be treated as a medical emergency. Children also have smaller circulating volumes and small losses can be significant.

The nervous system

Skull

The infant's skull has several unique characteristics:

- it is soft and pliable (because of incomplete ossification).
- it has an open anterior fontanel (until 18 months).
- it has relatively mobile cranial sutures.

This means the infant's head can expand in size and can accommodate varying degrees of raised intracranial pressure before becoming symptomatic. Complete ossification of the child's skull occurs by about 8 years of age. This means the older child with fused sutures and rigid skull will become rapidly symptomatic in the presence of RICP.

Spine

The gross anatomy of the spinal column and spinal cord is similar across all ages. However, there are some anatomical differences between adults and children which should be considered, particularly in the case of trauma patients:

- The interspinous ligaments are more flexible.
- The vertebral bodies are wedge-shaped and tend to slide forward with flexion.
- The facet joints are flat.
- The child has a relatively large head in proportion to the neck.
- The position of the caudal end of the spinal cord within the vertebral column changes with growth (e.g. in the neonate the cord extends to L2/L3 whereas by adulthood it extends to L1/L2).

⚠ **Although spinal cord injury in children is rare, two-thirds of those who do sustain a spinal cord injury present without abnormal radiological findings. Therefore, a significant spinal injury cannot be excluded until a full neurological assessment and MRI has been completed.**

Brain

The infant's brain doubles in size during the first 6 months of life and reaches approximately 80% of its eventual adult size by 2 years of age. The infant's pliable skull allows for this dramatic physical period of growth. The brain produces an immense number of synapses (synaptogenesis) in the first few years of a child's life and after this a prolonged period of 'pruning' or withering away of synapses occurs. The period of growth and development during the first 3 years is often referred to as the 'sensitive' or 'critical period' and is thought to be important for the emotional and social development of children. Myelination of the motor nerve pathways connecting the CNS with the PNS occurs by approximately 2 years of age. The lack of myelin in the younger brain results in the brain being more compressible which enables it to absorb more impact. Compared with adults, children have a higher water content, capillary density and cerebral blood volume, making them more susceptible to developing cerebral oedema after diffuse brain injury.

Neurological assessment in children

Background

A full neurological examination of an infant or child is usually performed with the aim of achieving a diagnosis. It will usually involve careful history taking from the parents (or carers), an assessment of nerve function (cranial, motor and sensory nerves), reflexes, behaviour, gait, coordination and will be supported by diagnostic investigations such as MRI, CT and EEG. In contrast to this, a neurological assessment carried out by the nurse or junior doctor will include the assessment of consciousness (brain dysfunction), the assessment of focal signs (pupil and limb responses) as well as observing heart rate, respiratory rate, and blood pressure.

The GCS is suitable for older children, but is not easily applied in the very young and therefore the GCS has been modified to suit paediatric patients to account for their neurological immaturity. For instance, the motor activity of infants is dependant on the myelination of nerve fibres (between the cortex, thalamus and the peripheral nerves) which is not complete until approximately 2 years of age.

The following are examples of modified paediatric coma scales:
- Adelaide scale.
- Pinderfield scale.
- James coma scale.

In children the verbal responses and motor responses will vary according to age. For instance, a frightened 7-year-old child may not cooperate during the assessment although neurologically unimpaired; a normal infant will not talk or obey commands to move his limbs; a neonate is unable to respond vocally or locate painful stimulus and the best motor response for a 6-month infant is flexion with spontaneous movement. Only eye opening can be measured in the standard way. Nurses are expected to apply their knowledge of normal development during the neurological assessment particularly when observing verbal and motor activities of children under 5.

Neonates

In newborn infants, changes in respiratory activity, jitteriness, and oculo-motor signs such as nyastagmus are often more significant than impaired alertness. Observations such as these should be reported separately because they are important signs of neurological deterioration for this age group.

Rapid neurological assessment

The initial assessment of the child with a sudden decreased conscious level should include initiatives to support airway, breathing and circulation prior to assessing their neurological status.

AVPU score

A rapid initial assessment of an infants or child's conscious level can be made using the AVPU method. This method is particularly useful for pre-hospital and emergency room setting. Patients are assessed as alert (A), respond to voice (V), responds to pain (P), or unresponsive (U). Children assessed as P or U will have a GCS of 8 or less.

Modified GCS

In circumstances where a child's condition needs ongoing assessment (e.g. following a head injury) a modified version of the GCS is used to record their progress.

Like the adult GCS, the modified version of the GCS is based on the observation of three aspects of behaviour (eye opening, verbal response, best motor response).

This enables clinicians to monitor the patient's condition by comparing a series of recorded observations over time to observe a trend in their condition.

Painful stimulus

Several methods can be used in applying a painful stimulus in the paediatric setting and the method of choice should depend on local policy, personal preference and the expertise of the practitioner. No one method is regarded as the gold standard, however the principle which governs all is to do no harm!

Methods of eliciting a painful response:
- Fingernail pressure
- Side of fingernail pressure
- Trapezium squeeze
- Supraorbital pressure
- Jaw margin pressure
- Squeezing the ear lobe

Other

Head circumference and palpating the anterior fontanelle.

Seizures in children

Approximately one-third of people newly diagnosed each year with epilepsy are children, who are most prone to developing epilepsy in early childhood or at adolescence. Epilepsy can however develop at any age in children or adults.

Seizures are brief malfunctions of the brain's electrical system resulting from cortical neuronal discharge. They are determined by the site of origin and can occur for the following reasons:

- Febrile convulsions
- Seizure disorders—epilepsy
- Space-occupying lesion
- Infections (encephalitis, meningitis, cerebral abscess etc.)
- Metabolic disorders
- Acidosis
- Head injury
- Hypoxia
- Electrolyte disorders

Presentation/types of seizure

Partial seizures

Partial seizures start in one lobe or one hemisphere and can be:

- *Simple partial seizures*, where there is no loss of consciousness, but the child often suffers an aura such as a change of taste or smell, numbness of face and body or a feeling of déjà vu.
- Complex partial seizures, may be a change of consciousness and the child may behave in a dazed or unusual way.

Generalized seizures

Both hemispheres are affected and can be one of the following:

- Tonic–clonic seizure (formerly Grand Mal)
- Tonic or clonic individually
- Atonic (drop attack)
- Myoclonic
- Absence seizures (formerly Petit Mal)

Diagnosis

A detailed history can lead to a diagnosis; an EEG is required and a CT/MRI scan is often undertaken; blood tests may be taken as an exclusion criteria.

Aims of care

The aim is to reduce/stop seizure activity whilst minimizing the side effects of treatment. This includes the following options:

- Pharmacological
- Anticonvulsant medication
- Surgery
- Vagal nerve stimulator (VNS) implant

Surgery for epilepsy

The aim of surgery is to remove the underlying cause of epilepsy, so reducing the number of seizures and increasing the child's quality of life. Surgery is only appropriate for a small number of children with intractable epilepsy and the selection process involves multiple investigations including MRI scanning, video-telemetry, EEG, SPECT scanning, neuropsychology, neuropsychiatry and more.

Difficulties arise when assessing these young children who often have behavioural or developmental issues and paediatric specialists are essential in these assessments.

Types of surgery

Hemispherectomy

Removal of part/the majority of one cerebral hemisphere is used for children with refractory epilepsy and extensive unilateral hemisphere disease (e.g.: hemimegaencephaly, Sturge–Weber syndrome).

Corpus callosotomy

Disconnection of the corpus callosum is used to prevent the propagation of seizures rather than the initiation of them and is most commonly used for the treatment of 'drop' attacks.

Multiple subpial transactions

This involves making surgical transactions horizontally at 5cm intervals in the cortex, the supposition being that this interrupts the horizontal spread of seizures, while preserving the vertical integrity of the functional cortex. It is used to treat unresectable areas of cortex such as the speech centres, for syndromes such as Landau–Kleffner.

Temporal lobectomy

Focal resection is undertaken in children with uncontrolled focal epilepsy, where a resectable lesion has been identified.

Outcomes following surgery for epilepsy are variable and individualized and should only be undertaken in specialized centres.

Multidisciplinary team should ensure

- Seizure management/reduction.
- Good communication between hospital and community teams.
- Good support and advice to family and child.

Further information for health professionals and the public

National Society for Epilepsy http://www.e-epilepsy.org.uk
National Institue for Health and Clinical Excellence http:// http://www.nice.org.uk/guidance/

Cerebral palsy

Definition and incidence

Cerebral palsy (CP) is a term used to describe a group of conditions which occur during early childhood. This includes children with motor impairment as a result of brain damage suffered either before or after birth. The motor disorders of CP are often associated with a range of additional problems including learning disabilities, global developmental delay and seizure disorder. CP is referred to as a non-progressive pathology. This is because it is characterized as having a changing clinical picture (until late teens) associated with continued brain development. In the UK, approximately 1 in 500 infants are born with CP and approximately 10,000 new cases are diagnosed each year in the European Union. Approximately 50% of children with cerebral palsy are born before 36 weeks gestation.

Types

Depending on which part of the brain has been damaged, CP can be classified as spastic, athetoid, ataxic or a combination of these, sometimes referred to as a mixed CP.

Spastic CP (70%)

Damage to the motor pathways in the cerebral cortex cause an upper motor neuron syndrome (hypertonia, jerky movements, increased reflexes, weakness of movement, loss of selective movement)

Athetoid CP (10%)

Damage to the motor pathways in the basal ganglia cause dystonic movements (sudden unwanted, involuntary movements)

Ataxic CP (20%)

Damage to the motor pathways in the cerebellum cause ataxic movements (clumsy and unintentional movements, lack of coordination, general difficulties in maintaining posture)

Mixed CP

Children with CP sometimes have a combination of the three types.

Causes

- Congenital—genetic, congenital brain malformations, maternal infection (80%)
- During labour and birth—birth trauma, asphyxia (10%)
- After birth—brain haemorrhage, meningitis, head injury (10%)

Pathophysiology

The primary pathology can occur in the subcortical white matter, basal ganglia, cerebellum and/or brainstem. In pre-term infants, damage to the periventricular white matter can be caused by either haemorrhages into the ventricles and the surrounding white matter or hypoxic brain injury. Damage to these regions cause major disruptions to the motor pathways which run between the brain and spinal cord.

Motor problems include:
- Difficulty in using and controlling muscles (e.g. walking, writing, eating, talking)
- Feeding difficulties (these generally increase with age)
- Dysarthric speech (their pronunciation is often unclear)

Non-motor (sensory disturbance) problems include:
- Vision (approximately 30% have squints), hearing loss (approximately 20%)
- Bladder dysfunction and incontinence, constipation, touch, drooling

General problems

Epilepsy (approximately 30%), hydrocephalus, learning difficulties (approximately 60%), however some people with CP have only moderate or mild difficulties while others are extremely intelligent), behaviour problems (approximately 30%).

Management

There is no cure for CP. However, CP can be effectively managed by the MDT. One of the main aims of care is to alleviate the effects of the condition by reducing symptoms. The general approach is for the MDT to work with the parents or carers to maximize child's potential to lead an independent life. Life expectancy for children with cerebral palsy is not much lower than the normal population.

Physiotherapy helps to promote good posture, comfort, and the prevention of contractures.

Occupational therapy helps to promote independence.

Speech and language therapy can help with speech development, eating, drinking, and swallowing.

Surgery

Orthopaedic surgery, rhizotomy, deep brain stimulation (in patients with primary dystonias).

Medication

Systemic: baclofen (oral or intrathecal), diazepam, dantrolene, tizanidine, levodopa.

Focal: botulinum toxin (helps relax limbs with contractures by blocking the release of acetylcholine when injected into the muscle).

Further information for health professionals and the public

SCOPE http://www.scope.org.uk
International Cerebral Palsy Society http://www.icps.org.uk

Congenital abnormalities

Spinal cord abnormalities

Encephalocoeles

Posterior encephalocoeles protrude the occipital bones and occasionally through the foramen magnum and the atlas.

Anterior encephalocoeles involve the frontal lobes, with a skin covering and hypertelorism.

Surgery is undertaken where appropriate and the outcome is dependant on the structures involved.

Arachnoid cysts

Abnormal development of the arachnoid membrane that requires surgical intervention.

Dandy–Walker complex

This describes a cystic enlargement of the fourth ventricle with foraminal atresia and atrophy of the surrounding brain. Treatment is surgical management of the cyst and associated hydrocephalus.

Arnold–Chiari malformation

This describes a spectrum of abnormalities of increasing severity and mainly involves the hind brain. Chiari II is associated with spina bifida, with associated hydrocephalus and may require a foramen magnum decompression.

Spina bifida

- Myelomeningocoele—the spinal cord is exposed or sometimes covered by a thin membrane.
- Meningocoele—there is a lumbar sac containing meninges but the neural tissue is not exposed.
- Spinabifida occulta:
  - Diastametomyelia—splitting of the spinal cord by a bony spur or fibrous band.
  - 'Tethered cord'—the spinal roots are tethered by a thickened filum terminale.
  - The presence of a lipoma or epidermoid cyst.

Aims

- Surgical management of the abnormality where appropriate.
- Management of kidney and bladder by a urodynamic team; also bowel management.
- Multidisciplinary management, including physiotherapy, OT.

Further information for health professionals and the public

Association for Spina Bifida and Hydrocephalus http://www.asbah.org

Vascular abnormalities

Occlusive arteriopathies

Moya Moya syndrome, where there is progressive narrowing or obstruction of major cerebral arteries, with resulting collateral blood supply.

Can be treated by revascularization from the extracranial to the intracranial circulation, with some effect.

Neurovascular abnormalities

Arteriovenous malformations and aneurysms are rare in children and their management is similar to adults, including coiling and embolization.

Vein of Galen malformations are congenital malformations which often result in heart failure at birth and the outcome for this malformation is variable.

Cerebrovascular

Acute stroke is a clinical syndrome, with an acute focal neurological deficit and can be defined as:
- Arterial ischaemic stroke—often due to sickle cell disease.
- Cerebral venous thrombosis.

Aim

The aim for the child following stroke is to stabilize the child and start rehabilitation.

Treatment

- Anticoagulation should be commenced where appropriate, except for children with sickle cell who should receive regular blood transfusions to maintain an HbS of < 30%.
- Early disability and assessment management for all children with neurovascular abnormalities should include.
  - Speech and language therapist (SLT) assessment/feeding/ communication
  - Pain management
  - Physiotherapy and OT
  - Liaison with community team
  - Psychology

Further information for health professionals and the public

Royal College of Physicians http://www.rcplondon.ac.uk/pubs/books/childstroke

Neurodegenerative disorders

Neurodegenerative disorders of childhood incorporate diseases of the central nervous system, peripheral nervous system or a combination of the two. Different conditions can cause symptoms to appear at or pre-birth, or at any stage during the childhood years. The condition may be one that is rapidly fatal (within months) or very slowly progressive with long periods of stability over many years. The majority are genetically inherited, many following a very classical pattern whilst others, even within siblings, present in different ways and at different ages.

Classification
- Neurometabolic
- Spinocerebellar
- Neuromuscular
- Acquired

Neurometabolic (examples)
Neuronal storage disorders
- Batten's diseases—autosomal recessive
- Niemann–Pick disease—autosomal recessive
- Tay–Sachs disease—autosomal recessive
- Mucopolysaccharidoses—most autosomal recessive

Leucodystrophies
- Krabbe's leucodystrophy—autosomal recessive
- Metachromatic leucodystrophies—autosomal recessive
- Adrenoleucodystrophy—X-linked recessive
- Pelizaeus–Merzbacher disease—X-linked recessive
- Vanishing white matter disease—autosomal recessive
- Megalencephalic (cystic) leucoencephalopathy—autosomal recessive

Mitochondrial
- Leigh's disease—autosomal or X-Linked recessive
- Alper's disease—autosomal recessive

Spinocerebellar (examples)
- Friedreich's ataxia—autosomal recessive
- Ataxia–telangiectasia—autosomal recessive
- Huntington's disease—autosomal dominant
- Infantile neuroaxonal dystrophy—autosomal recessive
- Multiple sclerosis—sporadic

Neuromuscular (examples)
- Duchenne muscular dystrophy—X-linked recessive
- Spinal muscular atrophy—autosomal recessive

Acquired (examples)
- Rasmussen's encephalitis—sporadic
- Subacute sclerosing panencephalitis—sporadic

Investigations

Investigations are aimed primarily at diagnosis, prognosis and genetic counselling, which may also lead to the possibility of future pre-natal testing.

Curative treatment is very rarely possible but in some cases disease progression can be delayed, e.g. dietary manipulation, replacement co-enzymes, vitamins, bone-marrow transplantation.

Diagnosis will be made following a combination of the following:

- MRI scans
- EEG, EMG
- Blood/urine/CSF biochemistry
- Muscle/nerve/ skin biopsy

Symptoms and management

Presenting features are loss of function: motor, intellectual or a combination.

The intrinsically progressive nature of the condition should be remembered when medication, interventions and therapies are proposed, and that the goals are maintaining and improving quality of life and preventing secondary complications.

Many of the following symptoms are common in neurodegenerative disorders and should be considered proactively and treated:

- Epilepsy
- Regression of skills
- Visual deterioration and loss
- Spasticity and muscle spasm
- Hypotonia/immobility
- Gastro-oesophageal reflux
- Feeding difficulties
- Aspiration
- Chest infections
- Constipation
- Sleep disturbance
- Excessive and distressing oral secretions
- Behaviour disturbances
- Intrinsic irritability

Support

Support from all members of the multidisciplinary team is essential to address the physical, emotional, educational, financial, and practical needs of the child, parents. and siblings.

Further information for health professionals and the public

Aicardi, J. (1998) *Diseases of the nervous system in childhood*. London: Mac Keith Press.

Brett, E.M. (1997) *Paediatric neurology*. Edinburgh: Churchill Livingstone.

Contact a Family, an organization that offers concise information on all conditions mentioned
http://www.cafamily.org.uk

Hydrocephalus in children

Hydrocephalus is by far the most common paediatric neurosurgical disorder. It is usually diagnosed during the first decade of life, particularly in infants under 1 year. Hydrocephalus in children shares many of the characteristics of the adult form, however there are some significant differences which are highlighted in this section.

Hydrocephalus in children (as in adults) is often described as a condition in which increased CSF pressure causes the dilatation of the ventricular system. It is caused by a diverse number of diseases where an imbalance between CSF production and its absorption leads to the overaccumulation of CSF. Incidence is reported between 3 per 1000 live births in the US to 1 per 1000 live births in Europe.

Non-communicating and communicating hydrocephalus

It is thought that hydrocephalus is either caused by an anatomical obstruction within the ventricular system (non-communicating hydrocephalus) or a functional obstruction to the sites of CSF reabsorption (communicating hydrocephalus). It is also thought that some infants (those with intraventricular haemorrhage) may have a combination of both types. It can be further classified into congenital and acquired causes.

Congenital causes	Acquired causes
Myelomeningoceles	Intraventricular haemorrhage
Aqueduct stenosis	Post-meningitis
Dandy–Walker syndrome	Brain tumours
Chiari malformations	Head injury
	Subarachnoid haemorrhage

Presentation

Signs and symptoms of hydrocephalus will vary according to age and cause.

Table 14.1 Signs and symptoms in infants

Acute onset	Gradual onset
Vomiting	Critical signs of raised intracranial pressure
Increasing head circumference	Developmental delay
Tense or bulging fontanelle	Changes to muscle tone
Open cranial sutures	Visual disturbances and papilloedema
Sun-setting eyes	
Lethargy and feeding intolerance	

Table 14.2 Signs and symptoms in older children

Acute onset:	Gradual onset:
Critical signs of raised intracranial pressure	Change in behaviour
Headache and vomiting	Poor concentration
Deteriorating conscious level	Increasing drowsiness (sleeping more)
Lethargy	Visual disturbances and papilloedema
Oculomotor dysfunction	
Increased muscle tone	

Investigations

Cranial ultrasound is the preferred method of imaging in infants with an open anterior fontanelle because the lateral and third ventricles can be easily viewed. Ultrasound also avoids the use of radiation and is relatively easy to use in the ward environment. CT is avoided as much as possible in the very young because of the dangers associated with radiation and the developing brain. CT remains the most effective way to view the ventricular system in older children and is commonly used for diagnosing hydrocephalus or a blocked shunt. MRI, as with cranial ultrasound, avoids the use of radiation and also produces higher resolution images.

Treatment

CSF shunts continue to be the main method of treatment in children; however the use of endoscopic third ventriculostomy is becoming more popular. This is due to the interest in developing new treatments which avoid the use of a shunt (and the associated complications) and also improved endoscopic techniques and outcome rates.

Complications

Similar to those seen in adults.

MDT

All patients and carers should be aware of possible symptoms of shunt or ventriculostomy failure at discharge. Follow-up care should include attendance at a dedicated hydrocephalus clinic at least every 3 years. Adolescent patients who may move from paediatric to adult services should receive vigilant transitional care.

Further information for health professionals and the public

Association for Spina Bifida and Hydrocephalus (ASBAH) http://www.asbah.org/

Brain and spinal tumours of childhood

Brain tumours

Paediatric brain tumours represent 20–25% of childhood cancers, being the second most common cancer in children under 15 years old and the most common solid tumour. Causes are largely unknown but a small number are genetic and there remains controversy regarding environmental factors. Nearly all brain tumours in children are primary tumours and rarely spread outside the CNS.

Outcome is dependent on:
- Age at diagnosis
- Location of tumour
- Tumour type
- Morbidity and mortality

The main groups of brain tumours in children include:
- *Astrocytomas*—can occur throughout the CNS and are classified by grades 1–4 or by histological description such as pilocytic, diffuse, anaplastic and glioblastoma.
  - Prognosis: good for totally resected low grade astrocytoma, poor for high grade tumours.
- *Medulloblastoma* (PNET: primitive neuroectodermal tumour of the posterior fossa): 20%, male predominance, peak age 5–8 years old and a second peak in adolescence.
  - Prognosis: although improving, prognosis remains poor for the infant and those with spinal metastases at presentation.
- *Ependymoma*—most commonly occurring in the posterior fossa
  - Prognosis: depends on child's age, degree of resection, histology and the presence of metastases at diagnosis.
- *Brainstem tumours*—a small number are cystic, focal and operative but the majority carry a poor outlook
- *Mid line tumours*—include craniopharyngioma, germ cell tumours, optic pathway tumours, hypothalamic, and pineal tumours.
  - Prognosis: difficult to resect and carry a high morbidity long term.

Presentation

Symptoms vary and are dependant on the presence of the following:
- Cerebral oedema
- Raised intracranial pressure
- Infiltration/compression of specific areas of brain

Early morning headache and vomiting are common symptoms and should always be investigated further. Focal neurological signs in line with the tumour location can include visual disturbances, endocrine disturbances, hemiparesis, seizures, cognitive changes, ataxia, and cranial nerve involvement. The child's age and development can make initial diagnosis difficult and delays in diagnosis are not uncommon.

Aims of care

- The overall aim is one of cure, but this may not be a long-term reality. The aim of surgery, radiotherapy, and chemotherapy must therefore be discussed with the family on an individual basis. Morbidity from adjuvant therapy can be high in the developing brain and consequently radiotherapy is avoided in the infant under three years old. Chemotherapy is consequently used in this age group and radiotherapy reserved until the child is older should recurrence occur.
- Relief from or control/management of symptoms such as headaches, seizures etc.
- Maintain QoL and dignity.
- Treatment of secondary hydrocephalus if required by insertion of ventricular peritoneal shunt or formation of a ventriculostomy.
- Psychological care of child and family.
- Long term concerns include neurocognitive, endocrinological, visual and personality changes, body image, family dynamics and mortality.

Spinal tumours

Primary spinal tumours in children are rare and comprise:
- Extradural: compression of spinal cord, commonly metastases
- Intradural: meningiomas (rare in children)
- Intramedullary: astrocytoma, ependymoma

Presentation

Symptoms may be difficult to diagnose in the infant with regard to dysfunction of bladder and bowel where the infant is not yet continent, and mobility and leg movement where the infant is not yet mobile/crawling.

Post-operative concerns with regard to spinal stability and bone growth may necessitate the use of a spinal jacket, to ensure safety and reduce the risk of scoliosis as the spine grows

MDT should have ensured

- Liaison between tertiary referral hospital and shared care hospital/DGH/GP, with regard to chemotherapy and ongoing surveillance.
- Local physio/OT assessment for adaptations/mobility aids.
- Local SLT input as required.
- Liaison with local social worker to ensure awareness of state benefits and Macmillan support.
- Liaison with school.
- Support needs addressed (extended family including siblings and grandparents).
- Effective communication between all parties.
- Appropriate, accurate information available to the family and to all disciplines involved with the child's care.

Further information for health professionals and the public

Brain and Spine Foundation. http://www.headstrongkids.org.uk
Brain and Spine Foundation. http://www.brainandspine.org.uk

Traumatic brain injury

Head injury is the commonest cause of acquired disability and mortality during childhood. Peak periods of incidence occur in children under 5 years old, and during mid to late adolescence. Mortality following head injury is lower in children than in adults, but the long-term sequelae in the former are often more devastating owing to the age and developmental potential of the child.

Significant effects of head injury in children are often unrecognized and it is not until the child is 'challenged' either academically or socially (and this may be several years in the future), that difficulties are recognized and these are usually behavioural (particularly as adolescence begins) or related to learning.

Physiological differences

The principles of optimising and controlling CPP in the child is similar to adults, but is age-dependent. In addition, hypovolaemia and thermo-regulation are poorly controlled in the acutely ill child and the unique characteristics of the young child's airway can prove challenging during resuscitation.

The scalp of an infant is thin compared with that of an adult and injuries may be difficult to identify by visual inspection only. In addition the infant's skull bones are thin and pliable with a degree of elasticity which often results in a more diffuse pattern of brain distortion than the adult skull.

The immature brain is relatively large with a highly mobile cervical spine, weakly supported by muscles and is therefore more easily injured.

Finally the immature brain is more susceptible to shear stress of acceleration—deceleration, due to incomplete myelination (normally completed around 2 years of age), higher water content and other phys-iological differences.

A diffuse brain injury prior to brain maturation may result in significant cognitive and performance deficits.

In the young child, head injury is mainly caused by falls from windows, stairs, trees and playground equipment; there is also a higher rate of pedestrian accidents because children have less road safety awareness than adults.

Prevention of injury is paramount, such as the use of car seats, the wearing of seat belts, the use of cycle helmets, and adequate supervision of children.

Non-accidental injury

In the child under 2 years of age, non-accidental injury (NAI)/shaken baby syndrome must always be considered, and the appropriate child pro-tection protocol instigated. There is a high level of mortality and mor-bidity resulting from subdural haematoma caused by shaking injuries in infants, especially those who have had significant and diffuse white matter hypointensity.

A multidisciplinary team is essential for the management of these children and families, who may have long-term care needs.

Presentation

Assessment of level of consciousness in babies and young children is difficult and an appropriate paediatric coma scale should be used. Clinical evaluation often proves difficult and there may be a normal neurological evaluation, in the presence of an intracranial injury in the infant.

Aims of care

- Stabilization of child and management of primary brain injury
- Stabilization of cervical spine
- Minimizing of secondary brain injury
- Rehabilitation of child and reintegration back into school
- Support to family and carers

Further information for health professionals and the public

Children's Brain Injury Trust http://www.cbituk.org

National Institute for Health and Clinical Excellence (2007) *Head injury: triage, assessment, investigation and early management of head injury in infants, children and adults.* Clinical Guideline 4. London: National Institute for Health and Clinical Excellence. http://www.nice.org.uk.

Acquired brain injury

Acquired brain injury (ABI) is by definition not hereditary, congenital or degenerative in origin.

Causes

- Cerebral tumour
- Toxins
- Metabolic abnormalities
- Infection—meningitis, cerebral abscess, encephalitis
- Hypoxic—ischaemic injury
- Cerebral haemorrhage

Presentation

Presenting signs may initially include signs of raised intracranial pressure and may also relate to the underlying cause—which may be global (e.g. hypoxic–ischaemic injury) or focal (e.g. cerebral tumour) in origin.

Aims of care

Immediate management of A,B,C,D (airway, breathing, circulation and disability) and of raised intracranial pressure.

Early detection of secondary complications to reduce the effects of secondary brain injury in the acute stage—hypoxia, hypercarbia, hypotension anaemia or ↑serum glucose levels.

Prompt diagnosis and referral to specialist services for management of their illness is imperative to optimise eventual recovery and prognosis.

Longer-term management presents unique challenges to the multidisciplinary team and includes early rehabilitation in terms of physical and psychological care provision and support and advice to the family.

The effects of acquired brain injury affect the whole family and not just the patient. All management must be patient-focused taking into consideration their preferences and maintaining their dignity, self-respect and decision-making abilities.

Care must be provided on an individual basis as no two patients will present with the same motor, cognitive, physiological or psychological responses to the insult.

Children and young people will need additional support reintegrating into their homes, school or possibly workplace. This includes addressing some environmental issues that may prevent them returning to their normal life, e.g. wheelchair access, bathroom facilities.

Some of the symptoms relating to less severe ABI may present as cognitive and behavioural problems after obvious physical problems have resolved. The school nurse is an invaluable resource and must be included in future management plans.

A neuropsychological assessment is important for children experiencing memory or psychosocial difficulties that are frequently under-estimated, compounding difficulties with new learning and behaviour.

Access to resources, funding or the development of 'packages of care', particularly if the individual is highly dependent on professional or carer support, can be a lengthy process. Early planning and anticipation of short- and long-term care needs is essential.

Further information for health professionals and the public

Cerebra, an organization for brain injured children and young people http://www.cerebra.org.uk

Contact a Family, an organization that offers concise information on all conditions mentioned http://www.cafamily.org.uk

National Institute for Health and Clinical Excellence http://http://www.nice.org.uk/guidance

Index

NEUROLOGICAL OBSERVATION CHART

Name:

Date of Birth: *Do not affix patient label*

Hospital No:

NHS No:

Consultant:

Date:													
Hour:													
Minutes:													
EYES OPEN **C** = eyes closed by swelling	Spontaneously	4												
	To speech	3												
	To pain	2												
	None	1												
BEST VERBAL RESPONSE **T** = ETT or Tracheostomy	Orientated	5												
	Confused	4												
	Inappropriate words	3												
	Incomprehensible sounds	2												
	None	1												
BEST MOTOR RESPONSE Record best response from arms **P** = Paralysed	Obey commands	6												
	Localises to pain	5												
	Flexes/withdraws to pain	4												
	Abnormal flexion	3												
	Extension	2												
	None	1												
TOTAL GLASGOW COMA SCORE														
PUPILS **+** = Reacts **-** = No reaction **S** = Sluggish	RIGHT	Size												
		Reaction												
	LEFT	Size												
		Reaction												
LIMB MOVEMENTS Record Right (R) and Left (L) separately if there is a difference	A R M S	Normal power												
		Mild weakness												
		Severe weakness												
		Abnormal flexion												
		Extension												
		No response												
	L E G S	Normal power												
		Mild weakness												
		Severe weakness												
		Extension												
		No response												